ENCEPHALITIS

Edited by **Sergey Tkachev**

Encephalitis
http://dx.doi.org/10.5772/46041
Edited by Sergey Tkachev

Contributors

Zakareya Gamie, Almas Khawar Ahmed, Mohammed M Hassoon, Karunamoorthi Annamalai Kaliyaperumal, Resat Ozaras, Ilker Balkan, Shailendra K Saxena, Hiroshi Shoji, Natalia Plekhova, Larisa Somova, Galina Leonova, Yurii Kaminsky, Anna Fisenko, Yongxin Yu, Durga Datt Joshi, Justin Jang Hann Chu, Wei-June Chen, Guey-Chuen Perng, Sergey Tkachev, SEREFNUR Oztürk, Hakan Ekmekci, Fahrettin Ege, Chieko Kai, Tomoyuki Honda, Misako Yoneda, Hiroki Sato, Halyna Biletska, Ihor Lozynski

Published by InTech
Janeza Trdine 9, 51000 Rijeka, Croatia

Publishing Process Manager Ana Pantar
Technical Editor InTech DTP team
Cover InTech Design team

Additional hard copies can be obtained from orders@intechopen.com

Encephalitis, Edited by Sergey Tkachev
p. cm.
ISBN 978-953-51-0925-9

For EU product safety concerns:
IN TECH d.o.o., Prolaz Marije Krucifikse Kozulić 3, 51000 Rijeka, Croatia,
info@intechopen.com or visit our website at intechopen.com.

Meet the editor

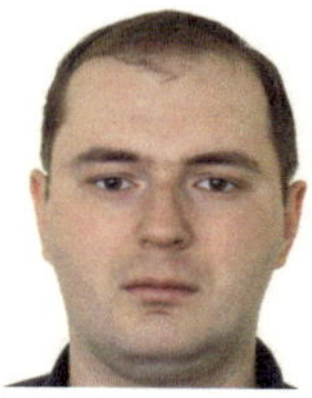

Dr. Sergey Tkachev graduated from the Faculty of Natural Sciences, Novosibirsk State University, Russia in 1998. From 1996 till the current time he has been the employee of the Institute of Chemical Biology and Fundamental Medicine SB RAS, Novosibirsk, Russia. The current research and scientific interests include virology, molecular genetics, biology and epidemiology of virus pathogens and especially – arboviruses (including Flaviviruses) and Rabies virus. He is the lecturer and instructor of Big Biochemical Workshop at the Faculty of Natural Sciences of Novosibirsk State University. In 2010 he attended a 2-week practice in Niigata Medical University, Japan. He is also the member of the editorial board of "Ticks and tick-borne diseases" journal (Elsevier) and the author of more than 40 articles and chapters in Russian and international journals and books.

Contents

Preface

Encephalitises are a group of inflammatory human and animal diseases of brain caused essentially by different pathogens. In spite of evident success in approaches for prevention, diagnostics and treatment during the last decades, the encephalitises of different etiology still constitute a menace for thousands of people all around the world.

Recently, three-volume book was published by InTech, including the first "Flavivirus Encephalitis" (edited by Daniel Růžek), the second "Non-Flavivirus Encephalitis" (edited by Sergey Tkachev) and the third "Pathogenesis of Encephalitis" (edited by Daisuke Hayasaka) parts, which can be found on InTech site (http://www.intechopen.com). But a lot of different aspects and information were not included in these volumes so we decided to publish the additional book.

The first part of this book is devoted to encephalitis clinical diagnostics and treatment. Proper diagnosis definition is an important step in encephalitis treatment so the 1st chapter considers the questions of clinical management of the patient and includes step-by-step instructions for encephalitis diagnostics.

In some cases the abnormalities in encephalitis clinical course or symptoms similar to encephalitis can be observed so the physicians should pay special attention to such patients. The 2nd and 3rd chapter describe the cerebrospinal fluid abnormalities that could be seen in some cases during the viral encephalitis and the cases of spontaneous intracranial hypotension that could be erroneously taken for encephalitis.

One of the important questions of any pathogen study is the epidemiology and monitoring and prediction of the epidemiological situation. Chapters 4 and 5 give the example of such monitoring of the encephalitis cases caused by viral pathogens in Japan and Nepal.

The members of different virus species are known to be the causative agents of encephalitis, so the second part of the book is devoted to viral pathogens, their epidemiology, pathology and diagnostics. Probably, the arboviruses (and especially members of the genus Flavivirus) are known to be one of the most known and frequent causative agents of encephalitis, so the following chapters are about arboviruses-induced encephalitises. The short review on causative agents of arboviral encephalitis is presented in Chapter 6. Chapters 7-12 are devoted to flaviviruses, their epidemiology, pathology and vaccine design. The attention should be paid to chapter seven which presents new tick-borne encephalitis virus group that was demonstrated to cause focal forms of tick-borne encephalitis with lethal outcome and has high pathogenic potential.

Other virus species are also known to be the causative agents of encephalitis, so the last chapters are devoted to non-arbovirus pathogens. Chapter 13 describes the fatal case of

Lissavirus encephalitis on the Russian Far-East. The detailed characteristics of the genetic, biological and pathological properties of isolated virus strain were determined. Chapter 14 is devoted to issues of pathogenesis of encephalitis caused by measles virus. The last chapter of the book focuses on encephalitis caused by enteroviruses which (especially Enterovirus71 (EV71)) have been documented to cause epidemics.

The authors and editors of the book hope that this work might increase the interest in this field of research and that the readers will find it useful for their investigations and clinical usage. Also I would like to thank my family, parents and colleagues who gave me a lot of support during the work on this book.

Sergey Tkachev
Laboratory of Molecular Microbiology,
Institute of Chemical Biology and Fundamental Medicine SB RAS,
Novosibirsk, Russia

Section 1

Encephalitis Clinical Diagnostics and Treatment

Chapter 1

The Clinical Management of the Patient with Encephalitis

Almas Khawar Ahmed, Zakareya Gamie and Mohammed M. Hassoon

Additional information is available at the end of the chapter

http://dx.doi.org/10.5772/55171

1. Introduction

1.1. Initial approach

It is important to follow a structured systematic approach to ensure good clinical care of the patient and to aid diagnosis. In an acute situation, the patient's airway, breathing and circulation must be assessed. Therefore, a Primary survey is undertaken and for this an ABCD approach is employed.

Determining the patency of the airway is crucial for the survival of the patient. In the general assessment of airway patency a clinician must observe the face and the neck. Abnormalities in the jaw mouth and neck must be noted as these could lead to airway compromise and future complications. Speaking to the patient for example by asking their name and observing their response, such as able to communicate in full sentences is a good indicator of unobstructed airways. Changes in vocalisation can be due to Asthma, COPD, emboli, oedema or even pneumonia. If any of these conditions are suspected a definitive diagnosis must be obtained as any of these could lead to further deterioration of the patient.

The second stage of the primary survey is the assessment of breathing. We begin with observation of the patient. Looking for signs of respiratory distress is important and failure to recognise this can lead to fatal consequences. Signs of respiratory distress can be the use of accessory muscles or changes in chest movement and in some cases even both.

Observation of the chest for any deformity is important but systemic observation is crucially important as well because it can show signs of cyanosis. At this point the respiratory rate needs to me measured. Then proceed to auscultate the chest and then end in percussion. Oximetry is also undertaken to determine the patient's oxygen saturations.

The third step in the process is an assessment of the circulatory system. This is a multidimensional assessment and many factors must be taken into account. As part of the circulatory assessment, examination of the extremities is undertaken to determine if they are warm or cool as a way of assessing perfusion. Next press the nail bed for 5 seconds and if the refill is less than 2 seconds the capillary refill time is normal[1]. Now position the patient at a 45 degree angle and observe the filling of the jugular vein. This is an indicator of the Jugular Venous Pulse (JVP) and in a healthy person the filling should be less than 3cm[2].

The clinician should then proceed to measure the blood pressure and auscultate the heart for murmurs; if an abnormality is suspected an ECG should be performed. After these vital steps are done the clinician should move to the lower extremities. The clinician should start with palpating the peripheral pulses; femoral, popliteal and posterior tibial artery as well as the arteries of the upper limbs. Examination of the calf muscles should also be undertaken for DVT[3]. IV access should be obtained as soon as possible if there are signs of haemodynamic compromise.

Assessment of disability is the last step of primary assessment. The AVPU score can be calculated or a calculation of the Glasgow coma scale. Pupillary light reflex and posturing can indicate if there is neurological damage and the severity of encephalitis. A measurement of capillary glucose can also be performed in this stage.

2. Clinical interview

The clinical interview can be divided into presenting complaint, history of presenting complaint, past medical history, family history, medication history and social history. Each part can give insight into the likelihood of encephalitis and the important signs to look for while performing the clinical examination.

2.1. Personal history

We commence by obtaining the basic demographic details of the patient, confirming you have the correct patient by verifying the name, age and sex of the patient. These basic details can also give some insight into aetiological agents of encephalitis as different aetiological agents have their own archetypes in transmission regarding age and sex.

2.2. Chief complaint

The onset of symptoms can give an indication of the aetiology of encephalitis; however the incubations period of the pathogens vary and overlap so it can be difficult to determine the aetiology from the onset of the symptoms (table 1).

Fever is a common complaint in encephalitis. Fever characteristics can be significantly different in various causes of encephalitis (table 2). However caution must be taken as fever is pathognomonic for various illnesses ranging from infections to autoimmune or even malignancy.

Pathogen	Incubation
HSV	2-12 days[1]
West Nile virus	1-6 days[2]
JE	5-15 days[3]
EBV	30-50 days[4]
Mycoplasma	7-21 days[5]
Bartonella henselae	7-14 days[6]
syphilis	9-60 days[1]

1. INCUBATION PERIOD OF DISEASE Epidemiology Review (1983) 5(1): 1-15. Oxford Journals
2. Vector Competence of California Mosquitoes for West Nile virus : Laura B. Goddard,* Amy E. Roth,* William K. Reisen,* and Thomas W. Scott* :Emerg Infect Dis. 2002 December; 8(12): 1385–1391.
3. The Epidemiology of Japanese Encephalitis: Prospects for Prevention : David Vaughn, Charles Hoke : Oxford Journals Medicine Epidemiologic Reviews : Volume 14, Issue 1 : Pp. 197-221.
4. Epstein-Barr Virus-specific Serology in Immunologically Compromised Individuals[1] : Werner Henle, and Gertrude Henle : Accepted March 6, 1981. : Cancer Res November 1981 41; 4222
5. Epidemiology of Mycoplasma pneumoniae Infection in Families : Hjordis M. Foy, MD; J. Thomas Grayston, MD; George E. Kenny, PhD; E. Russell Alexander, MD; Ruth McMahan, MN : JAMA. 1966; volume 197(number11): pages 859-866
6. The expanding spectrum of Bartonella infections: I. Bartonellosis and trench fever: BASS, JAMES W. MD; VINCENT, JUDY M. MD; PERSON, DONALD A. MD : Paediatric Infectious Disease Journal: January 1997 - Volume 16 - Issue 1 - pp 2-10

Table 1. There is an overlap in the incubation period of the various aetiological agents of encephalitis.

Aetiology	Fever characteristic
HSV	Mild pyrexia[2]
West Nile virus	Mild pyrexia[3]
JE	Mild pyrexia[4]
EBV	38 - 40°C in the first week [1:pages 871-872]
Mycoplasma	Morning temperature spikes [1: page 871]
Tick borne encephalitis	Relapsing- biphasic[5]
Toxoplasmosis Gondi	Relapsing [1:page 873]
Bartonella henesle	Mild pyrexia [1: page 872]

1. Fever of Unknown Origin: Clinical Overview of Classic and Current Concepts: Burke A. Cunha, MD, MACP : Infectious Disease Clinic of North America 21 (2007) Pages 867–915.
2. Herpes simplex virus infection: Dr Richard WhitleyMD, Bernard Roizman ScD: the Lancet : volume 357: Issue 9267, May 12 2001, pages 1513-1518
3. West Nile virus fever :Lásiková S, Moravcová L, Pícha D, Horová B. : Epidemiol Mikrobiol Imunol. 2006 Apr;55(2): 59-62
4. Transplacental Infection with Japanese Encephalitis Virus : Dr. U. C. Chaturvedi, A. Mathur, A. Chandra, S. K. Das, H. O. Tandon and U. K. Singh : Oxford Journals, Journal of Infectious Diseases : Volume 141, Issue 6 : Pp. 712-715
5. Tick-Borne Encephalitis : Uga Dumpis, Derrick Crook, and Jarmo Oksi : Oxford Journals , Clinical Infectious Diseases : Volume 28, Issue 4 : Pp. 882-890

Table 2. Fever characteristics of the various aetiological agents of encephalitis.

Cephalgia is another common symptom of encephalitis. The cerebellum, Dura Mater and bones of the skull are insensible to pain[4]. Cephalgia is usually due to vasculature or sinus pain so a differential diagnosis must be sought to eliminate other causes of cephalgia. A cognitive change within a patient requires further assessment. We need to consider if there are focal signs or if it a general deterioration of consciousness. There are no specific patterns of cognitive dysfunctions identified within any specific aetiological group nor are cognitive changes exclusive to encephalitis. Consequently a definitive diagnosis is required in such circumstances where the patient is obviously unstable and the clinician must determine a course of action to reach a diagnosis. This can be achieved by examination of the patient and thorough diagnostic tests. General cognitive changes[5] which can be encountered in an encephalitic patient would range from personality changes, mood disorders, amnestic disorders, hallucinations, and seizures.

Seizures and status epilepticus are a major concern in a patient with encephalitis. Depending on the aetiological agent seizures can be very common. In HSE virus encephalitis eliptogenic centres are located in the temporal and frontal cortices[6]. A seizure in a patient with HSV encephalitis is an indication of a poorer prognosis. In JE encephalitis periods of seizures alternating to periods of altered consciousness are common, they are however not as common in WN encephalitis and Murray Valley encephalitis[7].

2.3. Past medical history

Past medical history can demonstrate key risk factors of the patient suffering from encephalitis. For example any conditions which would leave the patient with an immunodeficiency like HIV, cancer or even a primary immunodeficiency in patient exhibiting symptoms of encephalitis would merit immediate diagnostic procedures. It is important to consider if the patient is up to date with their vaccinations. In an unvaccinated patient the most common cause of encephalitis would be due to a varicella virus[8]. The most common cause in a vaccinated patient is Herpes Simplex Virus[9] Others facts which need to be considered are a previous episode of fever as some causes of encephalitis have a pattern of remitting fever. It is also important to ask the patient is if they have any recollection of being bitten by mosquitoes or tics as this can indicate possible aetiological agents.

2.4. Family history

Primary immunodeficiency can predispose a patient to the risk of encephalitis as well as other infections. So if a history of immunodeficiency is obtained the patient should immediately commence treatment with immunglobulins[10].

An instance wherein family history is vital is if the aetiology of encephalitis is contagious and other members of the family experiences symptoms of an infection or has shown symptoms of encephalitis. This may be useful in reaching the diagnosis of encephalitis or even determining the aetiology of encephalitis. However the expression of symptoms in any illness is highly variable amongst individuals and that is something which should be kept in mind.

2.5. Medical history

Medications can cause cognitive changes and fever so a medication history should be obtained to ensure that the symptoms are not due to a chemical disturbance. Prescription drugs, non-prescription drugs and even recreational drug use should be noted.

2.6. Lifestyle history

Different continents have different common aetiological agents of encephalitis so a history of travel should be documented. If a person is inclined to an outdoor lifestyle this should also be taken into account as they are at a higher risk of being bitten by tics or mosquitos depending on their demographics. Seasons affect behaviour pattern for example mating pattern in mosquitos, so the season should also be noted.

3. Physical examination

After performing the primary survey and the clinical interview, the secondary survey can be undertaken. Some manifestations of encephalitis, which may be encountered, are discussed below.

3.1. General observation

During general observation we can start by assessing the skin. Some etiological agents which can cause encephalitis also cause dermatological lesions. A prime example is the most common viral cause of encephalitis which is HSV, HSV also causes herpetic skin lesions[11], which should been noted and is a good means to reach a fast diagnosis. Other aetiological agents which may also have dermatological signs are EBV[12] in which jaundice and oral petechiae can be observed. A patient infected with WNV occasionally will display a rash[13]. Basciliar angiomatosis[14] a vascular lesion of the skin which can extend to other organs is described as a Chancre and it is a diagnostic sign of primary syphilis. Untreated syphilitic patients can progress to encephalitis and observing skin changes can aid in diagnosis [15]

3.2. Examination of the eye

Many Etiological agents of Encephalitis can cause ocular symptoms. During a HSV infection the patient can develop keratoconjunctivits[16]. For a patient with an EBV infection a periorbital oedema may be noted[17]. Chorioretinitis[18] is a rare sequelae of West Nile Virus, Being rather uncommon it should still be excluded. Ocular manifestations of Mycoplasma pneumoniae infection other than conjunctivitis are uncommon[19]. The most frequent ocular manifestation of bartonella is neuroretinitis which is usually unilateral[20]. Interstitial keratitis is frequently reported in patients with syphilis[21].

3.3. Examination of the oral cavity

Oral involvement is common in many viral disorders. For example in HSV, ulcers on the buccal mucosa and the tongue are observed[22]. During a bout of EBV infection pharyngitis occurs in 80 - 90% of patients and is usually mild in nature and clears in 7 - 14 days[23]. WNV patients suffer from lymphadenopathy so the tonsils should be examined for any indications of tonsilitis[24]. Oral manifestations of primary syphilis are usually a solitary ulcer on the lip or tongue. Mucous patches and maculopapular lesions are the 2 principal features of secondary syphilis. Gumma formation and syphilitic leukoplakia are the manifestations of tertiary syphilis[25].

Periauricular lymph nodes are enlarged during West Nile Virus infection[26] Peripheral lymphadenopathy is a manifestation of tuberculosis[27]. Bartonella Henselae, the main causative agent of cat-scratch disease (CSD), appears to be the most common organism responsible for lymphadenopathy in adults and children[28].

3.4. Examination of the abdomen

After observation now palpations of the abdomen may be undertaken. Mycoplasma is a very rare cause of ascites more commonly cutaneous lesions upon the abdomen should be noted[29]. Other causes of ascites may be Bartonella Hensele and Syphilis. After general palpation the clinician may want to assess if individual organs can be palpated. Ascites can be evaluated by palpation and percussion. A first clue that there is a possibility of ascites is a rounded symmetrical abdomen with bulging flanks. Undulation test[30] is the gold standard in demonstrating ascites and within this test the clinician should feel for a fluid wave, which would account for a positive test. The clinician may also test to see if there is shifting dullness which is indicative of more than 500ml of ascetic fluid[31].

The clinician should then start with the liver. We position the patient in the recumbent position with the right-handed examiner on the right side of the patient[32]. EBV can cause significant hepatomegaly but it is not as common as splenomegaly[33]. HSV can cause hepatomegaly however it is rare. TB[34] causes hepatomegaly as it infiltrates most organs. Next we can perform the examination of the spleen. We position the patient in the supine position with the knee flexed. We begin below the left costal margin using the right hand firmly pushing down and then releasing[35]. Viral aetiologies in with splenomegaly can occur quite often is an EBV[36] infection. Another viral aetiology of encephalitis is WNV[37] and it is not as common as EBV in causing encephalitis coupled with splenomegaly. A very rare bacterial cause of encephalitis is TB[38], this bacteria infiltrates most organs so splenomegaly should not be ruled out. In order to complete a full physical examination you can perform a renal examination. However common aetiological agents for encephalitis do not usually cause renal disorders.

3.5. Neurological exam

Next we can perform a thorough neurological exam. This will not only indicate a possibility of encephalitis but also the extent of destruction within the cerebrum. To help differentiate meningitis from encephalitis, we can assess for nuchal rigidity by asking the patient to place their chin on their sternum. Inability to do so is a sign of meningitis. Kerning's sign can also be performed.

3.6. Examination of cranial nervs

We move on to a comprehensive assessment of the cranial nerves (table 3).

Cranial nerve	Test
Olfactory nerve	Smell [1 :page 111]
Optic nerve	Visual acuity, visual fields, ocular fundi[1 : page 116]
Optic nerve and oculomotor nerve	Pupillary reactions [1 : pages 116-149]
Oculomotor nerve, Trochlear nerve, Abducens nerve	Extraocular movement, including opening of the eye [1 :pages 149-208]
Trigeminal nerve	Facial sensation, movement of jaw, corneal reflexes [1 : pages 208-226]
Facial nerve	Facial movement, gustation [1 :pages 251-262]
Vestibulocochlear nerve	Hearing and balance [1 :Pages 263-269]
Glossopharyngeal nerve, Vagus nerve	Swallowing, elevation of palate, gag reflex, gustation [1 :pages 251]
Trigeminal nerve , Facial nerve, Vagus nerve , Hypoglossal nerve	Voice and speech [1 :pages 208 - 276]
Accessory nerve	Shrugging shoulders and turning of head [1 :pages 263-269]
Hypoglossal nerve	Tongue protrusion [1 :pages 270 - 276]
1. Adapted from: The neurologic examination: Dejong, Russell N. pages 111 to 270	

Table 3. Methods to test cranial nerve function.

3.7. Motor system

Now we can assess the motor system to discover if any damage has been done to the motor system. We first start off by testing strength. Strength is tested by having the patient resist your force as you attempt to move their body part against the direction of pull of the muscle that you are evaluating. This is graded on a scale of 0-5, with "0" representing absolutely no visible contraction and "5" being normal[39]. Strength testing is used to decide whether there is a neurogenic weakness and to determine which muscles/movements are affected. In correlation with the remainder of the motor exam, it should be possible to determine the particular part of the nervous system that is responsible for producing the weakness.

Testing reflexes is an important part of differentiating whether weakness is of an upper or lower motor neuron type. A reflex can be abolished without damaging motor axons[40]. In the setting of the patient with known weakness, reflex testing is a powerful tool to investigate the cause.[41] Symmetry of the reflexes needs to be considered in determining pathology. Pathological "spread of reflexes" is another objective sign of hyperactivity e.g. sustained clonus. Babinski reflex is a pathological reflex seen in upper motor neuron damage. However the validity of this reflex clinically argued as changes in foot tapping have been shown to more efficiently show upper motor neuron (UMN) lesions[42].

Muscle bulk can be primarily assessed by inspection. Symmetry is important, with consideration given to the dominance of the hand and overall body habitus. Generalized wasting or cachexia should be noted and may reflect systemic disease, including neoplasia. Severe atrophy strongly suggests denervation of a muscle, such as with lower motor neuron (LMN) lesions. The most common method is assessing muscle tone is passively moving the patients limb. Tone can either be decreased or increased. The two common patterns of pathologically increased tone, spasticity and rigidity[43]. We should consider the difference between spasticity and rigidity. Spasticity [44] is manifested as an increased resistance to ignition of movement proceeded with a rapid passive movement. Rigidity is an increase in tone which is seen throughout a variety of movements[45].

Coordination is tested as a part of a sequence of movements. Typically the patient is asked to hold his/her hands in front with the palms up, first with the eyes open and then closed (as when examining pronator drift, above). Now we should consider posture, gait and any abnormal movements. The patient should be able to stand erect with eyes open and closed to see if doing so incites abnormality in movements. Then you should ask the patient to walk and assess if there are any abnormalities in gait[46].

Now we can compare the differences between upper motor neurons and lower motor neuron lesion signs (table 4)

Comparison	UMN	LMN
Location of symptoms	Contralateral[2: pages 254]	Ipsilateral [2: pages 254]
Reflexes	Absent [1: page 46]	Present [1: page 50]
Fasciculation	Absent [3: chapter 9]	Present[3: chapter 9]
Spasticity	Present[1: page 46]	Absent[1: page 50]
Flaccidity	Absent [2: pages 250]	Present[1: page 50]

1. Adapted from: Reinhard Rohkamm, M.D., Color Atlas of Neurology, 2004 Thieme Pages 46 to 50.
2. Neuroanatomy text and atlas : john H. Martin third edition : 2003 McGraw-Hill
3. Merritt's Neurology 10th Edition (June 2000): by H. Houston Textbook of Neurology Merritt (Editor), Lewis P. Rowland (Editor), Randy Rowland By Lippincott Williams & Wilkins Publishers

Table 4. A comparison between Upper Motor Neurons and Lower Motor Neuron lesion signs

3.8. Sensory system

Somatic sensation can be tested using the dermatomes. However this is completely subjective to the patient's perception. It is up to the examiner to determine if indeed there is a loss of sensation and if the patient has the capacity to convey the results accurately. Changes in sensation and the symmetry of the changes should be noted. A comprehensive examination of the sensory system must be carried out.

4. Diagnostics

The principal goal in diagnostics is to identify if the patient is indeed suffering from encephalitis and then the aetiological agent of encephalitis. The most common causes of viral encephalitis are HSV and VZ encephalitis and they are the only curable causes also.

4.1. EEG

EEG changes in encephalopathies are similar to any encephalitis aetiological agent. There is a progressive increase in slow wave activities[47], the degree of which parallels the severity of brain dysfunction. A diffuse slow-wave background followed by the rapid development of periodic complexes in may be diagnostic of herpes-simplex encephalitis[48]. None of these patterns is specific to a particular pathophysiological process or diagnosis, but periodic epileptiform discharges are most likely to occur in an acute course of the disease[49].

4.2. Radiography

MRI is the most sensitive non-invasive test in early diagnosis of HSE due to its high sensitivity to inflammatory increased brain water content. The classical findings in herpes encephalitis are periodic lateral epileptiform discharge and hyper intense T2-weighted signal in the temporal lobe on MRI however these findings are nonspecific[50]. Japanese encephalitis MRI clues would be bilateral thalamic involvement; hemorrhagic involvement can be occasionally seen. Locations in which lesions can be seen are cerebrum, the midbrain and cerebellum, the pons and the basal ganglia. The locations in which hemorrhagic lesions can be seen are cortex, the midbrain, cerebellum, and pontine lesions[51]. Eastern equine encephalitis produces focal radiographic signs what distinguishes it from HSV encephalitis involvement of the basal ganglia and thalami[52]. An MRI preformed on a patient with Epstein-Barr virus encephalitis could show focal lesions in the basal ganglia[53]. The tick-borne encephalitis MRI revealed pronounced signal abnormalities in the basal ganglia and thalamus, without contrast enhancement[54]. Meningovascular syphilis can manifest T2-weighted hyper intense signal abnormalities, which are thought to represent cerebral infarctions[55].

4.3. Lumbar puncture

Lumbar puncture is indicated in a patient with suspected CNS infections (table 5).

Contraindications of lumbar puncture should be kept in mind. If the patient is showing signs of papilledema or an intracranial mass is suspected an urgent CT should be performed[56]. Local skin infections are an absolute contraindication and so are spinal deformities. Uncontrolled bleeding diathesis is also a contraindication.

Steps	Procedure
1	Obtain consent
2	Position the patient in the lateral decubitus position[1]
3	Locate landmarks: between spinous processes at L4-5[1]
4	Prep and drape the area after identifying landmarks. Use lidocaine 1% with or without epinephrine[2]
5	Assemble needle either an A-traumatic or Quincke and manometer. A-traumatic can reduce a post lumbar puncture headache. Attach the 3-way stopcock to manometer[3]
6	Insert needle through the skin and advance through the deeper tissues. A slight pop or give is felt when the Dura is punctured.[4]
7	When CSF flows, attach the 3-way stopcock and manometer. Measure the intracranial pressure which should be 20 cm or less.[5]
8	If CSF does not flow, or you hit bone, withdraw needle partially, recheck landmarks, and re-advance[1]
9	Once the ICP has been recorded, remove the 3-way stopcock, and begin filling collection tubes 1-4 with 1-2 ml of CSF each[5]
10	Remove needle, and place a bandage over the puncture site. Instruct patient to remain lying down for 1-2 hours before getting up[1]

1. Lumbar puncture: Anatomical review of a clinical skill : J.M. Boon[1,*], P.H. Abrahams[2], J.H. Meiring[1], T. Welch[3] Article first published online: 16 SEP 2004 : Clinical Anatomy : Volume 17, Issue 7, pages 544–553, 2004
2. Role of Local Anesthesia During Lumbar Puncture in Neonates : Joaquim M.B. Pinheiro, Sue Furdon, Luis F. Ochoa :Pediatrics Vol. 91 No. 2 February 1, 1993 pp. 379 -382
3. Choosing the best needle for diagnostic lumbar puncture : Damien Carson, MB BCh, FRCA and Michael Serpell, MB BCh, FRCA : Neurology July 1, 1996 vol. 47 no. 1 33-37
4. Lumbar Puncture : Miles S. Ellenby, M.D., Ken Tegtmeyer, M.D., Susanna Lai, M.P.H., and Dana A.V. Braner, M.D. New England Journal Med 2006; 355:e12September 28, 2006
5. Lumbar Puncture Technique: Thomas A. McLennan Canadian Medical Association Journal (1962) Volume: 86, Issue: 17, Pages: 789

Table 5. A step by step method of performing a lumbar puncture.

Once CSF is obtained test tube one sample is usually used for detecting protein and glucose levels. Test tube 2 is used to establish a possible etiological agent so can be used for serology and bacterial cultures. Test-tube 3 is used to establish cell count and finally test-tube 4 is reserved for any specifics tests.

4.4. Serology

Once you have a CSF sample it can be used to preform serology tests in order to identify any possible viral causes of encephalitis.

As the most common causes of encephalitis are viral, serology is a useful tool for diagnosis the aetiological agents of encephalitis. Routine PCR diagnosis of HSE type 1 and 2 is a highly sensitive and specific method for diagnosing encephalitis[57]. The identification of West Nile virus immunoglobulin M in cerebrospinal fluid is the recommended test to document central nervous system infection, but this test may not be positive in spinal fluid collected less than 8 days after the onset of symptoms[58].For the diagnosis of JE virus (JEV) infection an immunoglobulin M capture dot enzyme immunoassay can distinguish JEV from dengue infection[59]. The TaqMan assay was specific for WN virus and demonstrated a greater sensitivity than the PCR method [60].

5. Treatment

The treatment is mainly focused on medical treatment as surgery is rarely required. Medical treatments rely on the assessment of the patients' needs. Prioritising clinical care is crucial as encephalitis can be life threatening so focusing treatment on jus the aetiological agent is a flaw in the clinician's judgement. Ensuring the patient's vital signs stay within a physiological range and if an aetiological agent is discovered then treatment specified for that agent should be deployed.

5.1. Medical treatment

Encephalitis is a medical emergency. Initially as we discussed the ABCD guidelines should be followed. Then after the diagnostic steps are undertaken the patient should be isolated until the aetiology is determined as most viral causes are airborne (table 6).

Virus	Treatment
HSV-1 and HSV-2	Acyclovir[1]
Varicella-Zoster Virus	Acyclovir is recommended. Gancyclovir or adjunctive corticosteroids [2]
Cytomegalovirus	Gancyclovir [3]
EBV	Acyclovir initially or cidofovir once EBV identified[4].
Herpes B virus	No drug has been shown to be effective, although valacyclovir is the preferred agent[1]
Human herpes 6	Gancyclovir or foscarnet should be used in immunocompromised patients[1]
Measles	Steroid therapy [5]
St. Louis Encephalitis	Interferon alfa-2a [6]

1. Herpes simplex virus infections of the central nervous system: encephalitis and meningitis, including Mollaret's.
2. Antiviral Therapy of Herpes simplex and Varicella-zoster Virus Infections Peter Wutzler Institute for Antiviral Chemotherapy, Clinicum of the University of Jena, Erfurt, Germany
3. Cytomegalovirus infection of the central nervous system. Griffiths P. Source Department of Virology, Royal Free and University College Medical School, London, UK
4. Diagnosis and treatment of viral encephalitis : A Chaudhuri, P G E Kennedy
5. Treatment of measles encephalitis with adrenal steroids : John E. Allen
6. Interferon-α protects mice against lethal infection with StLouisencephalitis virus delivered by the aerosol and subcutaneous routes : T.J.G Brooks, R.J Phillpotts

Table 6. The treatment modalities for viral aetiological agents of encephalitis.

The next most common aetiological cause of encephalitis is bacterial. Neurosyphillis treatment is based on administering Penicillin at the same levels of treponemicidal levels found in

CSF[61]. Mycoplasma pneumonia encephalitis therapy most frequently deployed is erythromycin or minocycline. A high cerebrospinal fluid cell count, cerebrospinal fluid protein elevation, and higher age were associated with an unfavourable outcome[62].

We have to consider systemic complications as well as CNS complications. Monitoring vital signs continuously is essential in ensuring no sequelae develop and if they do they are swiftly treated. In patients with elevated intracranial pressure (ICP), management with corticosteroids and mannitol should be considered[63]. Corticosteroids are thought to decrease cerebral oedema. Now we should consider treatment targeted to specific symptoms. For example seizures are treated by anticonvulsive therapy. Analgesics may be needed to relieve headaches. Antipyretics may be needed for temperature control. Sedatives may be prescribes for irritability or restlessness.

Rare forms of encephalitis include acute disseminated encephalitis and paraneoplastic encephalitis. Acute disseminated encephalomyelitis is treated with high-dose corticosteroids. Plasma exchange can be considered when corticosteroids have not shown any benefit. We can also use treated with high-dose intravenous immunoglobulin (IVIG) [64]. Paraneoplastic encephalitis responds to immunotherapy with IVIG or plasma exchange.

5.2. Surgical treatment

In patients who have failed to respond to therapy to control elevated intracranial pressure or are inevitable at risk of uncal herniation a decompressive craniectomy is indicated. Surgical decompression may reduce changes of serious morbidity and mortality[65].

5.3. Prognosis

Cerebral inflammation is an indicator of mortality initial leucocytosis and development of severe hyponatremia is an indicator or increased morbidity and risk of mortality. In Japanese encephalitis a virus-specific immunoglobulin response is a marker for low risk of mortality[66]. Even though acyclovir reduces risk of mortality a high rate of patients still have morbidities[67].

Author details

Almas Khawar Ahmed, Zakareya Gamie and Mohammed M. Hassoon

Mid Yorkshire Hospitals NHS Trust, Wakefield, West Yorkshire, UK

References

[1] Exact determination of the central venous pressure by a simple clinical method. Borst Jg, Molhuysen Ja. : Lancet. 1952 Aug 16; 2(6729):304-9.

[2] Internal Jugular Venous Pressure In Man : Its Relationship To Cerebrospinal Fluid And Carotid Arterial Pressures : A. Myerson, M.D.; J. Loman, M.D. : Jama Vol. 27 No. 4, April 1932

[3] Homans J. Diseases of the veins. New England Journal of Medicine 1944:231:51–60.

[4] Innervation of brain intraparenchymal vessels in subhuman primates: ultrastructural observations : L Briggs, JH Garcia, KA Conger, H Pinto de Moraes, JC Geer and W Hollander: journal of American Heart association: Stroke Volume 16, No 2, 1985

[5] The textbook of pychosomatic medicine: James L Levenson :page 624: American psychiatric publishing incorporated.

[6] Seizures in encephalitis Usha Kant Misra DM, C T Tan MD, Jayantee Kalita DM : Neurology Asia 2008; 13 : pages 2-4

[7] Seizures in encephalitis Usha Kant Misra DM, C T Tan MD, Jayantee Kalita DM, Sanjay Gandhi PGIMS, Neurology Asia 2008; 13 : 1 – 13

[8] Viral Etiology of Acute Childhood Encephalitis in Beijing Diagnosed by Analysis of Single Samples : Xu, Yunhe Md; Zhaori, Getu Md; Vene, Sirkka Msc; Shen, Kunling Md, Phd; Zhou, Yongtao Md; Magnius, Lars O. Md, Phd; Wahren, Britta Md, Phd; Linde, Annika Md, Phd : Pediatric Infectious Disease Journal: November 1996 - Volume 15 - Issue 11 - pp 1018-1024

[9] Viral Encephalitis Richard J. Whitley, M.D. : New England Journel OF Medicine 1990; 323: pages 242-250 : July 26, 1990

[10] Enteroviral Infections in Primary Immunodeficiency (PID): A Survey of Morbidity and Mortality : E. Halliday, J. Winkelstein, A.D.B. Webster: science direct: Journal of Infection, Volume 46, Issue 1, Page 1

[11] Herpes Simplex Encephalitis Clinical AssessmentRichard J. Whitley, MD; Seng-Jaw Soong, PhD; Calvin Linneman Jr, MD; Chien Liu, MD; George Pazin, MD; Charles A. Alford, MD Journal of American medical association (JAMA 1982;247:317-320)

[12] Epstein-Barr Virus Infection : William A. Durbin, John L. Sullivan : Peadiatrics review volume 15 number 2, February 1, 1994, pages 63-68

[13] West Nile Virus: Epidemiology and Clinical Features of an Emerging Epidemic in the United States* Annual Review of Medicine Vol. 57: 181-194 (Volume publication date February 2006) First published online as a Review in Advance on September 1, 2005 DOI: 10.1146/annurev.med.57.121304.131418

[14] Relman DA, Loutit JS, Schmidt TM, Falkow S, Tompkins LS.The agent of bacillary angiomatosis. An approach to the identification of uncultured pathogens. New England Journal of Medicine. 1990 Dec 6;323(23):1573-80.

[15] Primary syphilis: Kathryn Eccleston, MRCP, Lisa Collins, MRCP and Stephen P Higgins, FRCP International Journal Of STD and AIDS March 2008 vol. 19 no. 3 pages 145-151

[16] Bilateral herpetic keratoconjunctivitis : Paula M.árcia F Souza, MD, Edward J Holland, MD, Andrew J.W Huang, MD, MPH, : Elsevier 4 March 2003

[17] Epstein-Barr virus infectious mononucleosis:M. Papesch[1], R. Watkins : Article first published online: 7 JUL 2008 DOI: 10.1046/j.1365-2273.2001.00431.x:Clinical Otolaryngology & Allied Sciences Volume 26, Issue 1, pages 3–8, January 2001

[18] West Nile Virus: Epidemiology and Clinical Features of an Emerging Epidemic in the United States Annual Review of Medicine Vol. 57: 181-194 2006

[19] Ocular Manifestations of Mycoplasma pneumoniae Infection : Mark B. Salzman, Sunil K. Sood, Michael L. Slavin, and Lorry G. Rubin : Oxford Journals : Medicine : Clinical Infectious Diseases : Volume 14, Issue 5 :Pp. 1137-1139

[20] Bartonella Neuroretinitis : Kenneth C. Earhart, M.D., and Michael H. Power, M.D. N England Journal of Medicine 2000; 343:1459 : November 16, 2000

[21] Secondary Syphilis with Ocular Manifestations in Older Adults :Ryan C. Maves1, Edward R. Cachay2, Maile Ann Young2, and Joshua Fierer: Oxford Journals, Medicine, Clinical Infectious Diseases, Volume 46, Issue 12 Pp. e142-e145

[22] Infection with Herpes-Simplex Viruses 1 and 2: André J. Nahmias, M.D., and Bernard Roizman, Sc.D., New England Journal Of Medicine 1973; 289:781-789October 11, 1973

[23] Acute and chronic symptoms of mononucleosis. Lambore S, McSherry J, Kraus AS : Journal of Family Practice 1991 Jul; 33(1):33-7.

[24] Clinical findings of West Nile virus infection in hospitalized patients, New York and New Jersey, 2000.D. Weiss, D. Carr, J. Kellachan, C. Tan, M. Phillips, E. Bresnitz, M. Layton, and West Nile Virus Outbreak Response Working Group: Emerging Infectious Disease. 2001 Jul-Aug; 7(4): pages 654–658

[25] Oral syphilis—re-emergence of an old disease with oral manifestation : C.M. Scott, S.R. Flint : International Journal of Oral and Maxillofacial Surgery: volume 34, issue 1, January 2005, Pages 58-63

[26] Isolation of West Nile Virus in Israel: B. Benkpof, S. Levine, R. Nerson : Journal of Infectious Disease. (1953) 93 (3): pages 207-218. doi: 10.1093/infdis/93.3.207

[27] Peripheral lymph node tuberculosis: a review of 80 cases. Dandapat MC, Mishra BM, Dash SP, Kar PK. Department of Surgery, M.K.C.G. Medical College, Orissa, India. British Journal of Surgery Volume 77, Issue 8, pages 911–912, August 1990

[28] Human Case of Bartonella alsatica Lymphadenitis : Emmanouil Angelakis, Hubert Lepidi, Atbir Canel, Patrick Rispal, Françoise Perraudeau, Isabelle Barre, Jean-Marc

Rolain, and Didier Raoul : Emerging Infectious Disease. 2008 December; 14(12): 1951–1953.

[29] Abdominal tuberculosis : still a potentialy lethal disease: Lingenfelser T; Zak J; Marks I. N; Steyn E; Halkett J; Prince S. K; American journal of Gastroenterology: 1993 : 88:744

[30] Undulation diagnosis of ascites. :Holldack K, Heller A Journel Arztl Wochensch. 1956 Mar 16;11(11):241-2.

[31] Emanuel LL, Ferris FD, von Gunten CF, Von Roenn J. EPEC-O: Education in Palliative and End-of-life Care for Oncology. © The EPEC Project,™ Chicago, IL, 2005: Pages 3-4

[32] Clinical Methods: The History, Physical, and Laboratory Examinations. 3rd edition. Walker HK, Hall WD, Hurst JW, editors. Boston: publisher Butterworths; : Chapter 4 : 1990

[33] Epstein-Barr Virus Infection : William A. Durbin, John L. Sullivan : Pediatrics in Review Vol. 15 No. 2 February 1, 1994 pp. 63 -68

[34] Gastrointestinal tuberculosis Todd A. Sheer and Walter J. Coyle : Current Gastroenterology Reports : Volume 5, Number 4 (2003), 273-278, DOI: 10.1007/s11894-003-0063-1 : Springer link

[35] Clinical Methods: The History, Physical, and Laboratory Examinations. 3rd edition. Walker HK, Hall WD, Hurst JW, editors. Boston: publisher Butterworths chapter 4 : 1990

[36] Epstein-Barr Virus Infectious Mononucleosis: MARK H. EBELL, M.D, M.S., Athens, Georgia, Ammerican Family Physician. 2004 Oct 1;70(volume 7):1279-1287.

[37] West Nile Virus Detection In The Organs Of Naturally Infected Blue Jays (Cyanocitta Cristata),Samantha E. J. Gibbs, Angela E. Ellis, Daniel G. Mead, Andrew B. Allison, J. Kevin Moulton, Elizabeth W. Howerth, David E. Stallknecht. : journal of wildlife diseases

[38] Hepatitis Complicated with Mycoplasma pneumoniae Infection in Children Lee SM, Tchah H, Jeon IS, Ryoo E, Cho KH, Seon YH, Son DW, Hong HJ.: Korean Journal of Paediatrics. 2005 Aug; 48(8):832-838. Korean.

[39] A Proposed Standard Procedure for Static Muscle Strength Testing Lee S Caldwell[a], Don B Chaffin[a], Francis N Dukes-Dobos[a], K. H. E. Kroemer[a], Lloyd L Laubach[a], Stover H Snook[a] & Donald E. Wasserman

[40] Clinical Methods: The History, Physical, and Laboratory Examinations. 3rd edition. Walker HK, Hall WD, Hurst JW, editors. Boston: publisher Butterworths chapter 4 : 1990

[41] Tendon-reflex testing in chronic demyelinating polyneuropathyH. R. Kuruoglu MD, Dr. Shin J. Oh MD* : Muscle & Nerve Volume 17, Issue 2, pages 145–150, February 1994

[42] Should the Babinski sign be part of the routine neurologic examination? Timothy M. Miller, MD, PhD and S. Claiborne Johnston, MD, PhD : American academy of neurology page 1147 June 17, 2005

[43] Reliability of the tone assessment scale and the modified ashworth scale as clinical tools for assessing poststroke spasticity :Janine M. Gregson, MRCP, Michael Leathley, PhD, A.Peter Moore, MD, Anil K. Sharma, FRCP, Tudor L. Smith, MCSP, Caroline L. Watkins, BA(Hons)- 1999 Published by Elsevier Inc Archives of Physical Medicine and Rehabilitation : Volume 80, Issue 9, Pages 1013-1016, September 1999

[44] Spasticity: a review. Department of Neurology, University of California, Irvine 92717-4275.Neurology [1994, 44(11 Suppl 9):S12-20] Type: Journal of Neurology. 1994 Nov;44(11 Suppl 9):S12-20.

[45] Spasticity And Rigidity: An Experimental Study And Review: Geoffrey Rushworth : Journal Of Neurology, Neurosurgery and Psychiatry. 1960 May; 23(2): pages 99–118.

[46] Movement, Posture And Equilibrium: Interaction And Coordination: Jean Massion: Progress in Neurobiology Volume. 38, pp. 35 to 56, 1992

[47] A characteristic EEG pattern in neonatal herpes simplex encephalitis : Eli M. Mizrahi, M.D. and Barry R. Tharp, M.D. : Neurology November 1, 1982 vol. 32 no. 11 1215

[48] Electroencephalography In Diagnosis Of Herpes-Simplex Encephalitis . Adrian Upton, John Gumpert The Lancet, Volume 295, Issue 7648, Pages 650 - 652, 28 March 1970

[49] EEG in neurological conditions other than epilepsy: when does it help, what does it add?S J M Smith : British Medical Journal: May 11, 2012 : cited Journal Neurology, Neurosurgery and Psychiatry 2005 page 76

[50] Early diagnosis of herpes simplex encephalitis by MRI: G. Schroth, MD, J. Gawehn, MD, A. Thron, MD, A. Vallbracht, MD and K. Voigt, MD : Neurology February 1, 1987 vol. 37 no. 2 179

[51] Diagnostic Neuroradiology MRI in Japanese encephalitis S. Kumar, U. K. Misra, J. Kalita, V. Salwani, R. K. Gupta and R. Gujral Neuroradiology (1997) 39: 180–184 Ó Springer-Verlag 1997

[52] Clinical and Neuroradiographic Manifestations of Eastern Equine Encephalitis Robert L. Deresiewicz, M.D., Scott J. Thaler, M.D., Liangge Hsu, M.D., and Amir A. Zamani, M.D. New England Journal Of Medicine 1997; Pages 336:1867-1874: June 26, 1997

[53] Paediatric Neuroradiology CT, MRI and MRS of Epstein-Barr virus infection: case report K. M. Cecil, B. V. Jones, S. Williams and G. L. Hedlund : Neuroradiology Volume 42, Number 8 (2000), 619-622, DOI: 10.1007/s002340000299 : springer link

[54] Diagnostic Neuroradiology MRI in tick-borne encephalitis H. Alkadhi and S. S. Kollias : Neuroradiology Volume 42, Number 10 (2000), 753-755, DOI: 10.1007/s002340000396 : springer link

[55] Neurosyphilis Presenting as Herpes Simplex Encephalitis : Illya Szilak, Francisco Marty, Joseph Helft, and Ruy Soeiro : Oxford Journals : Medicine Clinical Infectious Diseases: Volume 32, Issue 7 Pp. 1108-1109.

[56] Contraindications to lumbar puncture as defined by computed cranial tomography. : D J Gower, A L Baker, W O Bell, M R Ball : Journal Of Neurology and Neurosurgery and Psychiatry 1987; Pages 50:1071-1074 doi:10.1136/jnnp.50.8.1071

[57] Routine diagnosis of herpes simplex virus (HSV) encephalitis by an internal DNA controlled HSV PCR and an IgG-capture assay for intrathecal synthesis of HSV antibodies. Fomsgaard A, Kirkby N, Jensen IP, Vestergaard BF. Source Department of Virology Statens Serum Institut, Copenhagen S, Denmark. : Clinical and Diagnostic Virology, Volume 9, Number 1, January 1998, pp. 45-56(12)

[58] West Nile encephalitis and myelitis. Roos KL. Source Department of Neurology, Indiana University School of Medicine, Indianapolis, Indiana, USA. : Current Opinions in Neurololgy 2004 Jun; 17(volume3): pages343-6.

[59] Rapid Diagnosis of Japanese Encephalitis by Using an Immunoglobulin M Dot Enzyme Immunoassay :Tom Solomon, Le Thi Thu Thao, Nguyen Minh Dung, Rachel Kneen, Nguyen The Hung, Ananda Nisalak, David W. Vaughn, Jeremy Farrar, Tran Tinh Hien, Nicholas J. White, and Mary Jane Cardosa Journal of Clinical Microbiolology. July 1998 vol. 36 no. 7 2030-2034

[60] Rapid Detection of West Nile Virus from Human Clinical Specimens, Field-Collected Mosquitoes, and Avian Samples by a TaqMan Reverse Transcriptase-PCR Assay : Robert S. Lanciotti*, Amy J. Kerst, Roger S. Nasci, Marvin S. Godsey, Carl J. Mitchell, Harry M. avage, Nicholas Komar, Nicholas A. Panella, Becky C. Allen, Kate E. Volpe, Brent S. Davis, and John T. Roehrig : Journal of Clinical Microbiology. November 2000 vol. 38 no. 11 4066-4071

[61] Treatment of Syphilis 2001: Nonpregnant Adults : Michael H. Augenbraun : Oxford Journals : Medicine Clinical Infectious Diseases : Volume 35, Issue Supplement 2 :Pp. S187-S190

[62] Diagnosis, treatment, and prognosis of Mycoplasma pneumoniae childhood encephalitis: systematic review of 58 cases. : Daxboeck F, Blacky A, Seidl R, Krause R, Assadian O : Journal of Child Neurology. 2004 Nov;19(volume 11):865-71

[63] Effects of mannitol and steroid therapy on intracranial volume-pressure relationships in patients : J. Douglas Miller, M.D., Ph.D., F.R.C.S. (G. & E.), and Peter Leech, M.B.,

B.S., F.R.C.S. (E) : Journal of Neurosurgery March 1975 / Vol. 42 / No. 3 / Pages 274-281

[64] Intravenous immunoglobulin therapy in acute disseminated encephalomyelitis : Miki Nishikawa, MD, Takashi Ichiyama, MD, Takashi Hayashi, MD, Kazunobu Ouchi, MD†, Susumu Furukawa, MD : Paediatric Neurology: volume 21 issue 2, August 1999, Pages 583-586

[65] Craniectomy An aggressive treatment approach in severe encephalitis : S. Schwab, MD, E. Junger, MD, M. Spranger, MD, A. Dorfler, MD, F. Albert, MD, H. H. Steiner, MD and W. Hacke, MD: Neurology February 1, 1997 vol. 48 no. 2 412-417

[66] Fatal outcome in Japanese encephalitis. (PMID:3010752) Laorakpongse T : American Journal of Tropical Medicine and Hygiene. 1985 Nov; 34(6):1203-10.

[67] Herpes simplex encephalitis treated with acyclovir: diagnosis and long term outcome N McGrath, N E Anderson, M C Croxson, K F Powell : Journal Of Neurology, Neurosurgery and Psychiatry 1997;63:321-326 doi:10.1136/jnnp.63.3.321

Chapter 2

Cerebrospinal Fluid Abnormalities in Viral Encephalitis

Hakan Ekmekci, Fahrettin Ege and Serefnur Ozturk

Additional information is available at the end of the chapter

http://dx.doi.org/10.5772/54590

1. Introduction

1.1. Etiological factors for viral encephalitis

Encephalitis is defined as the presence of an inflammatory process of the brain in association with clinical manifestation of neurological system of the individual. In other words, onset of central nervous system (CNS) symptoms due to infections of the brain. Described pathogens reported as to be the causative agents for encephalitis, the majority of them are viral in origin, but sometimes bacteria or fungi or a postinfectious process. Inspite of the fact that molecular biology researches advance, new era of essentials elements in diagnosis commences, extensive tests are being used widely, the etiology of encephalitis remains unclear and unknown in a considerable degree of the patients [1-3].

Acute encephalitis includes a medical emergency. In most cases, the presence of focal neurological signs and mostly focal seizures will distinguish an encephalitic situation from an encephalopathic process. The diagnosis of encephalitis is suspected in a febrile patient who comes with altered conciousness and signs of cerebral dysfunction. The latters are so wise, therefore the dilemma of diagnosis starts with the beginning, and continues with the determination of the relevance of an infective agent. These agents may play a role in the neurologic manifestations of illness, but not necessarily by directly invading the CNS. Apart from this, there is a big challenge in distinguishing between infectious encephalitis and posinfectious encephalomyelitis. Vaccination programs were completed in the Western world already; therefore postinfectious or posimmunizative type encephalitis or encephalomyelitis (mainly acute disseminated encephalomyelitis [ADEM]) should be different in etiological aspect, since ADEM is mediated by an immunologic response to antigenic stimuli from infecting microorganisms or immunization. Noninfectious CNS diseases (e.g., fibroelastic tissue diseases, vasculitis, collagenous diseases, and paraneoplastic syndromes) can mimic encephalitis, or present with similar outcomes to those of encephalitis and should be account in the differential diagnosis. Herpes simplex encephalitis (HSE) is the commonest sporadic acute viral encehalitis in developed countries. The emergence of unusual forms of zoonotic encephalitis have an important public health problem all over the world. Vaccination and vector control measures are useful preventive strategies in the management of certain arboviral and zoonotic encephalitis [4].

Since the medical situation is emergent, in the approach to the patient with encephalitis, the main attempt should be carried out to build a reliable etiological diagnosis. Although, there are no definitive effective treatment – with few exceptions, no specific therapy is avaliable for most forms of viral encephalitis – in many cases, identification of a spesific agent – if possible – may be important for prognosis, potential prophylaxis, counseling of patients and family members, and public health issues [1].

Epidemiological clues that may help in directing the investigations for an etiologic diagnosis include season, geographical localization, travel history, occupational status, insect and animal contact, vaccinations, immunization of the insult. Therefore clinic approach should be carried out for etiology. Possible etiological agents of encephalitis – mainly viral – based on epidemiology and related risk factors are represented in Table 1. This table is revised from Infectious Diseases Society of America (IDAS) Guidelines 2008:

Epidemiology or risk factors	Possible infectious agent(s) for encephalitis
Agammaglobulinemia	**Enterovirus**
Age	
Neonates	Herpes simplex virus (HSV) type 2, Cytomegalovirus (CMV), Rubella virus,
Infant and children	Eastern equine encephalitis virus, Japanese encephalitis virus, Murray Valley encephalitis virus, Influenza virus, La crosse virus
Elderly persons	Eastern equine encephalitis virus, St Louis encephalitis virus, West Nile virus, sporadic Creutzfeldt –Jacob disease (sCJD)
Animal contacts	
Bats	Rabies virus, Nipah virus
Birds	West Nile virus, Eastern equine encephalitis virus,
Cats	Japanese virus,
Dogs	Rabies virus,
Horses	Rabies virus, Eastern equine encephalitis virus, Western equine encephalitis virus, Hendra virus
Skunks	Rabies virus,
Swine	Japanese encephalitis virus, Nipah virus
Immunocompromised persons	Varicella zoster virus (VZV), CMV, Human herpesvirus 6, West Nile virus, HIV, JC virus
Unpasteurized milk	Tick-born encephalitis virus,
Insect contact	

http://dx.doi.org/10.5772/54590

Epidemiology or risk factors	Possible infectious agent(s) for encephalitis
Mosquitoes	Eastern equine encephalitis virus, Western equine encephalitis virus, Venezuelan equine encephalitis virus, St Louis encephalitis virus, Murray Valley encephalitis virus, Japanese encephalitis virus, West Nile virus
Ticks	Tick-born encephalitis virus, Powassan virus,
Occupation	
Exposure to animals	Rabies virus,
Expoure to horse	Hendra virus,
Exposure to old World primates	B virus
Laboratory workers	West Nile virus, HIV,
Physicians and health care workers	VZV, HIV, Influenza virus, measles virus,
Veterinarians	Rabies virus,
Person to person transmission	HSV (neonatal), VZV, Venezuelan equine encephalitis virus (rare), Poliovirus, nonpolio Enterovirus, Measles virus, Nipah virus, Mumps virus, Rubella virus, Epstein-Barr virus (EBV), Human herpesvirus 6, B virus, West Nile virus (transfusion, transplantation, breast feeding), HIV, Rabies virus (transplantation), Influenza virus,
Recent vaccination	Acute disseminated encephalomyelitis,
Recreational activities	
Camping/hunting	All agents transmitted by mosquitoes and ticks (see above)
Sexual contact	HIV,
Spelunking	Rabies virus,
Swimming	Enterovirus,
Seasons	
Late summer/early fall	All agents transmitted by mosquitoes and ticks (see above), Enterovirus
Winter	Influenza virus
Travel	
Africa	Rabies virus, West Nile virus,
Australia	Murray Valley encephalitis virus, Japanese encephalitis virus, Hendra virus
Central America	Rabies virus, Eastern equine encephalitis virus, Western equine encephalitis virus, Venezuelan equine encephalitis virus, St. Louis encephalitis virus,
Europe	West Nile virus, Tick-born encephalitis virus,
India, Nepal	Rabies virus, Japanese encephalitis virus,
Middle East	West Nile virus
Russia	Tick-born encephalitis virus,
South America	Rabies virus, Eastern equine encephalitis virus, Western equine encephalitis virus, St Louis encephalitis virus,
Southeast Asia, China, Pasific Rim	Japanese encephalitis virus, Tick-born encephalitis virus, Nipah virus
Unvaccinated status	VZV, Japanese encephalitis virus, Poliovirus, Measles virus, Mumps virus, Rubella virus

Table 1. Possible Etiology of Viral Encephalitis [1]

Clinical findings (physical and specific neurological signs and symptoms) may indicate certain causative agents in patients with encephalitis (Table 2). This table is again revisely taken from the same guideline mentioned in the previous paragraph [1];

Clinical presentation	Possible infectious agent
General findings	
Lymphadenopathy	HIV, EBV, CMV, Measles virus, Rubella virus, West Nile virus,
Parotitis	Mumps virus
Rash	VZV, B virus, Human herpesvirus 6, West Nile virus, Rubella virus, certain Enteroviruses,
Respiratory tract findings	Venezuela equine encephalitis virus, Nipah virus, Hendra virus, Influenza virus, Adenovirus,
Retinitis Urinary symptoms	CMV, West Nile virus, St Louis encephalitis virus (early)
Neurological findings	
Cerebellar ataxia	VZV (in children), EPV, Mumps virus, St. Louis encephalitis virus,
Cranial nerve abnormalities	HSV, EBV,
Dementia	HIV, Human transmissible spongiform encephalopathies, sCJD and variant Creutzfeldt-Jacob disease (vCJD), Measles virus (Subacute sclerosing panencephalitis (SSPE))
Parkinsonism	Japanese encephalitis virus, St. Louis encephalitis virus, West Nile virus, Nipah virus,
Poliomyelitis-like flaccid paralysis	Japanese encephalitis virus, West Nile virus, Tick-born encephalitis virus, Enterovirus (enterovirus-71, coxsackieviruses), Poliovirus
Rhombencephalitis	HSV, West Nile virus, Enterovirus 71

Table 2. Possible etiological agents of viral Encephalitis based on clinical findings

2. CSF findings in viral encephalitis

Cerebrospinal fluid (CSF) is produced in choroid plexus of brain ventricules and in subarachnoid pial surface. Noninfective CSF contains maximum 5 wight blood cells (WBC) in a mm^3. The protein content in normal CSF does not exceed 50mg/dl and CSF glucose is 50-70 % of serum glucose levels. Central nervous system infections alter this normal content in varied degrees. Thus, knowing these alerations in various infectious and noninfectious situations is crucial for attaining veritable diagnosis. CNS infections should be born in mind in patients, who attain to emergency departments with fever, impaired consciousness and findings attributed to nervous system. Obtaining CSF with lumber puncture performed in early period leads to at once, differentiation of central pathologies from systemic ones, of infectious etiologies from noninfectious causes, and getting data concerning the character of a possible central nervous system infection; therefore CSF analysis maintains its importance as a valid method currently, for searching brain infections.

Lumbar puncture is performed generally from L4-5 intervertebral space. However L3-4 and L5-S1 intervertebral spaces are also utilized. Sufficient CSF sample should be obtained for routine laboratory tests, and a certain amount should be spared for advanced tests. Initially, protein and glucose levels are analysed from obtained sample, white blood cell count is done, and cultural analyses are performed. Opening pressure and protein concentration are increased, and glucose levels are decreased in bacterial menengitis. Polymorphonuclear cells (PNL) are usually found. Opening pressure is normal or mildly increased however in viral encephalitis and menengitis. In a classical viral encephalitis glucose levels are normal, but protein concentration is found to be mildly or moderatly increased. CSF findings in several infectious situations is summarized in Table 3.

	Bacterial menengitis	**Viral encephalitis**	**Fungal menengitis**	**Tuberculose menengitis**
Pressure	Increased	Normal-mildly increased	Normal-mildly increased	Increased
Glucose	Low	Normal	Low	Low
Cell count	PNL	Mononuclear	Mononuclear	PNL/mononuclear
Protein	High	High	High	High

Table 3. General characteristics of various CNS infections

In viral encephalitis, a more important problem is to find out the etiological agent and to apply therefore the appropriate antiviral agent beginning from the early period of the disease. Nevertheless, CSF findings, as they are analysed by routine tests, are not specific in viral encephalitis, and couldn't be heplfull to distinguish different etiological agents. These findings combined with radiological data could also not be assistant, and determination of etiology may be delayed. As a matter of fact, various serological methods, cell cultures and genom analyses are widely utilised currently. Methods to apply should be adapted to geographical factors, to epidemyological data, and to travel history in a specific individual. Negative results does not always rule out a certain agent, therefore repeated tests could be needed.

A hemorhagic CSF could be seen in Herpes simplex type I encephalitis [5]. Lymphositic pleocytosis (10-500 mononuclear cell/mm^3) and increased protein concentrations are usually found [6]. However, in immuncompromised patients especially, one could not encounter typical pleocytosis. Thus, CSF findings could be misleading in such situations; before ruling out the disease or an etiological agent, a wider CSF screen is needed in these patients. Determination of HSV-DNA with polymerase chain reaction (PCR) is a widely utilised method today. As a gold diagnostic standart currently, PCR's sensitivity is 95 % in Herpes simplex type I, and its specifity is 100 % [7]. Since the identification of HSV-I in the early period of the disease is an ongoing problem, the test should be repeated after 3-7 days in cases with negative results [1]. Studies searching for the association between HSV-DNA load and disease prognosis haven't revealed consistent results hitherto; hence, further studies are needed [8]. Isolation of the virus in cell culture is also possible, but methods sensitivity is quite low and is not invoked in clinical practice widely. Another method is to determine specific antibodies. Blood/CSF antibody ratio below 20/1 exposes the intratecal synthesis and is usefull in diagnosis of Herpes simplex encephalitis in a considerable degree. Positive PCR results are tend to diminish with the parenteral application of acyclovir, possibility of a positive test after second week is quite decreased; in contrast, in this period of the disease, specific antibodies are easily determined. The fact that patients with negative PCR and positive oligoclonal bands are frequently encountered in a specific period of the disease suggests that these two methods are sensitive to different stages of the diseases [9]. Recent studies displayed some inflamatory cytokine level alterations in CSF. While in the early period of the disease the IFN-γ and IL-6 levels are high, at the period of 2-6 weeks, TNF-α, IL-2 and soluable CD8 levels are found to be increased [10]. Maybe, these findings are reflecting the neuronal damage and inflamatory reaction, however the clinical importance of them are not well established currently.

A lymphocytic pleocytosis is seen in Varicella zoster virus (VZV) encephalitis (below 100 cells/mm^3), and increased protein concentrations and normal glucose levels are found. Opening pressure maybe increased [6]. In cell culture, the virus is rarely isolated. VZV-PCR is a usefull technique for determining the agent. Once again, negative results do not rule out the virus. In many cases, virus DNA is diminished in CSF after the first week, hence the way to be chosen is to analyze intrathecal antibodies at this period. Determining the ratio of IgG antibodies to blood content or IgM levels are helpfull. VZV glycoprotein E does not express antigenic resemblance with the herpes simplex virus, and is easily determined with performing ELISA. This method has a high specifity and sensitivity for VZV encephalitis, it may also be utilised for the differential diagnosis with herpes virus [11]. The test to be choosen in Ebstein-Barr virus and in Citomegalovirus encephalitis is again PCR. Negative results do not exclude the agents. Determining the alterations of IgM and IgG levels with serological analyses maybe usefull in EBV encephalitis. HHV-6 and HHV-7 PCR tests should be added to routine CSF screen in immuncompromised patients [5]. It should also be noted that HHV-6 PCR does not distinguish latent infection from active encephalitis. Diagnostic methods for encephalitis caused by herpesviridea family is shown in Table 4.

Besides HSV and VZV, PCR test is trusty also in JC virus. In immuncompromised patients in whom multifocal leucoencephalopathy is suspected, PCR technique is highly specific. Pleocytosis is charactheristic in Mumps encephalitis. Interestingly however, protein levels are generally normal and glucose concentrations are decreased. The disease should be differentiated from Lymphocytic choriomenengit virus, since decreased glucose levels are resulted also from that agent caused encephalitis (Figure 1). Cell culture and PCR are equally helpfull. Specific antibodies should be investigated if PCR is negative. Four fold increase in IgG levels or determining IgM are helpfull, but it should be born in mind that Mumps spe-

http://dx.doi.org/10.5772/54590

cific antibodies may express cross-reaction with Parainfluenza virus antibodies [6]. In the course of encephalitis caused by Enteroviruses, CSF cell count is generally normal, or a mildly mononuclear pleocytosis is present. Glucose levels are normal and protein concentration is increased. Method to be choosen is RT-PCR. Sensitivity and specifity are 86 % and 100 % respectively. Cell culture may also be helpfull. Despite Influenza encephalitis is rarely reported, it should be investigated in pandemic situations and/or in conditions, in which no other etiological agent is determined. Routine CSF screen is usually normal. The etiological analysis is performed by RT-PCR and cell culture in suspected cases.

HSV-1	PCR, quantitative PCR, routine serology
HSV-2	PCR, routine serology, culture
EBV	PCR, routine serology
CMV	PCR
HHV-6, HHV-7	PCR, routine serology, culture
VZV	PCR, routine serology, VZV Ge

Table 4. Diagnostic methods in herpesviridae family.

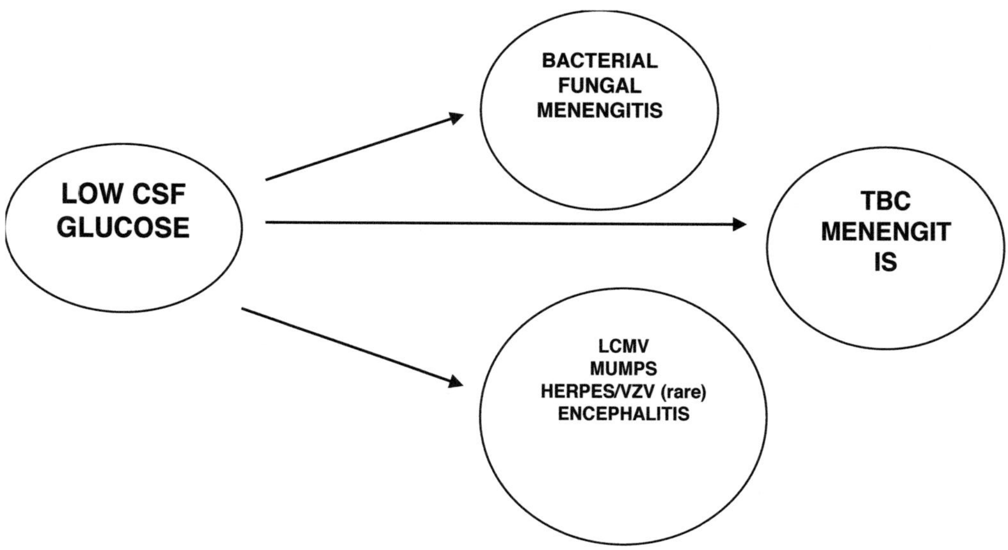

Figure 1. CNS infections, in which low CSF glucose levels are found.

In encephalitis caused by Flaviviruses, clinical suspicion maintains its importance. Methods that target Flaviviruses should be added to routine CSF analyses in endemic regions, or in patients who have a travel history; at times, repeated lumbar punctures are needed for determining the etiological agent. In West nile virus encephalitis, domination of polymorphonuclear leukocytes in hyperacute period, leaves its place to lympocytes afterwards. CSF protein concentrations are usually increased, glucose levels are normal. RT-PCR is assistant, but it is not possible in late stages of the disease to capture the virus RNA [12]. Virus isolation by means of CSF cultures is also utilised [13]. Today the most valid methods are serological approaches. The success of ELISA in detecting WNV-specific antibodies is increased in 8-21 days after the beginning of clinical symptoms. Similar serological methods can be used in other Flavivirus infections. In Japan encephalitis, for example, the valid method currently is ELISA capture of JE-IgM [14] (Table 5). Various biomarkers, which are detected in CSF in the course of WNV encephalitis may reflect the severity of disease and neuronal damage. In 58 % of cases with WNV, NfH-SM135 and GFAP-SM126 can be found positive, S100B positivity is seen in 90 % of this same group [15]. In Eastern equine encephalitis, leucocyte count is much more increased, and it can reach 1000-2000 cells per mm^3; it should also be noted that dominant cells are polymorphnuclear. CSF findings emerged from various encephalitic situations are summarized in Table 6.

As we mentioned above, a part of recent studies targets on inflammatory responses in CSF. Without question, these biomarkers are not etiology specific. However, they can be used for manifesting the severity of neuroinvasif disease. One of those markers is macrophage migration inhibitory factor (MIF) that increases in CSF in CNS infections [16]. Studies that investigate the association of these factors with possible etiological agents and disease severity is needed (Figure 2).

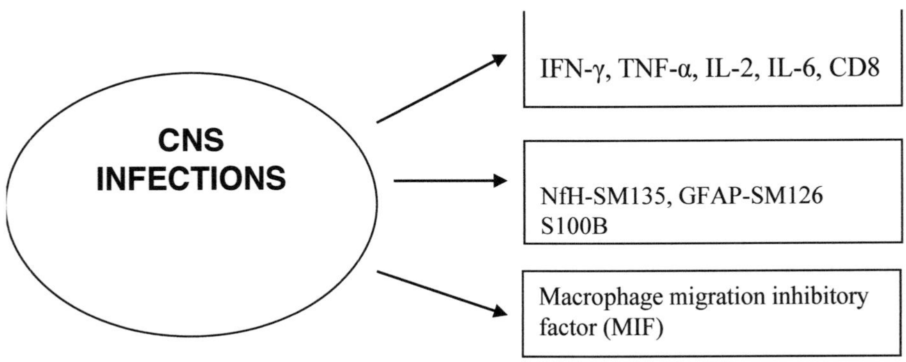

Figure 2. Several biomarkers elevating in CSF during the course of central nervous system infections.

FLAVIVIRUS INFECTIONS
Elevated protein, high cell count (initially neutrophilic; mononuclear pleocytosis after a certain time), normal glucose concentrations
RT-PCR, IgM ELISA capture
Virus isolation

Table 5. CSF characteristics and diagnostic methods in flavivirus encephalitides

CSF findings in all types of encephalitis may expose time dependent alterations. In cases with negative PCR, repeated lumbar punctures should be performed, differences in cell count should be observed, PCR studies should be repeated and new cell cultures should be made for virus isolation. This aproach is valid in patients receiving amprical antiviral treatment also. For example, it is known that PCR becomes positive several days after the onset of clinical symptoms in herpes encephalitis. PCR test becomes negative after a certain time in HSV and VZV encephalitis. This duration is shorter in patients receiving antiviral therapy. Once again, in herpes encephalitis, intrathecal antibody production commences beginning from the second week. In West Nile virus encephalitis, initial neutrophylic dominance gives way to a lymphocytic pleocytosis. Capturing specific IgM antibodies in the first week after syptom onset leads frequently to negative results. But the chance of detection increases in the following days. Therefore it is crucial to repeat lumbar puncture in such cases. On the other hand, WNV RT-PCR is positive in a narrow period, but the possibility of a positive result decreases as the disease progresses (Table 7).

	cell count	**Protein**	**Glucose**
HSV	MN	High	Normal-Low
VZV	MN	High	Normal-Low
CMV	MN	High	Normal
MUMPS	MN	Normal- High	Normal-Low
Enteroviruses	Normal-MN	High	Normal
WNV	PNL-MN	High	Normal
Influenza	Normal	Normal	Normal
JC virus	Normal	High	Normal

Table 6. CSF characteristics of encephalitis in various viruses.

	Cell count	**PCR**	**Antibody production**
HSV< 3 days	Normal-mononuclear	Negative	Negative
3-14 days	Mononuclear	Positive	**Negative-**Positive
"/>14 days	Mononuclear	**Negative-**Positive	**Positive-**Negative
WNV <2 days	Polymorphnuclear	Positive	Negative
2-7 days	Mononuclear	Positive-Negative	Negative
"/>7 days	Mononuclear	Negative	Positive

Table 7. Time dependent alterations of CSF findings in Herpes and WNV.

3. Future prospects of CSF studies for viral encephalitis

Current diagnostic methods which have been described above have been providing valuable proves for diagnostic process of the viral encephalitis but new approaches are needed with increased knowledge of pathogenesis of viral encephalitis. These are must be combined according to clinical picture and possible etiological agents. These promising methods are;

1. Detection of viral genomic materials

a. RT-PCR, IgM ELISA capture

b. Detection of viruses

c. Differentiation of lytic and lstent viral infectivity

2. Evaluation of inflammatory markers

a. IFN-γ, TNF-α, IL-2, IL-6, CD8

b. Macrophage migration inhibitory factor (MIF)

c. Determination of the antibodies

3. Evaluation of tissue and neuronal damage products

a. NfH-SM135, GFAP-SM126

b. S100B

4. Prognostic use of CSF findings in viral encephalitis [1, 3, 7].

Related to future prospects of diagnostic methods which will evaluate biomarkers in CSF must be improved as diagnostic and also prognostic methods.

Author details

Hakan Ekmekci[1], Fahrettin Ege[2] and Serefnur Ozturk[1*]

*Address all correspondence to: serefnur.ozturk@noroloji.org.tr

1 Selcuk University, Selcuklu Medical Faculty, Department of Neurology, Konya, Turkey

2 Ufuk University, Medical Faculty, Department of Neurology, Ankara, Turkey

References

[1] Tunkel Ar, Glasser CA, Bloch KC, Sejvar JJ, Marra CM, Roos KL, Hartman BJ, Kaplan SL, Scheld WM, Whitley Rj, Infectious disease society of America. The management

of encephalitis: clinical practice guidelines by the infectious diseases society of America, Clin Infect Dis 47 (2008) 303-327

[2] Rantalaiho T, Farkkila M, Vaheri A, Koskinemiemi M. Acute encephalitis from 1967 to 1991. Journal of the Neurological Sciences 2001; 184: 169 – 177.

[3] Steiner I, Schmutzhard E, Sellner J, Chaudhuri A, Kennedy PG. EFNS-ENS guidelines for the use of PCR technology for the diagnosis of infections of the nervous system. Eur J Neurol. 2012 Aug 6. doi: 10.1111/j.

[4] Chaudhuri A, Kennedy PGE. Diagnosis and treatment of viral encephalitis. Journal of postgraduate Medicine 2002; 78: 575 – 583.

[5] Ziai WC, Lewin III JJ, Update in the diagnosis and management of central nervous system infections, Neurol Clin 26 (2008) 427-468

[6] Romero JR, Newland JG, Diagnosis of viral encephalitides: Nonzoonotic-associated viruses, The pediatric infectious disease journal, 25 (2006) 739-740

[7] Jakob NJ, Lenhard TL, Schnitzler P, Rohde S, Ringleb PA, Steiner T, Wildemann B, Herpes simplex virus encephalitis despite normal cell count in the cerebrospinal fluid, Crit care med 40 (2012)1304-1308)

[8] Ziyaeyan M, Alborzi A, Haghighi AB, Moeini M, Pourabbas B, Diagnosis and quantitative detection of HSV DNA in samples from patients with suspected herpes simplex encephalitis, Braz J Infect Dis 15(3) (2011), 211-214

[9] Ambrose HE, Granerod J, Clewley JP, Davies NWS, Keir G, Cunningham R, Zuckerman M, Mutton KJ, Ward KN, Ijaz S, Crowcroft NS, Brown DWG, on behalf of the UK Aetiology of encephalitis study group, Diagnostic strategy to establishetiologies of encephalitis in a prospective cohort of patients in england, Journal of clinical microbiology 49 (2011) 3576-3583.

[10] Kamei S, Taira N, Ishikara M, Sekizawa T, Morita A, Miki K, Shiota H, Kanno A, Suzuki Y, Mizutani T, Itoyama Y, Morishima T, Hirayanagi K, Prognostic value of cerebrospinal fluid cytokine changes in herpes simplex virus encephalitis, Cytokine 46 (2009) 187-193

[11] Grahn A, Studahl M, Nilsson S, Thomsson E, Backström M, Bergström T, Varicella-zoster virus (VZV) glycoprotein E is a serological antigen for detection of intrathecal antibodies to VZV in central nervous system infections, without cross-reaction to herpes simplex virus 1, Clinical and Vaccine immunology, 18 (2011) 1336-1342

[12] LaSala PR, Holbrook M, Tick-Borne Flaviviruses, Clin Lab Med 30 (2010) 221-235

[13] Rossi SL, Ross TM, Evans JD, West nile virus, Clin Lab Med 30 (2010) 47-65

[14] Misra UK, Kalita J, Overview: Japanese encephalitis, Progress in Neurobiology 91 (2010) 108-120

[15] Petzold A, Groves M, Leis AA, Scaravilli F, Stokic DS, Neuronal and glial cerebrospinal fluid protein biomarkers are elevated after west nile virus infection, Muscle Nerve 41 (2010) 42-49

[16] Ostegaard C, Benfield T, Macrophage migration inhibitory factor in cerebrospinal fluid from patients wit central nervous system infection, Critical care 13 (2009)

[17] Crawford JR. Advances in pediatric neurovirology. Curr Neurol Neurosci Rep. 2010 Mar;10(2):147-54

Chapter 3

Spontaneous Intracranial Hypotension: What An Infectious Disease Physician Should Know?

Ilker Inanc Balkan and Resat Ozaras

Additional information is available at the end of the chapter

http://dx.doi.org/10.5772/53744

1. Introduction

Although the syndrome of spontaneous intracranial hypotension (SIH) is not an infectious disease, it is commonly involved in the differential diagnoses of meningitis and encephalitis. It is a clinical (headache, fever, even neck stiffness) and laboratory (cerebrospinal fluid (CSF) abnormalities) challenge for the physician. Considering this syndrome especially under some settings and taking care of the charactestic imaging findings would contribute to the diagnosis. We believe in that the physicians who care with these central nervous system (CNS) infections should be aware of this syndrome. Some patients under the suspicion of encephalitis have the SIH that could be diagnosed by approaches described in this chapter.

Patients presenting with fever, headache, stiff neck, nausea, vomiting and some other neurological signs suggesting meningeal irritation are always taken seriously and usually have a similar diagnostic algorithm. Differential diagnosis is usually based on the results of CSF analysis. In some cases, characteristics of the headache are the major factor determining the way to establish the diagnosis. Headache with a positional pattern, that occurs shortly after assuming an upright position and relieves by lying down, so called "orthostatic headache" is a distinctive symptom of SIH syndrome.

The spontaneous form of intracranial hypotension was first described by a German neurologist Georg Schaltenbrand in 1938 [1]. He recognized that "aliquorrhea," or as subsequently named "hypoliquorrhoea" a deficiency in cerebrospinal fluid, could result in headaches predominantly when upright. Since the introduction of magnetic resonance image (MRI) in daily diagnostic use in the early 1990s, much has been learned about SIH.

All or essentially all SIH cases are related with a spontaneous spinal CSF leak mostly at the cervicothoracic junction or along the thoracic spine [2].

SIH is an important and relatively frequent cause of newly onset daily persistent positional headaches in young and middle-aged individuals. Women are effected more frequently than men with a ratio of approximately 1.5/1. It is diagnosed about half as frequently as spontaneous subarachnoid hemorrhage and its incidence is estimated to be five per 100 000 [3].

Throbbing headache occurring or worsening in upright position and improving after lying down, so called "orthostatic headache", low CSF pressure, and diffuse pachymeningeal enhancement on brain magnetic resonance imaging (MRI) are the major features of the classic syndrome. Many other signs and symptoms may associate.

2. Diagnostic criteria of SIH

The diagnostic criteria used to verify the SIH cases are on shown on Table 1.

The clinical presentations and radiological findings may vary. Diagnosis is largely based on clinical suspicion, cranial MR findings and myelographic detection of dural leak. The positional characteristics of the headache should always be questioned in patients admitting with meningeal irritation signs. Orthostatic headache, characteristic imaging features on MRI and instantaneous improvement of symptoms with a successful blood patch are key points of differential diagnosis from viral meningoencephalitis or other causes of aseptic meningitis syndrome.

A. Diffuseand/or dull headache that worsens within 15 minutes after sittingor standing, fulfilling criterion D and with ≥ 1 of the following:
1. Neckstiffness 2. Tinnitus 3. Hypacusia 4. Photophobia 5. Nausea
B. At least1 of the following:
1. Evidence of low CSF pressure on MRI (eg,pachymeningeal enhancement) 2. Evidence of CSF leakage on conventionalmyelography, CT myelography, or cisternography 3. CSF openingpressure <60 mm H_2O in sitting position
C. No history ofdural puncture or other cause of CSF fistula
D. Headache resolves within 72 hours after epidural blood patching

Table 1. Diagnostic Criteria for Headache Due to Spontaneous Spinal CSF Leak and Intracranial Hypotension According to the International Classification of Headache Disorders, 2nd Ed42 (4)

3. SIH and aseptic meningitis

Patients admitted with fever, headache and CSF findings revealing lymphocytic pleocytosis, elevated protein concentration and normal glucose levels are prone to be misdiagnosed as viral meningoencephalitis or usually aseptic meningitis [5].

The clinical presentation of aseptic meningitis is generally nonspecific, with fever, headache, nausea and vomiting, occasionally accompanied by photophobia and a stiff neck. Physical examination typically reveals signs of nuchal rigidity

The syndrome of "aseptic meningitis" including differing etiologies and disorders, presents a diagnostic challenge to the clinician [6]. Although many infectious and noninfectious etiologies exist for this syndrome, viruses, especially nonpolio enteroviruses, are the most common (>85%) and most important agents encountered. Although seasonal variation is relative and not absolute, enteroviruses are most likely to be the cause of aseptic meningitis occurring during the summer or fall. The onset of symptoms is characteristically abrupt and typically includes headache, fever, nausea or vomiting, malaise, photophobia, and meningismus.

Because the presenting signs and symptoms of enteroviral meningitis are not distinctive, tuberculosis meningitis, herpes simplex encephalitis, HIV encephalitis and parameningeal infection that may mimic aseptic meningitis in their initial presentations must not be overlooked.

SIH may mimic aseptic meningitis. The main features of aseptic meningitis and SIH cases are compared in a case series newly reported form Turkey [7]. Various clinical and laboratory features of 11 consecutive cases of SIH and 10 consecutive cases of aseptic meningitis are given below (Table 2).

All of the 11 patients with SIH reported that their headache was occurring or worsening within minutes or hours assuming the upright position and improving by lying down, defined as "orthostatic headache". All met the diagnostic criteria defined by International Headache Society. The median duration of sudden-onset orthostatic headache was 10 days, ranging between 1 to 30 days. Five cases (5/11) had a previous diagnosis of migraine because of chronic headache. The newly onset orthostatic headache was throbbing and diffuse in all cases distributing from posterior neck (5/11), from frontal area (4/11), from left temporal region (1/11) and from left parietal region (1/11) to the whole cranium. The typical positional characteristics of the headache were noticed with further questioning of the patients.

Hearing changes, disturbed sense of balance, and nausea were noted in all patients. Posterior neck pain and vomiting were described in 9, tinnitus in 3 patients, and echoing in 1 case.

Stiff neck was detected in 5 patients, and fever (axillary; >37.3°C) in 7 patients. The highest temperatures of those with fever were measured as follows; 38.7 °C, 38.3 °C, 38.1 °C, 38 °C, 38.9 °C, 38.2 °C and 38.5 °C.

Eight of 11 cases had visual changes as blurring (5/11) and diplopia (5/11).

Among neurological disorders photophobia (8/11), phonophobia (8/11) were most frequent followed by subtle cognitive deficits (5/11), amnesia (4/11), confusion & syncope (3/11), dysgeusia (3/11), facial numbness (2/11), convulsion, hyperexcitability, dysarthria, ataxia, facial weakness, facial spasm (each 1/11).

	CLINICAL SIGNS & SYMPTOMS				CSF FINDINGS (Mean±SD)							
	Headache	**Fever**	**Nausea – Vomiting**	**Stiff Neck**	**Opening pressure (mmH_2O) (NR: 50-180)***	**Leukocyte (/ mm^3) (NR:0-5)****	**Lympho-cyte (/mm^3) (NR:0-5)**	**Protein concentra-tion (mg/dl) (NR:15-45) *****	**CSF Glucose /blood glucose (mg/dl) (NR: 40-80)**	**Enterovirus PCR positivity**	**HSV PCR positivity**	**TB PCR positivity**
SIH (n=11)	11/11	7/11	10/11	5/11	59 ±16.4	229±200	76 ± 5	55±49	61± 12/102 ±21	0/11	0/10	0/10
Aseptic Meningitis (n=10)	10/10	6/10	6/10	5/10	160±28.4	360±50	84±13	93±92	63±11/ 114±13	2/10	0/10	0/10

SIH: Spontaneous intracranial hypotension, CSF: Cerebrospinal fluid, NR: normal range, PCR: polymerase chain reaction, HSV: Herpes simplex virus, TB: tuberculosis

* Only five were measured.

** Pleocytosis was detected in only four SIH cases while all (n=10) cases of aseptic meningitis had lymphocytic pleocytosis varying between 32 and 1340 /mm^3.

*** Four SIH and seven aseptic meningitis cases had elevated CSF protein levels.

Table 2. Comparison of SIH and Aseptic Meningitis Cases

4. SIH and encephalitis

Despite the benign character of SIH, some rare cases may present with severe neurological findings. A few cases of SIH are reported whose chief clinical manifestation were diffuse severe encephalopathy with marked depression of consciousness, hyperexcitability or convulsion [7,8].

A 40 year old female [8] was admitted to Stanford University School of Medicine in California with a progressive cognitive decline of 2 to 4 weeks' duration. She developed a newly onset diffuse headache in orthostatic nature one month ago and she suffered a brief generalized seizure 2 weeks before admission. Her computerized tomography (CT) scan and electroencephalography (EEG) were normal and she was diagnosed as SIH with diffuse pachymeningitis on MRI, low CSF opening pressure (60 mm/H_2O) immediate clinical improvement responding to placement of epidural blood patch.

Two similar cases with SIH, with no defined preexisting comorbidities and newly pre-diagnosed as meningoencephalitis, were reported from Istanbul-Turkey. Both were young (29 and 21 years) males, brought to emergency departments of different hospitals in coma with a 3-year of time interval. One had a generalized tonic-clonic convulsion and the other who was evaluated as nonconvulsive status had hyperexcitability. Antiepileptic agents were administered for both before admission to the university hospital where the final diagnosis was established.

The first diagnostic steps for these cases were aimed to exclude Herpes encephalitis due to its high frequency and being a medical emergency. Although the patients were admitted with impaired conscious and convulsions, there were no signs of contrast enhancement (e.g. temporal, parietal or frontal lobe) suggesting HSV 1 involvement, the CSF opening pressures were slightly low (60 and 90 mmH_2O consequently) and HSV 1 PCR results were negative.

The diagnosis of SIH was established on the basis of specific cranial MR images, negative CSF findings and the prompt response to blood patch within 72 hours.

The most common cause of non-epidemic (not affecting a large number of people at once) encephalitis in developed countries is the herpes simplex virus. The most common signs of acute viral encephalitis are fever, headache, and a change in level of consciousness. Other common signs are the eyes becoming sensitive to light (photophobia), confusion, and sometimes seizures.

Some people exposed to insect-borne encephalitis viruses do not develop symptoms of encephalitis. They may only experience low-grade fever, drowsiness, and flu-like symptoms of malaise (general feeling of illness) and myalgia (muscle aches). Headache, vomiting, and sensitivity to light may follow. The epidemiological relatedness and a history of a travel, recall of an insect exposure are useful to exclude this type of encephalitis.

Symptoms and signs of meningeal irritation (photophobia and nuchal rigidity) are usually absent with a pure encephalitis but often accompany a meningoencephalitis. Patients with encephalitis have an altered mental status ranging from subtle deficits to complete unresponsiveness. Seizures are common with encephalitis, and focal neurologic abnormalities can occur, including hemiparesis, cranial nerve palsies, and exaggerated deep tendon and/or pathologic reflexes. Patients may appear confused, agitated, or obtunded.

Results of imaging in patients with encephalitis may or may not demonstrate abnormal radiographic findings on CT or MRI modalities. CT scanning is useful to rule space-occupying lesions or brain abscess. MRI is sensitive for detecting demyelination, which may be seen in other clinical states presenting with mental status changes (eg. progressive multifocal leukoencephalopathy) and typical contrast enhancing (mostly temporal lesions).

Initial examination of the CSF, although not diagnostic, will usually confirm the presence of inflammatory disease of the CNS. The findings with encephalitis, aseptic meningitis and meningoencephalitis are generally indistinguishable.

5. SIH and fever

The fever seen in SIH cases those mimic meningoencephalitis might be explained by the release of pyrogenic cytokines by endothelial cells and astrocytes of blood-brain barrier secondary to a drop in CSF pressure [10]. These cytokines are the main mediators of inflammatory response in infectious and non-infectious disorders. Another suggested mechanism for fever would be an impaired hypothalamic thermoregulation secondary to mechanical distractions and venous engorgement in cavernous sinus and diencephalic region.

6. Neurologic manifestations of SIH

Hearing changes including disturbed sense of balance, tinnitus and echoing; visual changes including visual blurring and diplopia; various neurological symptoms including photophobia, phonophobia, amnesia and facial numbness are common [11]. A significantly decreased level of consciousness might be observed in cases with SIH and even they would admit with confusion and syncope [7]. Subtle cognitive deficits are common particularly during episodes of headache [2].

Symptoms in SIH patients related to the vestibulocochlear system such as disturbed sense of balance, tinnitus and sense of echoing may be explained by direct transmission of the abnormal CSF pressure to that in the perilymph [21]. Visual impairment was probably due to stretching of the cranial nerves due to downward displacement of the brain [12].

7. Radiological manifestations of SIH

CNS imaging is key in the differential diagnosis. Essentially no MRI findings are seen in aseptic meningitis and imaging is not needed in most of the cases. Cases with encephalitis have special MRI findings varying due to the etiology, being the temporal lobe involvement of HSV 1 encephalitis the most common. In contrary, MRI findings are characteristic and imaging with contrast material is preferred in SIH. With the widespread and increasing use of MRI, SIH is more frequently recognized in recent years as an important cause of new onset persistent, daily, positional headaches. Diffuse pachymeningeal (dural) contrast enhancement is the main feature on cranial MRI. Some other findings of SIH have been described: Enlargement of pituitary, tenting of the optic chiasm, subdural fluid collections, engorged cerebral venous sinuses and findings due to sagging of the brain such as obliteration of subarachnoid cisterns, crowding of posterior fossa and descent of cerebellar tonsils [5].

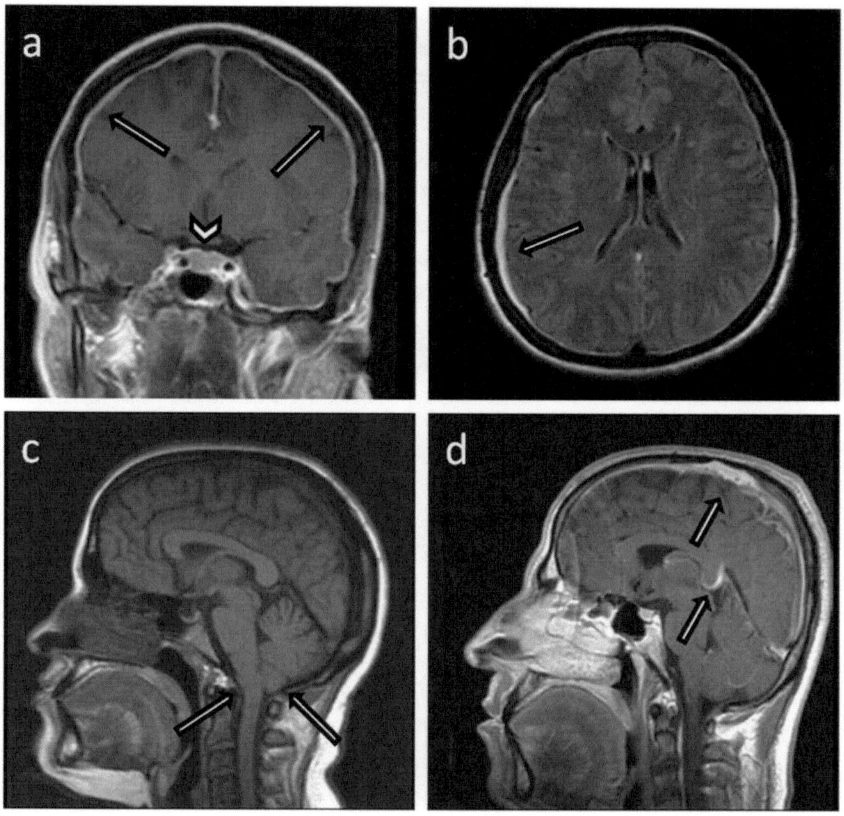

Figure 1. Thickening in meninges demonstrating pachymeningeal contrast enhancement (arrows) and enlargement of the pituitary gland (arrowhead)in a 36 years old female patient [7], presenting with orthostatic headache, stiff neck and fever. **b.** Axial FLAIR image of the same case showing bilateral thin subdural collection (arrow). **c.** Findings of sagging brain (arrow) in a 37 year old female (case 1] presenting with fever, severe headache, nausea and vomiting. **d.** Engorgement in cerebral veins (arrows) of a 44 year old male presenting with fever and meningeal irritation signs whose LP revealed a marked lymphocytic pleocytosis[450 / mm^3]. *(Derived from ref. 7. Photo courtesy of Sait Albayram, with permission)*

8. Management and follow up

The treatment of SIH is controversial. In some, bed rest, hydration, caffeine intake, and steroids are effective, while in other an epidural blood patching may be needed [2,5]. Epidural blood patch is performed by obtaining a small amount of the patient's venous blood and injecting into the epidural space close to the site of the leakage; the resulting blood clot then patches the meningeal leak by forming a dural tamponade [9]. Although the outcomes have been poorly studied, epidural blood patch is the preferred modality for a better treatment outcome in those that do not improve with conventional supportive treatment [13].

9. Conclusion

Fever, headache, and meningeal irritation findings are generally accepted as the clinical features of meningitis syndrome. When CSF findings are not characteristically compatible with bacterial or tuberculosis meningitis, it is usually defined as aseptic meningitis. Some cases with SIH, those admitting with signs of meningeal irritation, decreased cognitive levels, and various neurological signs and symptoms including hyperexcitability and status, may mimic meningoencephalitis. The characteristic features of SIH should promptly be searched in those cases. If the headache is in orthostatic nature, CSF opening pressure is low and characteristic MRI findings are present, the diagnosis would be established as SIH. The diagnostic criteria defined by International Headache Society would be suggested to exclude SIH in the differential diagnosis.

Author details

Ilker Inanc Balkan and Resat Ozaras

Istanbul University, Cerrahpasa Medical School, Infectious Diseases Department, Istanbul, Turkey

References

[1] Schaltenbrand G. Neuere Anschauungen zur Pathophysiologie de Liquorzirkulation. Zentralbl Neurochir 1938;3:290–9.

[2] Schievink WI. Spontaneous spinal cerebrospinal fluid leaks. Cephalalgia. 2008;28(12): 1345-56.

[3] Schievink WI, Maya MM, Moser F, Tourje J, Torbati J, Torbati S. Frequency of spontaneous intracranial hypotension in the emergency department. J Headache Pain 2007; 8:325–8.

[4] Headache Classification Subcommittee of the International Headache Society. The International Classification of Headache Disorders: 2nd edition. Cephalalgia 2004; 24(Suppl 1):9.)

[5] Mokri B, Low cerebrospinal fluid pressure syndromes. Neurol Clin. 2004;22(1):55-74.

[6] Connolly, KJ, Hammer, SM. Acute aseptic meningitis syndrome. Infect Dis Clin North Am 1990; 4:599-622

[7] Balkan II, Albayram S, Ozaras R, Yilmaz MH, Ozbayrak M, Mete B, Yemisen M, Tabak F. Spontaneous intracranial hypotension syndrome may mimic aseptic meningitis. Scand J Infect Dis. 2012;44(7):481-8.

[8] Beck CE, Rızk NW, Kiger LT, Spencer D, Hill L, Adler JR. Intracranial hypotension presenting with severe encephalopathy. J Neurosurg 89: 470-473, 1998.

[9] Berroir S, Loisel B, Ducros A, Boukobza M, Tzourio C, Valade D, Bousser MG. Early epidural blood patch in spontaneous intracranial hypotension. Neurology. 2004 Nov 23;63(10):1950-1.

[10] Johnson KS, Sexton DJ. Cerebrospinal fluid: Physiology and utility of an examination in disease states. In: Ed. Calderwood SW. UpToDate 19.1version, last updated 3rd May 2010.

[11] Mokri B. Low cerebrospinal fluid pressure syndromes. Neurol Clin. 2004;22(1):55-74.

[12] Horton JC, Fishman RA. Neurovisual findings in the syndrome of pontaneous intracranial hypotension from dural cerebrospinal luid leak. Ophthalmology 1994; 101: 244-51.

[13] Mokri B, Krueger BR, Miller GM, Piepgras DG. Meningeal gadolinium enhancement in low pressure headaches. Ann Neurol 1991; 294-5.

Chapter 4

Acute Viral Encephalitis/Encephalopathy in an Emergency Hospital in Japan: A Retrospective Study of 105 Cases in 2002 – 2011

Hiroshi Shoji, Masaki Tachibana,
Tomonaga Matsushita, Yoshihisa Fukushima and
Shimpei Sakanishi

Additional information is available at the end of the chapter

http://dx.doi.org/10.5772/54605

1. Introduction

Herpes simplex encephalitis (HSE) has come to be widely recognized as diagnosable and treatable at early stages of the disease. The incidence of encephalitis/encephalopathy resulting from other members of herpesvirus group such as varicella-zoster virus (VZV), Epstein-Barr virus (EBV), cytomegalovirus (CMV), and human herpes virus (HHV)-6 has also tended to increase in both healthy and immunocompromised patients (Shoji et al, 2002). In sharp contrast, the incidence of Japanese encephalitis (JE) in Japan has dramatically decreased to a few patients per year. However, JE remains a threat among the elderly and individuals with decreased or absent immunity to the JE virus (Ayukawa et al, 2002). Influenza-associated encephalopathy (FluE) is a threat for adults as well as children (Lee et al, 2010, Umemura et al, 2011, Watanabe et al, 2012). In the present study, we retrospectively analyzed the cases of 105 mainly adult patients with acute viral encephalitis/encephalopathy at our emergency hospital, St. Mary's Hospital, Kurume City during a recent 10-years period from 2002 to 2011.We present here our preliminary report of the changing patterns in HSE, JE and FluE during the past 10 years.

2. Objectives and methods

We extracted the clinical records of the 105 patients diagnosed with acute viral encephalitis/encephalopathy in 2002—2012 from the medical records of St. Mary's Hospital, Kurume

City. Our hospital is located in southwestern Japan and provides emergency medical care for approximately 500,000 local residents. The diagnostic criteria for each viral agent in the patients' clinical charts were, in principle, dependent on polymerase chain reaction (PCR) positivity in cerebrospinal fluid (CSF) or serologic four fold increases in pair sera or CSFs. HSE was diagnosed by clinical symptoms, CSF, magnetic resonance imaging (MRI), electroencephalogram (EEG), and virologic tests such as herpes simplex virus (HSV) PCR in CSF and enzyme immunoassay (EIA) IgG IgM antibodies. VZV-associated encephalitis was mainly diagnosed by characteristic skin eruptions. JE in Japan is seen from August to September. The diagnosis of JE is established by complement fixation (CF) or hemagglutination inhibition (HI) test in pair sera, or PCR for JE virus. FluE is defined as persistent consciousness impairment over 24 hours following an influenza infection; delirium or convulsive seizures due to high fever and metabolic disorders are excluded (Japanese guidlines for FluE, 2009).The clinical forms of FluE are divided into the status epilepticus type, thalamic type, acute necrotizing encephalopathy, hemorrhagic shock and encephalopathy, Reye syndrome, and others in which no CSF pleocytosis, high concentration of IL-6 and negative PCR in CSF for influenza virus are usually observed. Non-herpetic limbic encephalitis is identified by MRI findings in bilateral limbic systems and negative HSV PCR or EIA antibodies (Ichiyama T, 2008, Shoji et al, 2012). As for anti-N-methyl-D-aspartate receptor (anti-NMDAR) encephalitis or encephalopathy, ovarian teratoma is usually found, except for pedriatric cases (Dalmau et al, 2007, 2011). Patients with viral-related acute disseminated encephalomyelitis (ADEM) were diagnosed as having disseminated neurologic lesions following suspected viral infections.

3. Results

The following acute viral encephalitis/encephalopathy cases were identified among the 105 cases (Table 1): HSE, 14 cases; herpes zoster related encephalitis, 4; HHV-6 encephalopathy, 1; JE, 4; FluE, 20, mumps encephalitis, 3; and rotavirus encephalopathy, 1. As 'other' types, non-herpetic limbic encephalitis and anti-NMDAR encephalitis/encephalopathy numbered 7, and there were 12 viral-related ADEM cases.

The remaining 42 cases of viral encephalitis had unknown etiology. Thus, the incidence of HSE was 1.4 persons per year for 500,000 persons, JE was 0.4 per year, and FluE was 2.0 per year. With regard to seasonale occurrence, the HSE cases were sporadic and uncorrelated to the seasons, whereas the JE cases occurred in September and October, and FluE was observed during the winters.

Regarding the outcomes and onset ages of the 14 HSE cases, one patient died of pneumonia, and two patients showed relapse. Five patients were more than 65 years old (Fig.1); the mean age at onset was 47.3 years, and the male to female ratio was 6:8. There were only two HSE patients under 20 years old; an infant and a 14-year-old boy. The oldest HSE patient, an 88-year-old man was admitted in late September in a delirious state with tonic seizures; his CSF showed 683 cells per mm^3 and protein at 186mg/dL. HSV PCR was negative in his CSF,

http://dx.doi.org/10.5772/54605

but the EIA IgG for HSV showed a significant increase, and his MRI DW revealed high intensities in the right limbic regions (Fig.2). Four patients with VZV-associated encephalitis were diagnosed by the characteristic skin eruptions. Of CMV, EBV, and HHV-6 associated with encephalitis or encephalopathy, the case of a one-year-old girl with probable HHV-6 encephalopathy was identified (Fig. 3). She was admitted to our hospital with a high fever, tonic seizures, and consciousness impairment. Although apparent clinical symptoms of exanthem subitum were not observed, her serum FA IgG titer in the recovery stage showed a high titer of 1280x for HHV-6.

	2002	2003	2004	2005	2006	2007	2008	2009	2010	2011	Total
HSE	2	1	1	2	2	1	0	0	3	2	14
H. zoster, HHV-6 encephalitis/encephalopathy	0	0	0	3	1	0	0	1	0	0	5
JE	0	0	1	0	0	1	0	0	0	2	4
FluE	3	0	1	4	2	3	0	7	0	0	20
Mumps encephalitis	0	1	0	0	0	1	0	0	0	1	3
Rotavirus encephalopathy	0	0	0	0	0	0	0	1	0	0	1
NHALE, Anti-NMDARE	1	1	1	0	0	0	1	4	0	2	10
Viral-related ADEM	1	1	0	1	2	2	1	0	2	2	12
Viral encephalitis	4	7	10	3	3	5	0	2	1	1	36
Total	11	11	14	13	10	13	2	15	6	10	105

HSE=herpes simplex encephalitis, HHV-6=human herpesvirus-6, JE=Japanese encephalitis, FluE=influenza encephalopathy, NHALE=non-herpetic limbic encephalitis, anti-NMDARE=anti--N-methyl-D-aspartate receptor encephalitis, ADEM=acute disseminated encephalomyelitis

Table 1. Acute viral encephalitis/encephalopathy, St. Mary's Hospital, Kurume, Fukuoka, Japan, 2002 - 2011 (n=105)

Four cases of JE were recognized, with one case from September 2005, one from September 2007 and two from September and October 2011, respectively (Fig.4). The patients' ages and genders were 79 years/F, 93/F, 76/M, and 69/M, and the mean age was 79.3 years. One patient died one month after admission, and the other three patients suffered from severe sequelae. The 69-year-old man was found after having fallen in September 2011, and was admitted to our hospital. He was initially diagnosed as having had a stroke due to the onset of an acute right hemiparesis, but his CSF and MRI findings suggested JE, and the diagnosis was serologically confirmed by a significant increase in JE virus in the acute and convalescent sera. For all four JE cases, steroid pulse therapy was performed, but the effects were minimal.

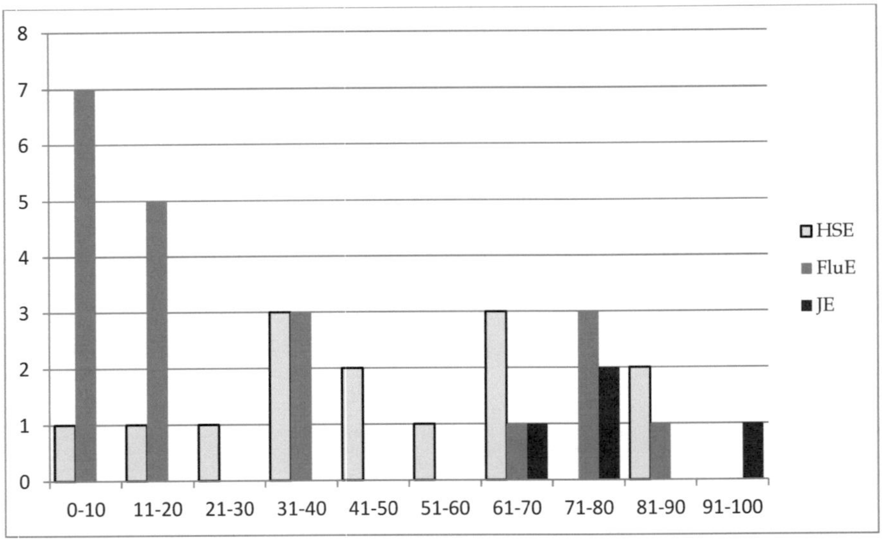

Kurume, Fukuoka, Japan, 2002 - 2011
HSE=herpes simplex encephalitis, FluE =influenza encephalopathy, JE=Japanese encephalitis

Figure 1. Age distribution of HSE, FluE and JE patients (HSE n=14, FluE n=20, JE n=4) at St. Mary's Hospital,

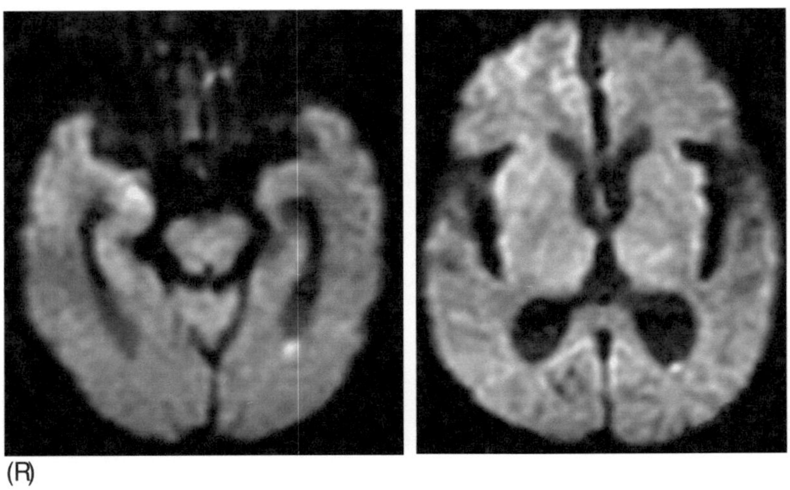

Figure 2. An 88-year-old man with herpes simplex encephalitis. MRI DW images on 4 days after onset revealed high intensities at the right amygdala, insula, and frontal lobe.

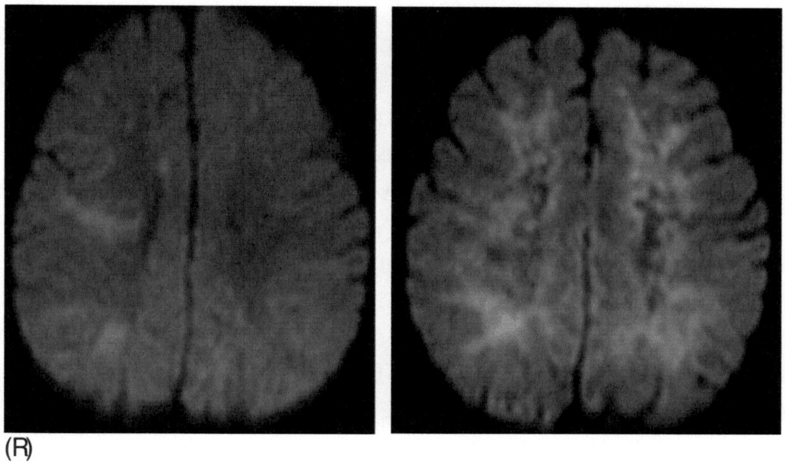

Figure 3. A 10-month-girl with HHV-6 encephalopathy; Lt, MRI DW on the 2nd day after onset showed high intensities at the right parietal and occipital lobes; Rt, 10 days later, the high intensities extended bilaterally into diffuse white matter.

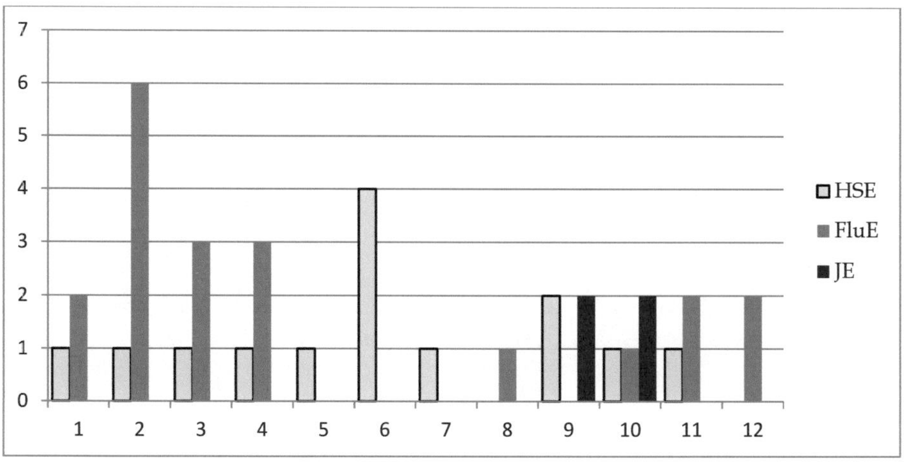

Figure 4. Monthly incidence of HSE, FluE and JE patients (HSE n=14, FluE n=20, JE n=4) at St. Mary's Hospital, Kurume, Fukuoka, Japan, 2002 – 2011

Ten pediatric and adult cases of FluE were identified, respectively. Seven FluE patients, including 4 adult cases, were seen consistent of the world epidemic of the new pig influenza H1N1 in 2009 (Fig.5).

The clinical forms of the pediatric cases (age under 15 years) included the status epilepticus type, the thalamic type, and the acute hemorrhagic shock and encephalopathy type. The clinical forms of the adult cases included several cases of the status epilepticus type, and one adult presented Reye syndrome. Among the status epilepticus-type cases of

FluE, a 32-year-old-man was admitted to our hospital with a fever of 39℃ and tonic seizures in August, 2009. A rapid test for influenza virus using a throat swab showed influenza type A, and his CSF exhibited no cell increase. An MRI revealed abnormalities of the cingulate gyri and basal ganglia (Fig.6), and an EEG showed diffuse slowness. The four adult status epilepticus type cases improved markedly after control for status epilepiticus and steroid pulse therapy, and they were all discharged without sequelae. An 83-year-old-man presented with influenza B in March 2005, then developed Reye syndrome with symptoms of consciousness impairment, hyperammonemia, and hepatic and renal dysfunction; he died one month after admission. Reye syndrome is characterized by acute non-inflammatory encephalopathy and fatty degeneration of the liver, usually after viral infection. Because this disease mainly affects children and teenagers, our case of the advanced age of 83 years old is a quite rare example.

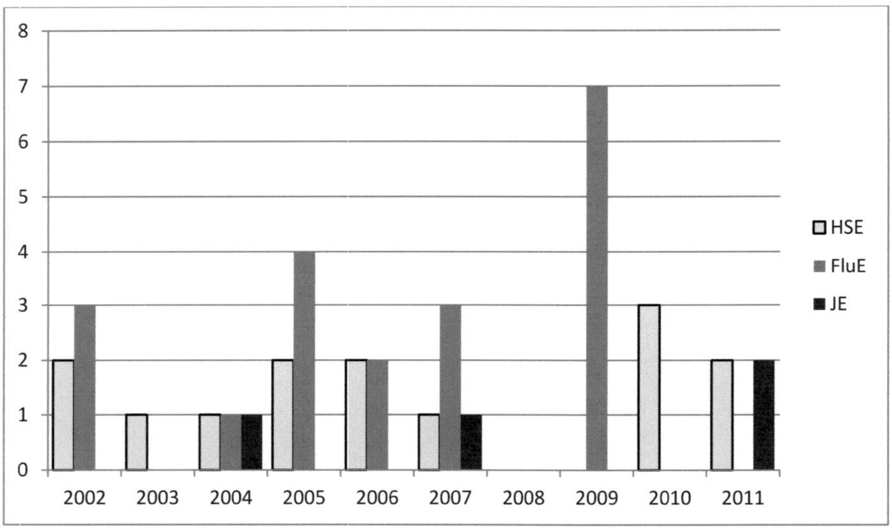

Figure 5. The occurrence by year of HSE, FluE and JE patients (HSE n=14, FluE n=20, JE n=4) at St. Mary's Hospital,Kurume, Fukuoka, Japan, 2002 – 2011

Next, a one-year-old boy with rotavirus encephalopathy was identified; he showed tonic seizures, consciousness impairment, hepatic and renal dysfunction, and disseminated intravascular coagulation following diarrhea and dehydration by rotavirus (acute hemorrhagic shock and encephalopathy type).

Low-temperature, steroid pulse and intravenous immunoglobulin therapies were performed, but he suffered from gait impairment and symptomatic epilepsy as sequelae.

Three cases of non-herpetic limbic encephalitis and four cases of anti-NMDAR encephalitis associated with ovarian teratoma were identified. The adult patient with anti-NMDAR encephalitis had a favorable outcome after resection of ovarian teratoma.

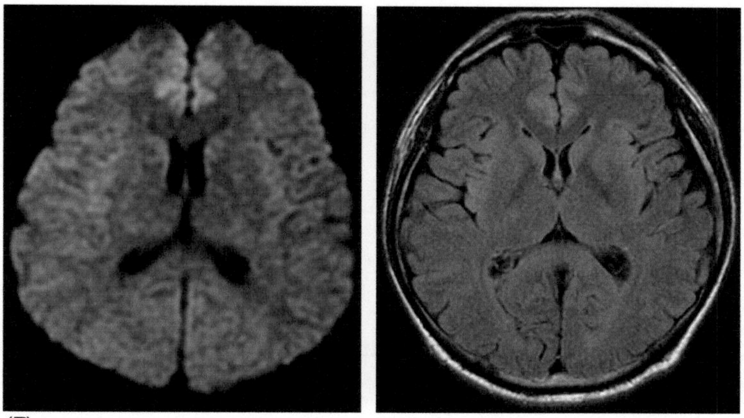

Figure 6. MRI DW & FLAIR images revealed high intensities at the cingulate gyri in a 32-year-old man with status epilepticus-type FluE (influenza-associated encephalopathy).

4. Discussion

The initial steps in emergency medicine for acute central nervous system (CNS) infections are to maintain a patent air-way, control convulsive seizures and protect the patient from brain edema, followed immediately by making a rapid etiological diagnosis and starting empiric therapy (Fitch et al, 2008, Solomon et al, 2010). Acute viral encephalitis/encephalopathy is non-invasively diagnosed by clinical symptoms, CSF, EEG, CT, MRI, and virologic tests such as PCR and EIA. The determination of the presence/absence of CSF pleocytosis is helpful for the differentiation of encephalitis and encephalopathy. Seasonable factors such as JE and FluE, and associated symptoms such as parotitis in mumps encephalitis should be considered for their diagnoses. Bacterial, fungal and tuberculous meningitis excluded on the basis of a decrease of glucose concentration in CSF and gram staining or bacterial latex tests.

The prevalence of viral and other types of encephalitis was estimated to be 17.7±3.2 per million person year, including 5.5±1.0 of viral, 1.2±0.07 of bacterial, and 8.9±0.7 of unknown etiology, in a nationwide questionnaire survey from 1989 to 1991(Kamei et al, 2000). HSE accounted for 63.9% of all identified cases of viral encephalitis, VZV for 8.0%, influenza virus for 1.3%, and Japanese B virus for 0.9% in this survey. The annual incidence with HSE was similar to that previously reported in the USA, 2.0 to 4.0 per million population (Whitley et al, 1998), while the incidence was 2.3 per million population in Sweden (Skoldenberg et al, 1984) and 1.0 per million population in the UK (Gulliford et al, 1984). According to this prevalence, the number of patients in our region over a 10-year period was estimated from 10 -18 for HSE, 0-2 for FluE, and 0-1 for JE, while we actually accumulated 14 HSE, 24 FluE, and 4 JE patients. The difference between the projected and actual numbers of adults with FluE in 2009 may have been caused by the new influenza A (H1N1) pandemic, in that year. Our hospital is located in southwestern Japan, and it is also likely that geographic factors such as higher possessing JE virus antibody in pigs or mosquitoes led to an increase in the number of occurrences of JE.

On the other hand, acute encephalitis/encephalopathy in children under 15 years of age has occurred in approximately 1,000 cases per year, as indicated in a large-scale survey of Japan. The etiology in order from most prevalent to least prevalent is influenza (25%), HHV-6 (11%), and rotavirus (4%) (Morishima, 2009). The incidence of HHV-6 encephalopathy, 7.0 per 100,000 infants, was estimated from the infant population of Japan, and severe neurological complications remained in half of these infants (Ohashi, et al, 2006).

Regarding the onset age of the 14 HSE patients, the under-30-year-old cases included one infant, a 14-year-old boy, and a 24-year-old man; the mean age of all 14 patients was 47.3 years. The peak onset age was in the 60s, although our past study identified two peaks at 20 and the 50s. The oldest HSE patient, an 88-year-old man, died of complicated pneumonia one month after admission, and another 80-year-old man suffered from severe memory impairment as a sequela, despite early acyclovir treatment. The upward trend of elderly patients with HSE may reflect the 'graving' of the Japanese populations, and also suggests that the reactivation of HSV can occur even in elderly people (Suzuki et al, 2012). All four of present patients with VZV-associated encephalitis had favorable outcomes after high-dose of intravenous acyclovir therapy.

All four of the JE patients we identified were elderly (including a 93-year-old), and their immunity to the JE virus was probably decreased or absent (Ayukawa et al 2002, Lee et al 2012). Presently, there is no specific therapy for JE, and thus JE vaccination might be advisable for elderly people in the epidemic area.

The incidence of FluE has increased in Japan since the 1997 winter influenza season. FluE affects mainly children under 10 years old (Okumura et al, 2012, Watanabe et al, 2012). In our hospital, 10 adult FluE cases were recognized in the 2002—2012 examination period, including four patients over 15 years old who were part of the epidemic of the new pig influenza variant in 2009 (Umemura et al, Lee N et al, 2010). For the pediatric patients, steroid pulse, intravenous immunoglobulin or low-temperature therapies were performed. The adult patients had favorable outcomes except for one case of Reye syndrome. Although hypercytokinemia has been contended to contribute to the pathogenesis, the IL-6 levels in our adult cases were in the normal range.

5. Conclusion

We analyzed the cases of 105 patients with acute viral encephalitis/encephalopathy who were treated at our emergency center, St. Mary's Hospital, Kurume City during the 10 years from 2002 to 2011. Fourteen HSE cases, 4 of herpes zoster-related encephalitis, 1 of HHV-6 white matter encephalopathy, 4 of JE, 20 of FluE, 3 of mumps encephalitis, and 1 of rotavirus encephalopathy were identified. As other types, 12 cases of viral-related ADEM and 7 cases of non-herpetic limbic encephalitis including anti-NMDAR encephalitis/encephalopathy were observed. The etiology of the remaining 42 cases of viral encephalitis was unknown.

http://dx.doi.org/10.5772/54605

Our results show an upward trend in HSE and JE toward patients over 65 years of age and an increase in adult-onset FluE. Although mortality rates of HSE and JE cases were low, the JE patients remained severe sequelae. The adult FluE patients had more favorable outcomes compared to the pediatric patients. Specific anti-viral drugs are still limited, and acute viral encephalitis/encephalopathy such as FluE overlaps into immunological pathogenesis. Thus, the rapid diagnosis of etiology and pathophysiology and initiation of empiric therapy are required.

Author details

Hiroshi Shoji[1], Masaki Tachibana[2], Tomonaga Matsushita[2], Yoshihisa Fukushima[2] and Shimpei Sakanishi[3]

1 Division of Neurology, St. Mary's Hospital, Kurume, Fukuoka, Japan

2 Cerebrovascular Department, St. Mary's Hospital, Kurume, Fukuoka, Japan

3 Pediatrics, St. Mary's Hospital, Kurume, Fukuoka, Japan

References

[1] Ayukawa R; Fujimoto H, Ayabe M, Shoji H, Matsui R, Iwata Y, Fukuda H, Ochi K, Noda K, Ono Y, Sakai K, Takehisa Y, & Yasui K (2004). An unexpected outbreak of Japanese encephalitis in the Chugoku district of Japan, 2002. *Jpn J Infect Dis* 57. 63-66.

[2] Belay ED; Bresee JS, Holman RC, Khan AS, Shahriari A, & Schonberger LB. Reye's syndrome in the United States from 1981 through 1997 (1999). *N Engl J Med* 340. 1377-82.

[3] Costa PS; Ribeiro GM, Vale TC, Casali TG, Leite FJ (2011). Adult Reye-like syndrome associated with serologic evidence of acute parvovirus B19 infection. *Braz J Infect Dis* 15. 482-3.

[4] Dalmau J; Lancaster E, Martinez-Hernandez E, Rosenfeld MR, & Balice-Gordon R (2011). Clinical experience and laboratory investigations in patients with anti-NMDAR encephalitis. *Lancet Neurol* 10. 63-74.

[5] Dalmau, J.; Turzen. E., Wu, H.Y., Masjuan, J., Voloschin, A., Baehring,J.M.,Shimazaki, H., Koide, R., King, D., Mason, W., Sansing, L.H., Dichter,M.A., Rosenfeld, M.R. & , D.R. (2007). Paraneoplastic anti-N-methyl-D-asparate receptor encephalitis associated with ovarian teratoma. *Ann Neurol* 61.25-36.

[6] Fitch MT; Abrahamian FM, Moran GJ, & Talan DA.Emergency department management of meningitis and encephalitis (2008).*Infect Dis Clin North Am* 22:33-52.

[7] Gulliford MC; Chandrasekera CP, Cooper RA, & Murphy RP (1987). Acyclovir treatment of herpes simplex encephalitis: experience in a distinct hospital. *Postgrad Med J* 63. 1037-41.

[8] Ichiyama, T.; Shoji, H., Takahashi, Y., Matsushige, T., Kajimoto, M., Inuzuka, T. & Furukawa, S. (2008). Cerebrospinal fluid levels of cytokines in non-herpetic acute limbic encephalitis: comparison with herpes simplex encephalitis. *Cytokine* 44.149-153.

[9] Japanese committee for influenza encephalopathy (2009): Influenza encephalopathy guidelines.

[10] Kamei S; Takasu T (2000). Nationwide survey of the annual prevalence of viral and other neurological infections in Japanese inpatients. *Intern Med* 39: 894-900.

[11] Lee DW; Choe YJ, Kim JH, Song KM, Cho H, Bae GR, & Lee JK (2012). Epidemiology of Japanese encephalitis in South Korea, 2007-2010. *Int J Infect Dis* 16:e448-52.

[12] Lee N; Wong CK, Chan PK, Lindegardh N, White NJ, Hayden FG, Wong EH, Wong KS, Cockram CS, Sung JJ, & Hui DS (2010).Acute encephalopathy associated with influenza A infection in adults. *Emerg Infect Dis* 16: 139-42.

[13] Morishima T; (2009). Infantile viral encephalitis and encephalopathy in Japan.*Virus* 59. 59-66

[14] Ohashi M; Yoshikawa T, Miyake F, Sugata K, Suga S, & Asano Y (2006). Nationwide survey of exanthema subitum associated encephalitis/encephalopathy in Japan. *J Pediatric Infect Dis & Immun* 18. 385-92

[15] Okumura A; Tsuji T, Kubota T, Ando N, Kobayashi S, Kato T, Natsume J, Hayakawa F, & Shimizu T. (2012). Acute encephalopathy with 2009 pandemic flu: comparison with seasonal flu. *Brain Dev* 34:13-9

[16] Shoji H; Kimura N, Kumamoto T, Ichiyama T, & Takahash Y(2011). Non-herpetic acute limbic encephalitis: A new subgroup of limbic encephalitis? Ed by Hayasaka D. Pathogenesis of Encephaitis. *INTECH* p267-78.

[17] Shoji H; Wakasugi K, Miura Y, Imaizumi T, & Kazuyama Y. Herpesvirus infections of the central nervous system (2002). *Jpn J Infect Dis* 55:6-13.

[18] Skoldenberg B; Forsgren M, Alesting K, Bergström T, Burman L, Dahlqvist E, Forkman A, Frydén A, Lövgren K, & Norlin K (1984). Acyclovir versus vidarabine in herpes simplex encephalitis: randomized multicenter study in consecutive Swedish patients. *Lancet II* 707-11.

[19] Solomon T; Michael BD, Smith PE, Sanderson F, Davies NW, Hart IJ, Holland M, Easton A, Buckley C, Kneen R, & Beeching NJ (2012); National Encephalitis Guidelines Development and Stakeholder Groups.Management of suspected viral encephalitis in adults--Association of British Neurologists and British Infection Association National Guidelines. *J Infect* 64:347-73.

http://dx.doi.org/10.5772/54605

[20] Suzuki K; Shoji H, & Hondo R (2012). An 89-year-old female with elderly-onset herpes simplex encephalitis, who, recovering with acyclovir therapy, relapsed two months later and died. *Brain & Nerve* 64:1063-8.

[21] Umemura S, Yamasaki M, Takahashi Y, Matsumoto K, & Miyamura M (2011). An adult case of pandemic (H1N1) 2009 influenza associated encephalopathy (2011). *Rinsho Shinkeigaku* 51. 422-5.

[22] Watanabe Y; Tsuji M, Sameshima K, Wada T, Iai M, Yamashita S, Hayashi T, Aida N, & Osaka H (2012). Clinical characteristics of acute encephalopathies associated with influenza H1N1-2009 in children . *No To Hattatsu* 44:35-40.

[23] Whitley RJ; (1998). Herpes simplex virus infections of the central nerve system. A review. *Am J Med* 85 (supple 2A): 61-7.

Chapter 5

Review on Japanese Encephalitis Outbreak Cases in Nepal During the Year 2011

Durga Datt Joshi and Jeevan Smriti Marg

Additional information is available at the end of the chapter

http://dx.doi.org/10.5772/52422

1. Introduction

Nepal is one of the richest countries in the world in terms of bio-diversity due to its unique geographical position and altitudinal variation. The elevation of the country ranges from 60 m above sea level to the highest point on earth, Mr. Everest at 8,848 m, all within a distance of 150 km resulting into climatic conditions from subtropical to artic mentioned by Nepal Tourism Board, 2006. JE cases are observed mostly in Terai area (The lowland plains of the Terai lie at an altitude of between 67 and 300 m (220 and 980 ft tropical climate) (Joshi, 1983). In Southeast Asia it is thought to cause up to 50000 clinical cases and 10000 deaths per year (WHO/SEARO, 1979). The earlier reports have shown that the case fatality rate (CFR) is high in Nepal, and nationwide it has ranged from 15% to 46% for the years 1978 to 1994. There are 75 districts, 14 zones and five development regions in Nepal. Out of 75 districts 36 districts are affected by Japanese encephalitis.

Japanese encephalitis (JE) has been occurring in the South-East Asia and Western Pacific Regions for a long time. In Nepal, it has occurred first time in Rupandehi district then in Sunsari, Morang and latter in all 23 districts of Terai and inner Terai (Joshi, 1983). Incidence of this disease has been recorded first time in different years in the following countries. Japan, China and Republic of Korea have reduced the incidence of this disease now (WHO/SEARO, 1979).

The entomological survey conducted in May/June, 1981 at the endemic areas of western region of Nepal, have recorded the prevalence of the following species such as (a) *Culex tritaeniorhynchus*, (b) *Cules vishuni*, (c) *Culex gelidus*, (d) *Culex fusecephalus*, (e) *Culex epidesmas* (f) *Culex bitaeniorhynchus* (g) *Mansonia annulefera* (h) *Mansonia indiana* (i) *Mansonia uniformis*, (j) few species of genus *Aedes*, genus *Armigeris* and genus *Anopheles* (Pradhan, 1981).

These mosquitoes can breed in sub-urban and peri-urban area provided the ecological conditions similar to rural area are present (Pradhan, 1981, Khatri et al., 1981, 1983). These mosquitoes can breed same environment wherever it is favourable.

Japan	1949 to 1950
Egypt	1977
Republic of Korea	1949 to 1958
China	1949
Malaysia	1955 to 1960
Indonesia	1955 to 1960
Philippines	1950 to 1955
Singapore	1955 to 1960
Bangladesh	1977
Vietnam	1958 to 1969
India	1955 (South), 1973
Burma	1974
(West Bengal), U.P. and Bihar	1978
Thailand	1969 to 1970
Sri Lanka	1968
Nepal	1978

Table 1. Historical reviews of JE outbreak worldwide.

2. Infected population and death cases from Japanese encephalitis (JE) disease in Nepal (EDCD/DHS)

High Risk Population: 12.5 million

High Risk Population: (Below 15 Years) 5.5 millions

JE Cases:26658 people during the year 1978-2003

Death Cases: 5370 people during the year 1978-2003

Mortality: 5 to 25%

Incidence: 50% (Below 15 Years)

In Nepal JE has been recorded and reported as a seasonal disease in Nepal. "Shrawan" (July and August) appears to have been the deadliest month for the Nepalese as far as human casualties from JE are concerned.

http://dx.doi.org/10.5772/52422

3. Japanese encephalitis distribution in Nepal

This JE virus is transmitted through a series of bites -when the mosquito bites a pig, for instance, it transmits the virus to the pig which acts as a host to the virus. The virus is further transmitted to humans when bitten by mosquitoes who have already bitten the pig.

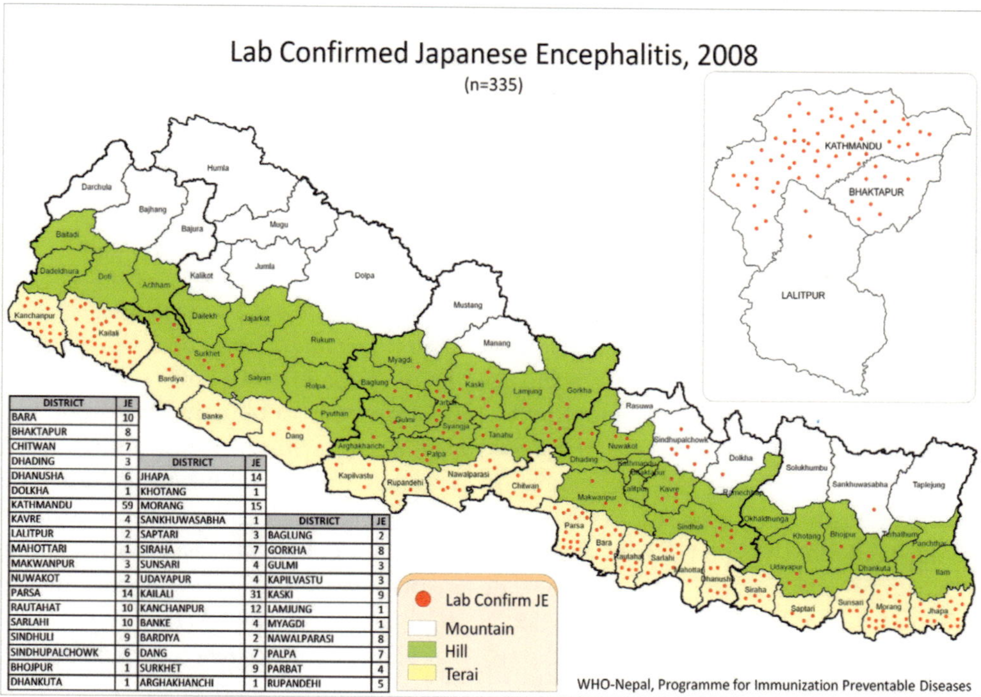

Scheme 1. Map 1.

The virus attacks the central nervous system of human, causing encephalitis-an infection of the brain. The patients starts vomiting, suffers severe headache and fever gradually becomes unconscious and nears death due to brain swelling. Even if the patients survive they remain with a lot of deflect- both physical and intellectual. Such a deadly disease, so wide spread in Nepal and without a cure. Preventing mosquito bite is thus so very important. But unlike for dengue virus, there is a vaccine for Japanese B virus which the government is trying to make available in mass. Japanese encephalitis virus also called Japanese B virus.

The mosquitoes that transmit this disease breed in and around dirty, stagnant water and in areas where the pigs are farmed. We all know that there are many places in and around Kathmandu that fits into this description, so I would urge you to hurry and get vaccinated. Another disease Filarisis- is also transmitted through the disease vector that is the female *Culex* mosquito. Filariasis is spread from infected persons to uninfected persons by mosquitoes that release large numbers of very small worm larvae, which circulate in an affected person's blood stream. The worms grow and live in an infected person's lymph vessels for about 7 years and divide in the lymphatic system. This causes inflammation and eventually blocks the lymphatic system and causes a lot of disfiguration.

The government is trying again to eradicate this disease by distributing the drug called Diethlcarbamazine- a three tablets-at-a-time treatment, and a single tablet treatment of Albendazole. However the medical fraternity is in doubt about its continuation. Saving the most important of all disease for the last, malaria, which is transmitted by the female Anopheles mosquito, causes febrile disease. One of the agents called Plasmodium Falciparum causes very severe malaria, which can lead to death. Again there is no vaccine against this agent. But effective drug prophylaxis has been in use to prevent the disease. Nonetheless mosquito prevention and control is the key against all these disease.

4. Epidemiological cycle of Japanese encephalitis

Japanese encephalitis (JE) is caused by a Flavivirus that, in a human case, causes severe encephalitis leading to death or permanent disablement. It is a zoonotic disease, transferred from animals (commonly domestic pigs but wild boars and migratory birds may also be important amplifier hosts and reservoirs) by a mosquito vector to humans. Important social factors may also play an important role in JE transmissions with the poorest sectors of the population most often affected (e.g. people sleep outside during hot humid months where the vector density is at peak, and often sleep close to pigs). JE has been occurring in the South-East Asia and Western Pacific Regions for a long time. In Southeast Asia it is thought to cause up to 50000 clinical cases and 10000 deaths per year (WHO, 1979). Japan, China and Republic of Korea have reduced the incidence of this disease now (WHO/SEARO 1979). These countries had very well developed long term plan to control the epidemicity of JE by regular vaccination in children and pigs they had also improved pig husbandry system and also vector control by draining the water from the rice field on a regular interval period.

JE cases are observed mostly in Terai region of Nepal (Joshi, 1983). The earlier reports have shown that the case fatality rate (CFR) is high in Nepal, and nationwide it has ranged from 15% to 46% for the years 1978 to 1994 (Joshi, 1983, 1986, 1987, Joshi et al., 1994). In Nepal, JE occurred first time during the year 1978 in Rupandehi district then in Sunsari, Morang and has since become endemic in all 24 districts of Terai and Inner Terai (Joshi, 1983). JE is a seasonal disease in Nepal, it occurs as an epidemic form only in the rainy (monsoon) season (July to October).

In Nepal, about 5000 people died due to JE from the year 1978 to 2006. Every year 3000 to 4000 people at risk and about 200-300 people die from complications associated with JE. About 12.5 million people in Nepal live in JE risk areas. Children who are less than 15 years of age are more likely to develop disease during a JE outbreak. Approximately 50% of JE survivors are left with chronic neurological syndrome and organ damage.

The highest morbidity 7.94% was seen in Kailali district. JE cases diagnosed, reported and recorded by Child Health Division of DHS, during the year 2011 in Nepal are shown in table no. 2.

1. District	Total JE Cases	Morbidity
2. Baitadi	1	0.79
3. Banke	7	5.56
4. Bara	2	1.59
5. Bardiya	2	1.59
6. Bhaktapur	1	0.79
7. Chitwan	4	3.17
8. Dang	3	2.38
9. Dhankuta	2	1.59
10. Dhanusha	7	5.56
11. Ghulmi	1	0.79
12. Gorkha	1	0.79
13. Illam	2	1.59
14. Jhapa	4	3.17
15. Kailali	10	7.94
16. Kanchanpur	5	3.97
17. Kapilbastu	2	1.59
18. Kathmandu	9	7.14
19. Kaski	1	0.79
20. Kavre	4	3.17
21. Lalitpur	2	1.59
22. Mahottari	5	3.97
23. Makwanpur	1	0.79
24. Morang	6	4.76
25. Nawalparasi	9	7.14
26. Palpa	3	2.38
27. Parsa	4	3.17
28. Pyuthan	1	0.79
29. Rautahat	6	4.76
30. Rupandehi	2	1.59
31. Saptari	1	0.79
32. Sarlahi	1	0.79
33. Sunsari	9	7.14
34. Surkhet	1	0.79
35. Syangja	3	2.38
36. Udayapur	4	3.17
37. 2011 total	**126**	**100**

Source: Child Health Division, IPD Section, WHO, 2011

Table 2. JE cases diagnosed, reported and recorded by Child Health Division of DHS, during the year 2011 in Nepal

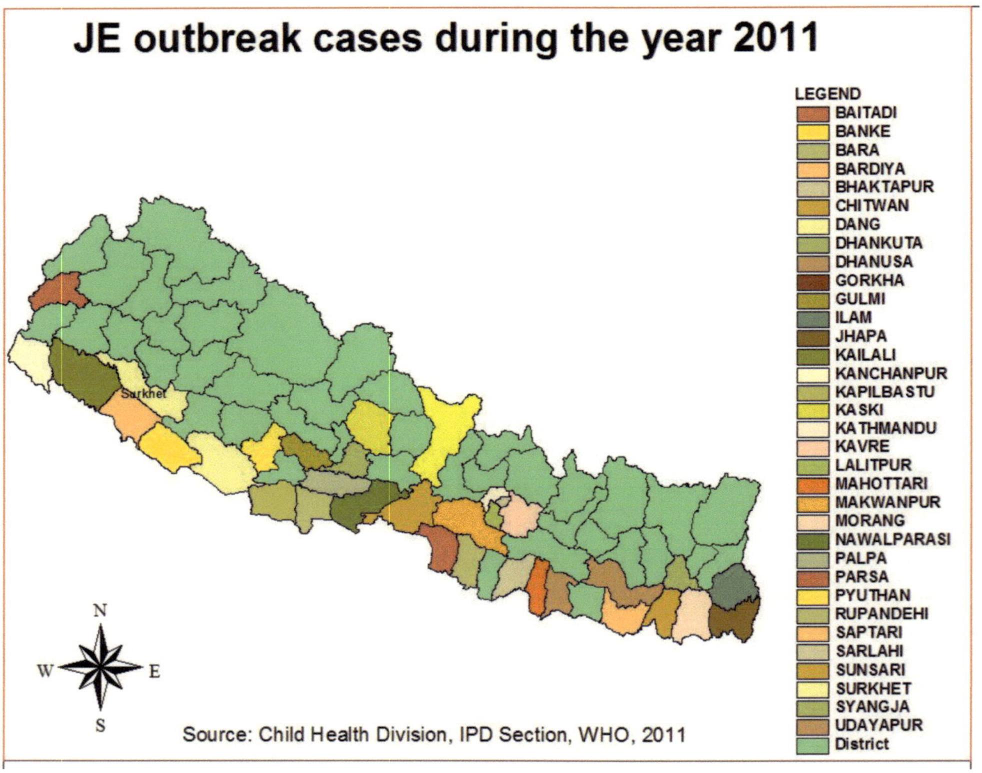

Scheme 2. Map 2. JE outbreak cases in Nepal during the year 2011; Source: Joshi, et al., 2012.

http://dx.doi.org/10.5772/52422

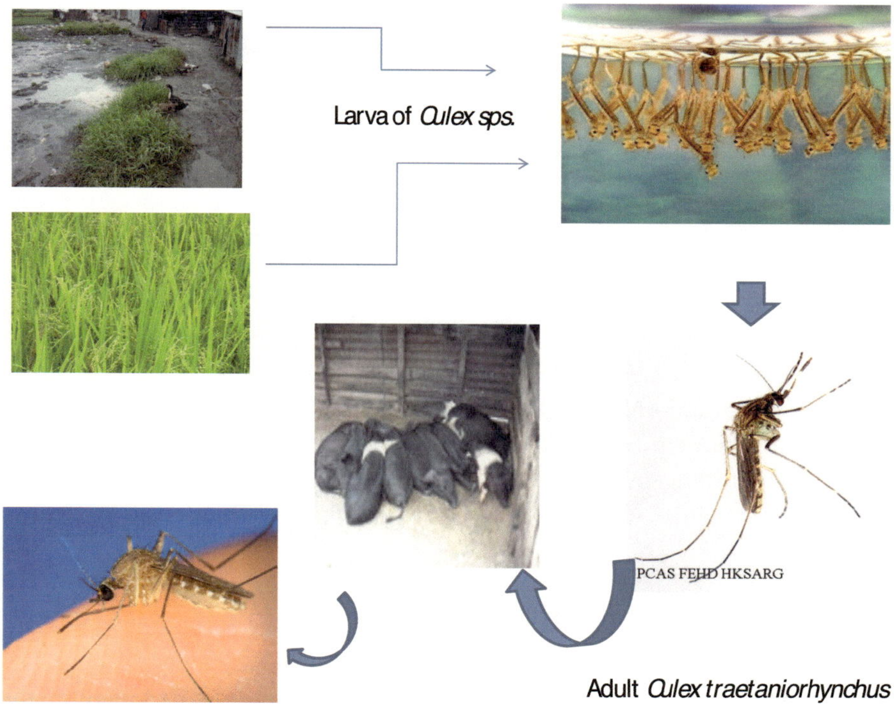

Figure 1. Epidemiological cycle of JE transmission. Source: Joshi, et al., 2012.

5. District (province) wise JE cases recorded during the year 2011:

Bhaktapur District

Bhaktapur hospital sees surge in Japanese encephalitis (viral fever) patients

The number of viral fever patients has increased in most of the hospitals in Bhaktapur district coinciding with the change in weather. Many people suffering from viral fever have been coming to the hospitals and health centre in the district. Along with the upsurge in the number of viral fever patients, the number of people suffering from typhoid and jaundice has also increased according to the District Public Health Office, Bhaktapur.

Superintendent at the Bhakatapur Hospital, Dr. Indra Prajapati said the diseases might take epidemic proportion if timely measures are not taken. Health Official in the district say the spread of viral fever is also because patients in the rural areas of the district have the habit of only taking paracetamol tablets that they buy at local drug stores instead of visiting the doctors for a thorough check-up. As many as 100 people suffering from fever come to the Bhaktapur Hospital daily for treatment, and many of them only after advanced stage of the disease. The District Public Health Offices said on an average 500 patients suffering from viral fever are said to come to the hospitals, medicals, health centre and drug stores throughout the district in a day. **(Sources: Rising Nepal 2011 August 15, 2068)**

Kathmandu District

Illness due to Japanese encephalitis Vaccine

Kathmandu: Debaki Bhandari, 48 yrs of 13 Kavre Panauti, became ill after taking vaccine. According to Doctor, she became ill after taking vaccine immediately. Shir Memorial Hospital of Banepa referred her to Kathmandu for treatment.

Student became ill due to viral (Japanese encephalitis) disease

Benighat 9, almost students of Orbang Primary School became ill. After unable to go to school, health assistant Kashiram and ANM SunitaThapa visited their home and treated them. According to health assistant, Kashiram Sharma of Beni Health Post, out of 77 sick students, 15 had neck problems, 12 had viral fevers and remaining was normal condition. This was due to climatic changes and poor sanitation, he added. **(Source: Kantipur, 20th October 2011)**

Chitwan District

Japanese encephalitis (viral fever) identified as influenza AH3

INFLUENZA AH3 virus has been linked with a viral fever outbreak in Chitwan, health officials said. Blood samples collected from various parts of the district tested positive for the Influenza AH3. Ram Kumar KC of the vector control programme of District Public Heath Office (DPHO) said apart from influenza AH3, Japanese encephalitis was also detected in some patients.

"We didn't have any encephalitis case last year," he said. According to the DPHO, over 1,500 people suffering from viral fever visited major hospitals in Chitwan in the last three weeks. Most of the patients were in the 16-50 years age bracket. Health officials warned that the number of patients could rise in the coming days. **(Sources: Kathmandu Post, August 19, 2011)**

Kaski District

Japanese encephalitis (viral fever) grips Pokhara

The pressure of patients at Western Regional Hospital and health posts in Pokhara is alarmingly increasing owing to flu of typhoid and viral fever for past few days. Among the total number of the patients visiting the health posts, 35-40 per cent of them are suffering from typhoid and viral fever, said the hospital.

Buddhi Bahadur Thapa, Medical Superintendent of the hospital said the number of typhoid and viral fever patients increased during the change of season. Most of the patients are suffering from fever, cough and common cold, he added.

As the infection of common cold and fever increasing across the district, the number of patients visiting the private hospitals and taking medicine from pharmacies are increasing from the past few days. Informing that some patients who suffer from the viral fever also picked up asthma, diabetes and heart related problems. Thapa said that the people who got infected the immediate medical treatment.

Doctors informed that Padam Nursing Home, Charak Hospital and Fewa City Hospital registered the large number of patients. Thapa said that as the viral fever was a communicable disease, many persons were easily infected with the flu. Since last few days the people of Syangja, Tanahu, Parbat, Lamjung and other adjoining districts have been suffering from the viral fever and typhoid and the flu is developing into the pandemic.

When the local hospitals of these districts couldn't stand the pressure of the patients, they recommended patients for the hospital of Pokhara. Likewise, the number of viral flu patients is increasing in Dolakha. Especially the children and elderly people are infected with the flu.

GauriShanker Campus of the district remained close for Sunday when the principal vice-principal of the campus caught the flu of viral fever. Health worker at the Primary Health Centre Charikot Shanti Neupane said that viral fever was pandemic in both the urban and rural areas of the district this year. **(Sources: Rising Nepal, August 15, 2011)**

Bara District

Two children dead due to Japanese encephalitis

Bara, 29 Mangsir, two children were dead in Bara last night. According to local person, Gajendra Kumar, son of Upendra Jaiswal and Aman Kumar of Lal Babu Prasad Jaiswal were dead during treatment at national medical college Birgunj. They were referred to national medical college. JE is caused by mosquitoes – borne viral fever. **(Sources: Annapurna Post December 16, 2011)**

Tanahun District

Japanese encephalitis (viral fever) regime in Damauli

Viral fever is said to be raging in Damauli and it's surrounding areas over the past few days. Damauli Hospital and private clinics are receiving an increasing flow of patients since the start of the Nepali month of Shrawan. Out of total 200 patients that the hospital receives daily, around 100 are the patients of viral fever. The situation inside the Damauli jail is worrisome. Out of 95 inmates serving jail sentence, 75 are suffering from viral fever. The spread of viral fever has prompted the Department of Health to send a team of health officials said the Districts Public Health Office. **(Source: Rising Nepal, July 23, 2011)**

Arghakhanchi District

Japanese encephalitis (viral fever) and Pneumonia outbreak

Arghakhanchi, District hospital was fully occupied due to large number of viral fever and pneumonia cases. Due to large number cases and lack of beds, patients are being treated on floor.

Patients have admitted forty to fifty within one week of time. There are only 15 beds but 40 to 50 patients are sick, hospital informed that more than 30 patients are being treated on the floor. Children are sicker than other age group; this age groups belong to 1 to 2 yrs. According to Chief,

Acting District Hospital Dr. Ram Prasad Sapkota, viral pneumonia patients are more in hospital. He told that it has been difficult to doctor and medical people because of full of patients in hospital. He added that more than 100 patients are being treated in OPD on Sunday. Patients complained that lack of bed, more patients treated and patients are brought for hospital for treatment and they have to stay in hotel. 25 pneumonia patients are admitted in hospital daily. Patients are coming from not only headquarter but also from urban areas for treatment. CMA told that patient flow rate is increased more in health and sub-health post in VDC. Four doctors complained that they are faced problem due to outbreak of disease. Dr. Sapkota told that lack of bed, pneumonia patients are treated lying on the floor. He added more that patients are increasing day by day and most of the patients are seriously due to form pneumonia and viral fever, they came to hospital for treatment. **(Source: Kantipur, September 26, 2011)**

Dang District

Pig farming ban in Dang

Pig farming has been banned inside the Tribhuvannagar Municipality area. The ban was levied by the municipality in wake of the spreading out of the Japanese encephalitis in the Terai region. The ban is effective within Chbhaisota in the north, Ratnapur-Bharatpur road in the South, Runway-Bharatpur in the east and Sewar River in the west. The municipality has also begun killing the stray pigs and ducks that are left unclaimed even after repeated request to the owners to get rid of them, said Mayor Amar BahadurDangi. The Nepal Bank Ltd., Agriculture Development Bank and other financial institutions have also been requested not to issue loans for pig farming in the region, adds Dangi. The municipality has so far killed 40 pigs and two ducks found unclaimed in various wards of the municipality, it is learnt **(Source: Rising Nepal, July 5, 2002).**

Banke District

JE stalks mid-western Terai district

Japanese encephalitis, a mosquito-borne viral disease, has stalked the mid-western Terai districts lately, claiming one life and taking scores others ill. Gumi Rana of Chaulahi from Dang district died of Japanese encephalitis on Monday while undergoing treatment at Nepalgunj based Bheri Zonal Hospital. The hospital sources said the flow of encephalitis patients is surging in recent days. According to Dr. Bimal Dhakal, the chief at the hospital, 11 Japanese encephalitis patients have been admitted to the hospital in the past one month and some of them are still receiving treatment. The hospital data shows that most of the patients are form Dang, Banke and Bardiya districts. Mid-western Terai districts come under the grip of fatal Japanese encephalitis during the monsoon every year. Last year, 105 Japanese encephalitis patients were admitted to Bheri Zonal Hospital and 23 of them died of the disease. Dr. Dhakal is of the opinion that the fatal disease is beyond control due to the lack of public health awareness. Ram Bahadur Chand of District Public Health Office Banke, however, claimed the office has been working to prevent the spread of the disease. **(Source: Kathmandu Post, August 17, 2011)**

One died from JE

Ram Bahadur Chand, Focal person of District Public Health claimed that awareness programme about JE activities is being disseminated. Bed nets were distributed for the consumers across Rapti river areas. Insecticides could not be sprayed due to heavy rains, he agreed. Insecticide will be sprayed after cease of rain. According the public health office, JE regular vaccine is giving under one year child to control the JE. JE is controlled due to vaccine. Doctor advised that, people have to use bed net regularly, clean and cut unnecessary bushy and make tidy filling water ditch to save from JE disease. Altogether 105 JE patients were admitted out of which 23 patients were died in Bheri Zonal Hospital last year. **(Source: Kantipur, August 17, 2011)**

Japanese encephalitis claims two lives

Two persons died of Japanese encephalitis, a viral disease transmitted by mosquitoes, while undergoing treatment at Bheri Zonal Hospital on Friday. Krishni Tharu, 40, of Kailali and Chandra Shahi, 13, of Surkhet died of the disease. A hospital source said that the number of patients suffering from the disease is surging in the mid and far western Terai districts in the past few days. On Monday, eight-years-old Gomi Rana of Dang succumbed to the ailment during treatment. **(Sources: Kathmandu Post 2011 August 21)**

Two persons died due to Japanese encephalitis

Two persons died of Japanese encephalitis on Friday. Krishni Tharu, 40, of Kailali and Chandra Shahi, 13, of Surkhet died of the JE disease while undergoing treatment at Bheri Zonal Hospital. On Monday, eight-years-old Gomi Rana of Dang Chailahi died. Number of JE patients are increasing. A total 15 patients are admitted till now.

Dr. Chudamani Bhandari, Director, Kathmandu Epidemiology and Disease Control Division told that he didn't get any information from that disease. Japanese encephalitis caused by Flavi virus. This virus is found in pig and bird. It is transmitted by culex mosquito. But JE isn't transmitted from one person to another person. We can save from mosquito in spite of there is no drug of JE. **(Sources: Kantipur, 2011 August 22)**

More one dead due to JE

Banke: more one kid dead due to JE, 7 - Sorhawa, Bardiya 7 - years old AsmitaChaudhari was dead during treatment period and 3 were dead due to JE before. JE cases are raised and 33 persons are admitted in Bheri Zonal Hospital till Tuesday. According to hospital source, patients are also admitted in Nepalgunj and Kohalpur.

According to Director Bimal Dhakal, patients flow like encephalitis disease is raising. Child ward is fully occupied. According to hospital source, most of patients have come from Bardiya districts. Nine patients from Berdiya, 7 from Banke, 7 dang, 1 Jajarkot, 8 Kailali, 1 Salyan and 1 from Surkhet are admitted.

Before this, 40 years Krishni Tharu of Baunia, 13 years Chandra Shahi, Tatopani of Surkhet, 8 years Goma Rana of Chaulahi of Dang were dead.

When rainy season begins, JE cases are seen in Western Terai district of Nepal. Last year, 105 patients were admitted for treatment, among them, 23 were dead.No. of total patients admitted – 33 (Bardiya – 9, Banke – 7, Dang – 7, Jajarkot – 1, Kailali – 8, Salyan – 1 and Surkhet – 1). **(Source: Kantipur, August 31, 2011).**

Three died due to Japanese encephalitis in Banke

Nepalgunj: Three persons died of encephalitis in Banke district during the Nepali month Saun. Five others are undergoing treatment in local Bheri Zonal Hospital and seven others returned after the treatment. The hospital has been providing the medicines Cyanula and Fluide at free of cost to the patients of encephalitis who as undergoing treatment in the hospital. **(Source: Rising Nepal 2011, August 20)**

Kailali District

Four deaths due to Japanese encephalitis

More than 36 persons are affected by JE in Dhangadhi in this year. According to DPHO Kailali, 36 were admitted for treatment, among them 4 were dead. Twenty six were returned to their home after recovery and 6 were referred to other place for treatment. Hasulia and Mashuria are highly JE affected area. JE outbreak after the 2nd week of Ashar in this year, said Karki.

Last year 5 persons were dead due to JE and more than 50 were affected by this disease. Since 2 years, JE cases are deceasing due to vaccination. According to DPHO officer Karki, JE cases seem till 3rd week of Ashoj. **(Source: Kathmandu Post, September, 2, 2011)**

Japanese Encephalitis claims four in Dhangadhi

Four persons died of encephalitis while receiving treatment at Seti Zonal Hospital, Dhangadhi. Hospital's official DilipShrestha said altogether four persons died since second week of July in this year. The deceased persons include Khagisar Joshi, 6 of Bauniya VDC, Sarita Chaudhary, 22, of Hasuliya VDC. Kamala Shahi, 11, of Pahalamnpur of Kailali district and Mani Ram Oli, 28, of Kanchanpur district, said the hospital. Altogether 36 persons have been admitted to the hospital for the treatment of encephalitis and six patients among them have been referred for further treatment. The hospital providing free treatment facility for the encephalitis patients, said Shrestha. **(Sources: Rising Nepal, September 2, 2011).**

Kanchanpur District

Four deaths due to Japanese encephalitis

Four people died due to Japanese encephalitis in Kanchanpur district. They died while undergoing treatment in Mahakali Zonal Hospital. Raju Chaudhari from Raikwar Bichwa VDC died while undergoing treatment in Seti Zonal Hospital. The deceased persons include Bindu Dhami – 24yrs., of Bauniya VDC-8, DalbirTamata 48 yrs. of Daiji VDC-5 and Dhani Budha – 60 yrs. from Badampur of Bhimdatt municipality said the hospital. According to Keshab Datt Awasthi, Medical Recorder Officer from Mahakali Zonal Hospital, JE patients are increased in the hospital.

He said that, altogether 35 persons have been treated of encephalitis and 15 patients went to home after treatment. 13 patients among them have been referred for further treatment and rest 2 patients went without information in the hospital.

More patients pressured in the month of Bhadra but only 2 patients have been admitted in the month of Asoj. Last year, 26 persons have been admitted, out of which 2 persons were died. According to Dr. Dipendraraman Singh, Chief of hospital, JE cases are seen in patients due to unvaccination. **(Source: Gorkhapatra, September 30, 2011)**

http://dx.doi.org/10.5772/52422

6. JE Vaccination in children

About 103% vaccination coverage in children population targeted were in Kailali and Banke districts and 100% coverage in Dang district, 73% in Bardiya district but in Rupandehi and Kanchanpur district 40 and 41% JE vaccine coverage respectively, which was very low coverage (See table no. 3).

Area	Age group	Total	Male	Female	Sex Ratio
Rupendehi	0-4 yrs	85964	43957	42007	1.05
	5-9 yrs	100724	51855	48869	1.06
	10-14 yrs	93215	48354	44861	1.08
	Total	279903	144166	135737	
Dang	0-4 yrs	59987	30284	29703	0.098
	5-9 yrs	67656	34279	33377	1.02
	10-14 yrs	65860	33411	32449	1.05
	Total	193503	97974	95529	
Banke	0-4 yrs	48809	24612	24197	1.06
	5-9 yrs	56410	28955	27455	1.02
	10-14 yrs	51041	26698	24343	1.03
	Total	156260	80265	75995	
Bardiya	0-4 yrs	47789	24246	23543	1.03
	5-9 yrs	58875	29670	29205	1.02
	10-14 yrs	52823	27215	25608	1.06
	Total	159487	81131	78356	
Kailali	0-4 yrs	79693	40843	38850	1.05
	5-9 yrs	95326	48698	46628	1.04
	10-14 yrs	86588	44590	41998	1.06
	Total	26160	134131	127476	
Kanchanpur	0-4 yrs	49777	25506	24271	.099
	5-9 yrs	55802	28545	27257	0.096
	10-14 yrs	52438	26790	25648	0.097s
	Total	158017	80841	77176	

Source: CBS 2001 population census.

Table 3. JE Risk six districts population of children between 1 to 15 age, sex and sex ration in Nepal

7. Discussion

The earlier reports have shown that the case fatality rate (CFR) is high in Nepal, and nationwide it has ranged from 15% to 46% for the years 1978 to 1994 (Joshi et al., 1981). It has been proved that JE virus causes encephalitis in humans and abortion in pigs while no symptoms in other animals and birds. Mostly children aged five to fifteen is victimized than adults. About fifty percent of the JE survivors are left with neurological syndrome and damage to the organs (Joshi, 1983, Pradhan, Khatri et al., 1981, 1983).

The people in the districts are dying due to Japanese encephalitis, and it threatens to assume epidemic proportions. The government has just started its second round of vaccination under mass vaccination program for the disease, which should have been completed by 2006. Because of the delay in vaccination, the number of patients suffering from Japanese Encephalitis may increase and take an epidemic form.

The vaccine "anti JESA-14-14-2 live attenuated" is produced in China and that it was found to be above 98 percent effective in Chinese children (RSS, 2006). In Nepal, some two million people live in the Terai regions considered to be highly affected areas. In order to prevent the epidemic, more than three million doses of vaccines had been arranged during the year 2005.

Vaccination campaign against Japanese encephalitis has been started in Banke district from 26 July 2006. It is said that all 422,000 people above one year of age from Banke district were vaccinated in the campaign, which would continue until August 18, 2006. The full doze vaccine has been provided by the district public Health office. According to the schedule, the campaign would remain until July 17, 2006 in Nepalgunj municipality and from July 27 to August 18, 2006 in 46 VDCs of the districts (JE vaccination report of Banke, 2006).

The reduction in case incidence of Japanese encephalitis, in some countries like China, Japan and Korea has been achieved by applying certain measures such as:

i. Mass vaccination of susceptible group of population,

ii. Vaccination of piglets of endemic areas,

iii. Anti-mosquito campaign, i.e. vector control measure both larva and adult.

3.5 million of JE vaccine doses was procured by the Ministry of Health during the year 2006/2007. The vaccine is made in China by Chengdu Institute of Biological Product. This vaccine will be used in children under 15 years of age of 24 districts of JE risk and high-risk areas of Nepal.

In Nepal twenty-four districts of Terai are declared as JE prone disease area. About 12.5 million people in Nepal are in JE risk category. Children who are less than 15 years of age are more prone to suffer in case of a JE outbreak. In China, JE vaccination in childrens has shown 98.4% immunity which is very encouraging (EDCD and IPD, 2006). During the year 2007 about 35,00,000 doses of JE vaccine is going to be procured. So far about 5000 people died due to JE from the year 1978 to 2006. Every year 3000 to 4000 people yet risk and about 200-300 people die due to JE.

http://dx.doi.org/10.5772/52422

8. Conclusion

For the reduction of JE cases in Nepal mass vaccination programme should be carried out every year for children in high risk districts of JE. Except symptomatic treatment there is no specific treatment for Japanese encephalitis. There is a Japanese encephalitis vaccine prepared in Japan, China and Rusia. There are two types of vaccines one liquid and other freeze dried. Vaccination can be done subcutaneously two doses of 1 ml each above 3 years of age and 0.5 ml. For children upto 3 years of age at an interval of 7-14 days. Third doses should be given before one year. This will protect for 3 years in the endemic zone. One more booster dose after 3 years has been recommended which will give life long immunity to an individual (Joshi et al., 2003).

To conclude, mosquito borne disease is on the rise. There are many methods for mosquito control and depending the situation, source reduction (e.g., removing stagnant water) biocontrol (e.g. importing natural predators such as dragonflies), trapping, using nets and using pesticides can be helpful. In endemic areas, there should be spraying of insecticides every day. People should stay inside between dusk and dark if possible. When outdoors, wearing pants and long-sleeved shirts is a must. Exposed skin should be sprayed with mosquito repellants (Neopane Arpana, 2011).

Acknowledgements

I would like to thank following staff of NZFHRC for their continuous help in preparing and translating notes and papers from Nepali to English language published in different media of Nepal on Japanese encephalitis; Ms. Minu Sharma, Ms. Meena Dahal, Dr. Anita Ale, Ms. Kabita Shahi, Ms. Indira Mainali during the year 2007 to 2011. This study was supported by International Development Research Centre (IDRC), Ottawa, Canada.

Author details

Durga Datt Joshi and Jeevan Smriti Marg

*Address all correspondence to: ddjoshi@healthnet.org.np/joshi.durgadatt@yahoo.com

National Zoonoses and Food Hygiene Research Centre (NZFHRC), Kathmandu, Nepal

References

[1] Annapurna National Daily News Paper 2011.

[2] Annual Report of Child health Division, Department of Health Services IPD Section WHO, 2011.

[3] Banke District Public Health Office.JE vaccination report for the year 2006.

[4] Gorkhapatra National Daily News Paper, 2011

[5] Japanese Encephalitis Campaign Central Plan.Epidemiology and Disease Control Division and Child Health Division, Immunization Unit Department of Health Services 2006.

[6] Joshi, D. D. and Gaidamovichs. Serological Surveillance of Virus Encephalitis in Nepal, II Serological survey of pigs, birds and other animal population for JE in the epidemic area following outbreak in 1970 and 1980. Bull. Vet. Sc. & A.H. Nepal. Vol. 10 and11 1981;82:8-12.

[7] Joshi, D. D., Bista, P. R. and Joshi, H. Japanese Encephalitis A Zoonotic Pubic Health Problem in Nepal.NZFHRC. 2003;1-3

[8] Joshi, D. D., Pant, D. K. Shah, Y., 2012. Review on Japanese Encephalitis Outbreak Records Reported by Different Media, News and Survey during the year 2007 to 2011 in Nepal. Published by NZFHRC. PP 39-50.

[9] Joshi, D.D. Incidence of Japanese Encephalitis in Children during 1978, 1979 and 1980 Outbreak.Nepas J. 1983, 2, 18-25.

[10] Kantipur National Daily News Paper. 2011.

[11] Khatri, I.B., Joshi D.D. and Pradhan, T.M.S. Epidemiological Study of Viral Encephalitis in Nepal.J. Inst. Med.,1981; 4: 2;133-144.

[12] Khatri, I.B., Joshi, D.D., Pradhan, T.M.S. and Pradhan S. Status of Viral Encephalitis (Japanese Encephalitis in Nepal).JNMA 1983;66:21;1:97-110.

[13] Neopane, Arpana, 2011. Mosquito Borne Disease.Published in Kathmandu Post. April 18, 2011.

[14] Pradhan, S. Role of mosquitoes in the transmission of JE, Seminar on VE. Siddhartha Jaycees Souvenir, 23 Jestha 2038, Bhairahawa, 1981;6-8.

[15] RSS Report published in the Rising Nepal June 19 2006.

[16] The Himalayan Times Daily News Paper. 2011.

[17] The Kathmandu Post Daily News Paper. 2011.

[18] The Rising Nepal, Daily News Paper. 2011.

[19] WHO/SEARO. Report Technical Information of Japanese Encephalitis and Guidelines for Treatment, New Delhi, India, 1979.

Section 2

Encephalitis Causative Agents

Chapter 6

Arboviral Encephalitis

Guey-Chuen Perng and Wei-June Chen

Additional information is available at the end of the chapter

http://dx.doi.org/10.5772/52327

1. Introduction

Arboviruses (arthropod-borne viruses) are a group of pathogens that are transmitted by hematophagous arthropods, mainly mosquitoes and ticks, between susceptible vertebrates [1]; many of them are also characterized by their movement through arthropod communities: vertical (or transovarial) [2] and venereal transmission [3]. Thus far, more than 500 arboviruses have been identified worldwide, particularly in tropical and subtropical areas [4-6]. Of these, some 80 species can cause human diseases with a broad spectrum of symptoms, including encephalitis, fever, and hemorrhaging [7]. Most arboviruses are classified into three families (the Togaviridae, Flaviviridae, and Bunyaviridae) in the current viral classification system. Minor groups of arboviruses include those belonging to the Rhabdoviridae (vesicular stomatitis Indian and bovine ephemeral fever viruses), Reoviridae (bluetongue virus and Colorado tick fever), and Asfarviridae (African swine fever virus; ASFV); all of which have trivial or no roles in causing human diseases.

Viruses belonging to the Togaviridae are enveloped and spherical with a size of 65~70 nm in diameter; they contain an icosahedral nucleocapsid within which is included single-stranded positive-sense RNA [8]. Viral RNA serves as both the genome and viral messenger (m)RNA. The entire genome encodes a non-structural polyprotein which is processed by host and viral proteases, while a structural polyprotein is expressed by subgenomic mRNA [9]. The genus *Alphavirus* in the family Togaviridae includes 29 virus species, all of which are transmitted by mosquitoes [10]. The Flaviviridae is composed of viruses that also contain single-stranded positive-sense RNA; however, their virions are smaller in size than Alphaviruses, usually 45~50 nm in diameter [11]. The genus *Flavivirus* contains about 70 members; a number of them are infectious to humans, *e.g.*, dengue virus and West Nile (WN) virus. Flaviviral RNA possesses a single open reading frame, encoding a polyprotein, which is then processed to three structural proteins (C, M, and E) and seven non-structural proteins (NS1, NS2A, NS2B, NS3, NS4A, NS4B, and NS5) by host and viral proteases [11].

The Bunyaviridae is one of the largest groupings of animal viruses, containing more than 300 viruses [12]. Except for the genus *Hantavirus*, all of them are transmitted by arthropods [12]. Viral particles are spherical with a size >100 nm in diameter, and are composed of four structural proteins encoded on its tripartite single-stranded negative-sense RNA genome consisting of the L, M, and S segments [13].

Various arboviruses belonging to those three major families can specifically cause encephalitis. Of these, Eastern equine encephalitis (EEE) virus, Western equine encephalitis (WEE) virus, and Venezuelan encephalitis (VEE) virus belong to the Togaviridae [14], Japanese encephalitis (JE) virus, St. Louis encephalitis (SLE) virus, WN virus, and tick-borne encephalitis (TBE) virus are from the Flaviviridae [15, 16], while California encephalitis (CE) virus and La Crosse (LAC) virus are members of the Bunyaviridae [7]. Recently, increasing evidence has shown that certain arboviruses such as dengue (DENV) and chikungunya viruses (CHIKV) may occasionally cause encephalitis in addition to their conventional symptoms,which usually involves headaches, muscle and joint pain, and rashes [17-19].

2. Epidemiology of encephalitic arboviruses

Arboviruses are usually transmitted through bites of blood-feeding arthropods (primarily mosquitoes and ticks) in two major cycles (Figure 1). The man-arthropod-man cycle is characteristic of dengue virus, while EEE, WEE, WN, JE, and CE viruses are transmitted by an alternative cycle involving non-human mammals and birds [10]. For the infections by arboviruses that cause encephalitis, humans or horses become an incidental or dead-end host, while animals such as birds and pigs serve as reservoirs or amplifying hosts [20].

Togaviridae. Viruses causing EEE, WEE, and VEE are all members of the Alphavirus genus in the family Togaviridae [21]. In fact, they are the only viruses in this group that commonly cause encephalitis and are restricted to the Americas. There are other Alphaviruses also with limited distributions, such as CHIKV (Asia and Africa), O'nyong-nyong virus (Africa), Sindbis virus (Africa, Europe, and Asia), Mayaro virus (South America), and Ross River virus (Australia), however these are expected to eventually become distributed worldwide [22]. Epidemiologically, all Togaviridae are similar in that these viruses have wild avian hosts, are transmitted from birds to mammals by mosquitoes, and may cause encephalitis in horses and humans [22].

Flaviviridae. At least 7 arboviruses including TBE, Kyasanur Forest disease (KFD), JE, Murray Valley encephalitis (MVE), SLE, Rocio, and WN viruses are reported to be associated with causing encephalitic symptoms [23]. Some of these are described below.

The TBE virus is a member of the family Flaviviridae, which is geographically distributed worldwide, usually in rural areas at temperate latitudes, including all over Europe and the Scandinavia, the former Soviet Union, and East Asia [24]. Incidences of human cases markedly increased in the early 1990s, mostly in Europe [25]. It was reported that the TBE incidence was 8690 cases during 1965~1992, while 8674 cases were documented in a smaller window of time between 1993 and 2006 in the Czech Republic, indicating a steep rise in this region [25]. Rodents are the primary reservoir hosts of this virus, which is transmitted by the bites of hard ticks (*Ixodes*) in nature [24].

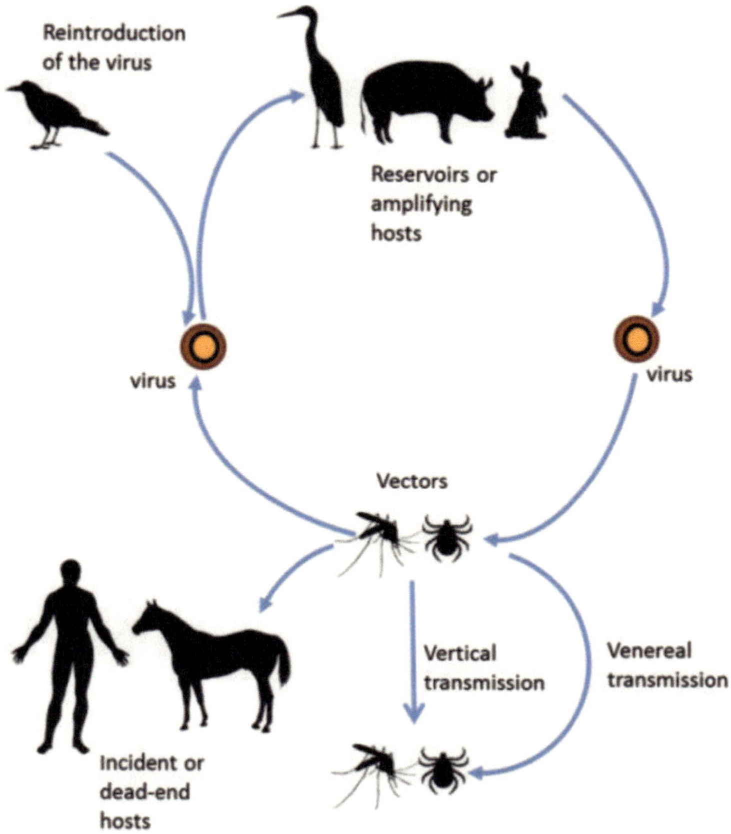

Figure 1. Transmission cycles of arboviruses in nature. Two major cycles cover the transmission of most arboviruses, one is mam-to-man and the other usually involves non-human mammals and birds.

The JE virus is mainly amplified in pigs and birds and are transmitted by *Culex* mosquitoes (primarily *Cx. tritaeneorhunchus*) between vertebrates [26]; it causes a significant number of human encephalitis cases in most areas of Asia, especially eastern, southern, and southeastern Asia, as well as the South Pacific regions [27]. It recently expanded to the Torres Strait of northern Australia in 1999, and has now become endemic in Australia [28, 29]. JE virus is estimated to cause about 30,000~50,000 cases each year worldwide [15, 30]; of which, 10,000~15,000 may be fatal [31].

WN virus was first isolated from a febrile patient in the West Nile region of Uganda in 1937 [32]. It has caused epidemics in Africa, Europe, the Middle East, Asia, and, more recently, in North America [33]. Since the emergence of WN virus in the United States in 1999, it has spread all over North America and caused more than 20,000 humans to be ill and 770 deaths (http://www.cdc.gov/ncidod/dvbid/westnile/surv and control.htm). Neuroinvasive disease due to WN virus infection can occur, 2946 and 2866 cases were reported in 2002 and 2003, respectively [34].

The SLE virus is a close relative to WN virus, and actually is a member of the Japanese encephalitis serocomplex [35]. Predominantly, SLE virus is naturally maintained in a transmission cycle between ornithophilic mosquitoes and birds, but occasionally these arthropods feed on mammalian blood, causing encephalitis in humans [36]. Nearly 5000 human infections were reported between 1964 and 2005, making it the major cause of epidemic encephalitis in association with flaviviral infections before the introduction of WN virus into the United States (http://www.cdc.gov/ncidod/dvbid/arbor/pdf/SLEDOC07132006.pdf).

Buynaviridae. In this family, viruses involving symptoms of encephalitis include Rift Valley fever (RVF), LAC, CE, and Jamestown Canyon [37]; all are mosquito-borne. RVF virus mostly occurs in Africa and the Middle East, while the other three, which are classified in the California serogroup, are restrictedly distributed in North America [37]. Of these, the LAC virus causes the most human disease, with dozens to hundreds of hospitalized cases reported each year in the United States [38]; unlike EEE, California serogroup including LAC is not dependent on avian hosts for natural transmission. Rodents usually serve as its major vertebrate host [37].

3. Mechanism of central nervous system (CNS) infection by arboviruses

Despite many years of intensive efforts and investigations on the pathways leading to infections of the CNS by arboviral families after the bite of an arthropod carrying an infectious agent, the exact mechanism remains to be further delineated. There are multiple routes that can be considered, depending on the characteristics of the virus. Some advocate the mechanism of direct viral spread from the periphery to the CNS [39], particularly for arboviruses involved in brain infections. It is thought that these viruses are amplified in dermal tissues and then in lymph nodes via migration of dendritic (Langerhans) cells before invading the CNS [40, 41]. However, the mechanism allowing for these viruses to perform the last step, to enter and invade the CNS, is less clear. The MVE, SLE, and JE viruses were speculated to enter the CNS via the olfactory pathway [42], while transcytosis across cerebral capillary endothelial cells was reported in JE [43]. In addition, virion-budding on the parenchymal cells after replication at the blood-brain barrier may also occur [44]. In experimental models, many infections by encephalitic arboviruses are diffusely spread throughout the brain [45, 46]. Furthermore, the absence of viral antigens in the choroid plexus or ependyma indicate that these viruses were not actively targeted to and replicated in this tissue but rather entered the CNS via a hematogenous route [47] (Figure 2), especially in patients with severe viremia [48].

http://dx.doi.org/10.5772/52327

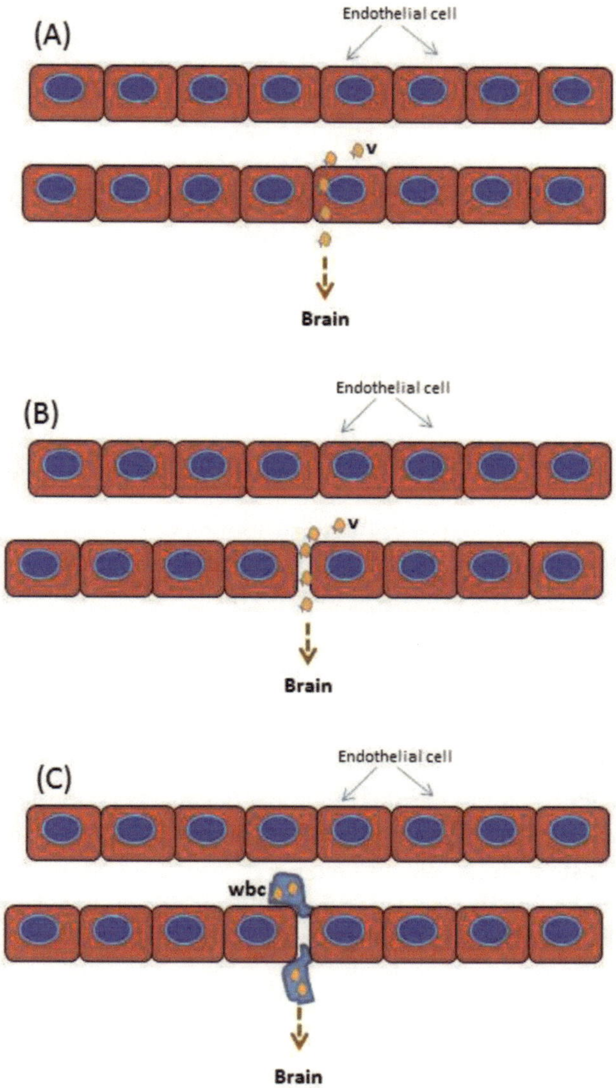

Figure 2. Hypothetic routes for arboviruses to infect the brain tissue hematogenously. (A) Infection of endothelial cells before the virion enters the brain tissue. (B) Virions enter the brain tissue through disrupted BBB. (C) Infected white blood cells enter the brain tissue by passing through the disrupted BBB.

In a study on JE, extensive infection of neurons resulting in cellular defects was shown in the cerebrum and cerebellum [49]. The cerebral and cerebellar capillary endothelial cells are responsible for maintaining the integrity of the blood-brain barrier (BBB) [50]. In both animals and humans, the BBB generally prevents viral invasion into the CNS [51], unless it has been disrupted, resulting in increased permeability and inflammatory cell infiltration [52, 53]. Disruptions in the BBB actually allows for peripheral blood mononuclear cells (PBMCs) to migrate from the circulation into brain tissues [54, 55].

Under normal circumstances, lymphocytes constantly enter the CNS, but in small numbers [56]. However their presence in the CNS may increase in response to viral infections [57]. In fact, infected PBMCs can be isolated in brains from mice inoculated with JE virus as early as 3 days post-infection [58]. Moreover, leukocytes were observed moving between endothelial cells of capillaries at sites in the BBB where tight junctions had been dissociated [49]. This suggests that at least some inflammatory leukocytes that had become infected in the periphery move along in the blood current and migrate to the CNS tissues [58, 59]. Furthermore, infection and resultant apoptosis of astrocytes, which serve as a protective component of the BBB and can defend against penetrated virions or virus-infected leukocytes, are frequently seen in the brain. This probably results in severe impairment of the BBB, facilitating the passage of more virus-infected PBMCs, using a "Trojan horse" strategy.

4. Pathogenesis of arboviral infections

Arboviral diseases start with a bite from an arthropod creature carrying infectious virus. The pathogen may be considered an innocent bystander or an unnecessary byproduct from an infected vertebrate host. The arthropod imbibes this blood for its own purposes, to facilitate ovulation, and takes up the accompanying virus in the meal. The presence of pathogen is not a critical event in the life cycle of the insect and may or may not cause it harm. The persistence of disease is none of these creatures' fault, since survival is the game plan for all organisms on earth. In many instances, arboviruses are capable of surviving inside the coming host without inducing any visible adverse effects. Given the opportunity, the pathogens will reentry and challenge a new host. If the host is capable of implementing a "survival strategy" in response to the viral infection, the host will be fine. Occasionally, these creatures may enter a host, such as human beings, in which the environment may not be as friendly as others, and a hostile survival race is engaged. The race tactics instigated by both sides are normally controllable and do not result in overt disease. But in some cases, the regulatory programs in the host do not coordinate well with each other or could also be disturbed and/or handcuffed by substances released from the pathogens. This can result in dysfunctional operational systems that are harmful to the host, leading to detrimental outcomes, including death. As a whole, the occurrence of the severe consequences is very rare. For instance, with JEV infection, the overall global incidence of cases annually is at 1.8 per 100,000 people [60].

Timing is critical in the diagnosis of acute arboviral encephalitis. The progression and variation in clinical manifestations among infected subjects may differ, depending on the individual's age and geographical habitat, the arthropod's feeding behavior, genetic differences in the viral strain, and the immune status of the affected patients. One of the common clinical features in arboviral infections is viremia. However, the duration and level of this viremia in humans is significantly different with each and every family of viruses. In a commensal arboviral-host relationship, one may expect high levels of viremia to cause too much pathogenesis in the host but too low levels to not facilitate transmission. One may expect a consistent middle range in viremia to be obtained. Extreme variation in or high titers of vi-

http://dx.doi.org/10.5772/52327

rus in the blood may be a sign that humans are an accidental or dead-end host to most arboviruses. Identifying the cellular sources responsible for viremia will likely help us uncover the underlying mechanisms leading to arboviral encephalitis and aid in the development of vaccines and anti-viral drugs. Because of this, finding the permissive cell lineages accounting for circulating virus in infected patients has been the central focus for several decades. In spite of these efforts, the answer remains elusive.

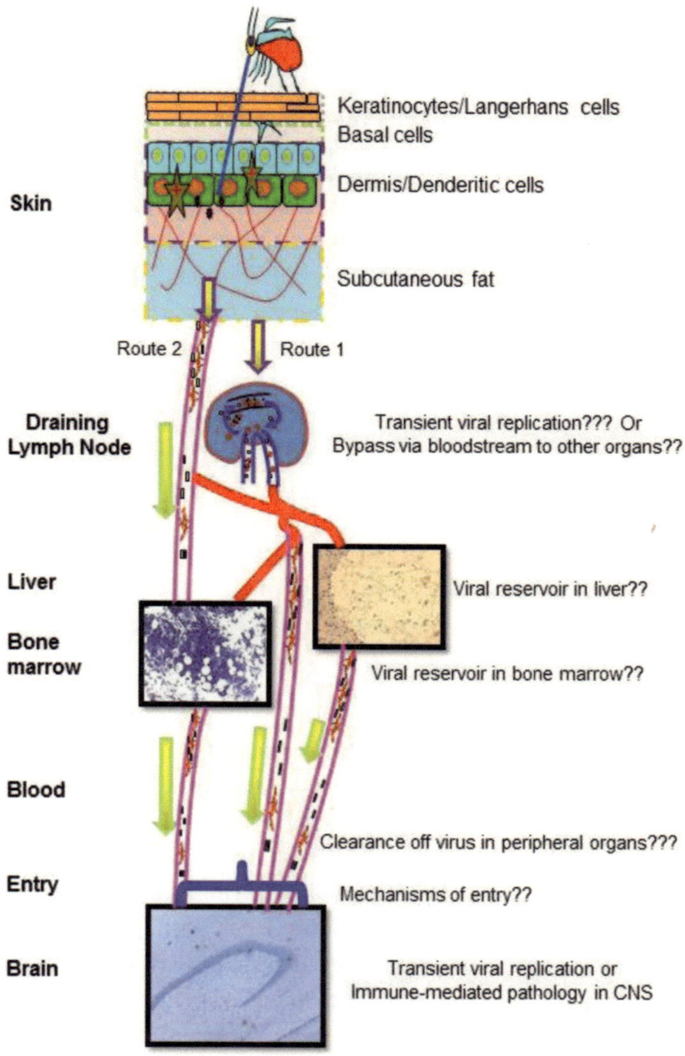

Figure 3. The possible route of the virus in vertebrates from peripheral tissues to the brain. Arboviral infections start with the bite of insects carrying an infectious virus. The exact location where the virus is deposited remains poorly understood. There are multiple ways a virus may spread and circulate before reaching to the brain. Please refer to the text for more details.

Arboviral infections are introduced into the hosts during the blood meals of arthropods carrying infectious virus. The first obstacle that the arthropod encounters is the physical barrier of the skin, which is composed of several layers of keratinocytes interspersed with a network of capillaries (Figure 3). There are two possible routes that the virus may use as a reservoir to amplify the progeny after its deposition by the mosquito. One passage way may be released into the blood pools of lacerated capillaries. In this situation, it is generally assumed that the initial target cell supporting the viral replication is Langerhans dendritic cells of the skin (Figure 3, route 1) [61]. The infected Langerhans dendritic cells migrate to draining lymph nodes where a brief viral replication may occur and the virus is considered to enter the blood stream through the lymphatic and thoracic ducts [61]. The virus may enter the bone marrow [62] or liver [63] where a secondary amplification may occur or directly disseminate to the brain inducing inflammation.

An alternate route would be direct deposition of the viruses into the blood stream (Figure 3, route 2), or so-called capillary feeding, during the engorgement of the arthropod. Results from RVFV suggest that the liver seems to be an early and dominant target of the virus [63]. The damage to the hepatocytes of the RVFV-infected liver is likely a result of apoptosis [63]. The evidence suggests that this virus may get deposit directly into the capillary and take a ride through the circulation to the liver compartment where permissive cells, likely hepatocytes, provide RVFV a means to produce progeny (Figure 3). In addition, studies investigating mosquito imbibing behavior with *Aedes aegypti* revealed that the mosquito's proboscis is flexible and predominantly obtains blood directly from the capillary and only occasionally from the blood pools formed in the tissues by the leakage from previously lacerated capillaries [64]. These results were later confirmed with the mouse's ear and human beings implementing the same experimental designs [65, 66]. In this route (Figure 3, route 2), the virus may gain access directly to the bone marrow where a brief viral replication can occur, extravasates into the circulation, disseminates to other parts of the body, and penetrates the brain via mechanisms discussed in Figure 2.

However, determining the first cells infected by the viruses subsequent to the bite remains a challenging event to investigators. The scenario via route 1 (Figure 3) is complicated by a number of issues. Keratinocytes on the outermost epidermal layer of the skin are endowed with toll-like-receptors (TLR) [67] and may be considered a component of the primary innate immune system. Langerhans cells mainly reside in the thin layer of the epidermis, which does not contain capillaries, while the dendritic cells are predominantly in the thicker dermis layer, which is filled with capillaries. Route 1 has been extensively investigated with diseases derived from mosquito-borne viruses. This pathway could be the true route for those viruses belonging to the human-is-dead-end-host group, since the virus titers from these cells are too low to permit transmission to new mosquitoes. In contrast, if human beings are the host for the virus, such as dengue virus, then the assumption that this virus takes this route should be reconsidered. Experiments have revealed that only a very short window period is available for dengue virus to be transmitted, during the high viremic stage, usually within 3-5 days after the onset of the clinical fever. Thus, if the mosquitoes imbibe the blood meal during this stage, the virus will spillover and infect the local Langerhans dendritic cells and the cycle of illness will resume. If this is the case, then we would observe a sinusoidal wave-like pattern for viremia in infected dengue patients. But in reality, this is not the case. Thus, this evidence indicates that an alternate route could exist, such as direct deposition of virus into the blood stream. Interestingly, it has been suggested that during imbibing, approximately 50% of the fascicle penetrates into the skin [68], suggesting that the location of the blood drawn by the vector is from the capillary-rich dermis layer, implicating that pathogens may be directly injected into the blood.

One of the puzzling issues is what cellular constituents are the protective components in asymptomatic cases. Interestingly, apoptotic keratinocytes and dendritic cells are observed in human skin explants when dengue virus is directly injected into the epidermis with a fine needle [69]. Considering the fact that a majority of dengue virus infections are asymptomatic, this evidence suggests that the role of dendritic cells at the site of fascicle penetration is to eliminate or temporarily contain the intruders and thereby prevent or reduce the dissemination of dengue virus. However, the role of keratinocytes and dendritic cells in clearance of dengue virus remains to be further investigated.

Although most persons bitten by an infected mosquito will experience no symptoms or will have a very mild presentation of the disease, approximately 1 to 2 percent will develop a recognizable illness. The clinical symptoms for the initial phase of arboviral encephalitis are very similar and similarly variable from person-to-person for all the virus families. Some individuals may have mild symptoms, such as a fever and headache, while others may have a more severe presentation. In this case, symptoms may include a rapid onset of severe headache, high fever, muscle aches, stiffness in the back of the neck, and problems with muscle coordination, disorientation, photophobia, convulsions and coma. The illness will usually occur five to 15 days after the bite of an infected mosquito or tick. However, the symptoms may resemble other common febrile illnesses. Thus, in order to diagnose correctly and determine the proper treatment in a timely manner, it is important to seek professional help immediately or as soon as clinical signs appear.

In order for an affected subject to have a risk for neurological disorder, the virus entering the human host has to possess two major criteria: neuroinvasiveness and neruovirulence. The term "neuroinvasiveness" means that the virus is capable of passing or crossing through the BBB, a structure that separates the immune privileged compartment of the brain from the peripheral system. The term "neruovirulence" refers to the capacity of viral replication in the CNS tissues. There are several mechanisms involved on the induction of neuroinvasion. The virus can either replicate and induced damage of the nearby endothelial cells [70] in the cerebral capillary or in striated muscle [71] surrounding the BBB. Alternatively, virus may enter the CNS by endocytosis via the olfactory bulb or the choroid plexus, for example, JEV [43], CHIKV [72] and VEEV [73]. In addition, high viremia is a major feature of only some of the arboviral infections, thus some viruses can cross the BBB via the vascular route by passive transfer carried by infected leukocytes [74]. Spreading virus to the CNS through the trigeminal nerve after local amplification of the virus has been proposed as well [73]. The neurological symptoms induced by some of these arboviruses, which are able to increase the permeability of vasculature and spillover into the CNS, are capable of disrupting cognitive biological processes. In order to differentiate the evasion strategies employed, animal models are required. Currently, there are only a limited number of animal models available for a few arboviruses; JEV [59], EEEV [75], LACV [71], WNV [76] and CHIKV [72]. However, the cardinal features of human clinical encephalitis induced by these arboviruses are hardly reproduced in these models. Therefore, what the exact mechanisms by which arboviruses cross the BBB remains poorly understood, as well as the precise mechanisms by which circulating peripheral pathogens induce the inflammation of the brain remain largely unknown.

Nevertheless, the best systems available that have been used to characterize the biological properties of arboviruses in animal models are the WNV [76, 77], LACV [71], EEEV [75], and CHIKV [72, 78]. Results revealed that viral strain variations, in addition to the host age and immune conditions, contribute a significantly to neuroinvasiveness and neurovirulence. Infection of the mice intradermally or subcutaneously leads to the robust replication of WNV, LACV, and CHIKV in the brain, particularly in newborn mice. But the mechanisms contributing to neurotropism of other viruses are less clear since suitable models are not available.

When viruses enter the CNS, a variety of cells are permissive for infection [46, 79]; some cells may be more susceptible than others, and the viruses may have their differential preferences [74, 75, 78, 80]. Regardless, the net consequence is the activation and/or damage to residential cells. This results in the recruitment of defense cells with immune system functions to the damaged site. An inflammatory response occurs due to the presence of an overproduction of multiple functional cytokines from the infiltrating cells [81-83]. The nature of the privileged environment of the brain bestows it with characteristics that make restoration to the default normal status far more complicated than other parts of the body. The most salient feature of the brain is that a large proportion of the cells are terminally differentiated. These cells are very difficult to renew and replace. Therefore, affected encephalitic patients suffer long-term neurological impairment as a result from the infection [18, 28]. These symptoms include short-term or long-term memory loss, seizures, and impaired judgment [28, 84, 85]. A neurological exam is performed to evaluate the mental status, detect neurological problems, such as motor dysfunction and seizures, and help determine which area of the brain is affected [18].

The causes of the dysfunctional circuitry in neurons are likely different among the arboviruses. Some viruses have the capacity of direct engagement with neurons by infection, while others may induce cell death or apoptosis in nearby cells, which shed releasates, likely triggering a cascade of events that damages the neuronal tissue [81, 82]. This may be why some viruses can be recovered from the CNS easier than others in autopsy specimens. For those viruses capable of infecting small animals, results also suggest the observed scenarios. In contrast, for the viruses with limited capacity to replicate in animal models, the actual causes of neurological symptoms are less clear.

The initial symptoms of the arbovirus infections that induced encephalitis are very similar, especially for those mild cases of encephalitis, which makes the correct diagnosis a challenge to physicians. In order for accurate diagnosis, in addition to the routine examination on the physical performance, specific tests are required, such as electroencephalogram, brain mag-

http://dx.doi.org/10.5772/52327

netic resonance imaging (MRI) and X-ray computed tomography (CT). These tests allow for a scan of the head to detect abnormalities, such as swelling (edema) and bleeding (hemorrhage) [86]. These sophisticated instruments are likely available in very advanced clinics and may not be very convenient or available for the majority of patients affected by arboviral encephalitis. Thus, alternate diagnostic methods are applied. These are biological approaches, which include virus isolation from cerebrospinal fluid, blood, and biopsy specimens, detection of viral genetic and/or antigenic materials, and specific antibodies to the virus. However, there are pros and cons for each of these diagnostic assays. Sensitivity and specificity, and antibody cross-reactivity are always a concern.

5. Treatment of arboviral infections

Currently used drugs to treat arboviral encephalitis. There is no cure for arboviral encephalitis and treatment is generally supportive, with maintenance of respiratory and circulatory systems while the infection runs its course. The purpose of the palliative care is to reduce the malfunctioning of critical organs and to relieve symptoms, while the body fights the infection. The priority of the treatment is to ensure the alleviation of pain, as well as to mitigate the swelling in the brain, reduce the fever and prevent dehydration and other chemical imbalances by administration of intravenous fluids. As a whole, the treatment for arboviral encephalitis depends on the cause. Some clinical cases of arboviral encephalitis can be mitigated successfully if medication is started as soon as possible. A number of therapeutic drugs specific to arboviral infections are under investigation for their potential antiviral and neuroprotective effects: minocycline and curcumin for JEV and other arboviruses [87-89], ribavirin for LACV [90], interferon (Omr-IgG-aM) and humanized monoclonal antibody (Mab E16) as a potential candidate for WNV treatment [61, 91, 92]. However, currently there is limited information available on the effectiveness of these therapeutic modalities in the clinical setting. Additionally, there are a number of reliable medicines that are commonly prescribed to treat the symptoms mentioned above; administration of benzodiazepines (*e.g.*, lorazepam [Ativan®) to prevent seizure, diuretics drugs (*e.g.*, furosemide or mannitol) to reduce brain swelling, sedatives to relieve irritability, antibiotics to prevent secondary infections, and acetaminophen to control fever and headache. For those patients whose brain functions may be severely affected, interventions like physical therapy and speech therapy may be needed after the illness is controlled.

6. New drug development

The life cycle of arboviruses *in vivo* is not well understood, even though a great amount of detail on the comprehensive biology of these viruses *in vitro* has been intensively investigated and uncovered. As aforementioned, the genetic material for a majority of the arbovriuses is positive-sense single-stranded RNA, which can function as mRNA and be infectious by itself. It has been proposed that this genomic viral RNA can become encapsulated within the biological material from the host cell to form an infectious vesicle.These particles may fuse with other biologically functional identities, potentially leading to the initiation of new infections, which can result in the formation of completed and perfect virions. Interference with the processes and network signaling involving classical virion formation has been a common target for drug development. However, in reality, the perfect virion *in vivo* has not been visualized, suggesting an alternate form of virion may exist *in vivo*. Consequently, the real structures needed to design the intervention remains elusive. Furthermore, diseases induced by arboviruses are acute illnesses where timing is critical. Infected individuals normally delay in seeking professional help, resulting in the subjects arriving at the hospital in a far worsen condition. Thus, the availability of intervention drugs, the timing of the administration and the effect of the drugs on the arboviral infections remain critical issues.

7. Prognosis

Prognosis depends on the particular type of arbovirus causing disease, and on the age and prior health status of the patient. The prognosis is worse in very young patients, elderly patients, and patients with compromised immune systems. LAC encephalitis most often occurs in children, while WNV and SLV encephalitis usually occur in persons older than 50 years of age [20]. Encephalitis caused by EEV and JEV carries a high risk for serious neurological damage and death. Death rates range all the way up to 20% for arboviral encephalitis, and the rates of lifelong effects due to brain damage can reach 60% for some types of arboviruses.

8. Vaccine prevention for arboviral infections

Infection with an arbovirus provides immunity to that specific virus, but not to other arboviruses, suggesting that arboviral infection is a vaccine preventable disease. Thus, the development of new, more effective vaccines and the appropriate animal models in which to test them are paramount. Although for many important arboviruses, there are currently no approved vaccines available for human use, while for some, safe and effective vaccines have been used for decades. For instance, a clinical approved inactivated vaccine against TBEV has been used in Russia, Germany, Austria, and China [93].

JEV is one of the few arboviruses for which a vaccine is available. The JEV vaccine made from infected mouse brain can achieve efficacies of at least 80% [94]. But because of the cost and safety concerns, development of a better JEV vaccine has been an ongoing project. For example, the development of a live-attenuated virus vaccine (SA14-14-2, for use in China and a part of Asia) and more recently, in March 2009, the FDA approved a new, inactivated cell-culture-derived JEV vaccine (IXIARO) for use in adult travelers over the age of 17 [95-98]. In addition, a live-attenuated yellow fever–Japanese encephalitis chimeric vaccine (IMOJEV™) was recently licensed in Australia and is under review in Thailand [98].

http://dx.doi.org/10.5772/52327

As for WNV, an approved and efficacious vaccine for humans is not available, even though equine WNV vaccines are in use [99]. However, it is anticipated that a WNV vaccine for human use will be available within a couple of years. In addition, inactivated TBEV vaccine is currently available in Europe [100].

For others, such as the Alphaviruses, human vaccines are available only as Investigational New Drugs, and thus are not in widespread use.The rest of the arboviral vaccines are currently undergoing clinical phase III trials, and are anticipated to be available for public usage within 5 years if everything goes as planned. While some of these vaccines have currently only received approval for animal usage, newer versions for human use are in the process of being evaluated or developed.

New challenges in vaccine development have been met with new technologies in vaccine research. Many of the newer vaccines are now being developed by recombinant DNA technology [100]. For example, chimeric virus vaccines have been developed using infectious clone technology for many arboviruses including, WNV, JEV, and TBEV. Other successful approaches have involved the use of naked DNA encoding and subsequently expressing the desired protective epitopes. Naked DNA vaccines have been used for TBEV and JEV and are currently under development for use against WNV. The development of less expensive, more authentic animal models to evaluate new vaccines against arboviral diseases will become increasingly important as these new approaches in vaccine research are realized.

However, technical issues do exist in the nature of these viruses. One of the unique biological features in a majority of arboviruses is the constitution of the genetic material. The positive-sense single-stranded RNA genome can function as mRNA, which is capable of producing an infectious virus if the RNA is inside a biologically functional identity. To add the second layer of difficulty in vaccine development, arboviruses may have multiple life cycles, since the physical morphology of these virions may be a mosaic form *in vivo* [62]. These features may be one of the reasons why developing a vaccine against arboviruses is such a difficult task. Despite the potential dilemma, there are some successes; though continued improvement in developing arboviral vaccines that are capable of preventing encephalitis is an urgently needed and challenging task.

Other foreseeable methods for areas where arboviral encephalitis is prevalent include insecticide spraying, which may be used to control outbreaks. Wearing insect repellent and avoiding outdoor activities when mosquitoes are active may also be helpful.

9. Conclusion and perspective

Arboviral encephalitis is a very significant human disease and is caused by a large group of viruses distributed across multiple virus families. The virus is introduced to human beings by hematophagous arthropods, mainly mosquitoes and ticks. With a wide spectrum of clinical manifestations, the diseases are very difficult to diagnose and treat. Although arboviral infections are vaccine preventable and treatable diseases, only a couple of anti-viral therapeutic drugs and vaccines are available. However, several new drugs are undergoing clinical trials and some will likely become available within 5 years. Animal models that can capture the cardinal features of disease seen in their human counterparts will be a very critical technological advance. Using adequate animal models can pave the way for understanding and uncovering the paramount host and viral factors responsible for breaking down the BBB and leading to the penetration of the virus into the CNS, as well as serving as a good platform to test for effective and preventive modalities.

Acknowledgements

This work was supported by a grant from Chang Gung Memorial Hospital (CMRPD190163) (WJC), Emory SOM startup fund, and from the Center of Infectious Disease and Signaling Research, Aim for The Top University Project (NSC99-2321-B006-008), National Cheng Kung University, Taiwan (GCP).

Author details

Guey-Chuen Perng[1,2,3] and Wei-June Chen[4,5*]

*Address all correspondence to: wjchen@mail.cgu.edu.tw

1 Department of Pathology and Laboratory Medicine, Emory Vaccine Center, Emory University School of Medicine, USA

2 Center of Infectious Diseases and Signaling Research, National Cheng Kung University, Taiwan

3 Department of Microbiology and Immunology, College of Medicine, National Cheng Kung University, Taiwan

4 Graduate Institute of Biomedical Sciences, Chang Gung University, Taiwan

5 Department of Public Health and Parasitology, College of Medicine, Chang Gung University, Taiwan

References

[1] Daniels, P. W. (2002). Emerging arboviral diseases. *Australian veterinary journal*, 80(4), 216, Epub 2002/06/11.

[2] De Foliart, G. R., Grimstad, P. R., & Watts, D. M. (1987). Advances in mosquito-borne arbovirus/vector research. *Annual review of entomology*, 32, 479-505, Epub 1987/01/01.

[3] Thompson, W. H., & Beaty, B. J. (1977). Venereal transmission of La Crosse (California encephalitis) arbovirus in *Aedes triseriatus* mosquitoes. *Science*, 196(4289), 530-1, Epub 1977/04/29.

[4] Davis, L. E., Beckham, J. D., & Tyler, K. L. (2008). North American encephalitic arboviruses. Neurologic clinics ix. Epub 2008/07/29, 26(3), 727-57.

[5] Gould, E. A., & Solomon, T. (2008). Pathogenic flaviviruses. *Lancet*, 371(9611), 500-9, Epub 2008/02/12.

[6] Zacks, M. A., & Paessler, S. (2010). Encephalitic alphaviruses. *Veterinary microbiology*, 140(3-4), 281-6, Epub 2009/09/25.

[7] Alatoom, A., & Payne, D. (2009). An overview of arboviruses and bunyaviruses. *LabMedicine*, 40, 237-40.

[8] Westaway, E. G., Brinton, M. A., Gaidamovich, S., Horzinek, M. C., Igarashi, A., Kaariainen, L., et al. (1985). Flaviviridae. *Intervirology*, 24(4), 183-92, Epub 1985/01/01.

[9] Ten Dam, E., Flint, M., & Ryan, M. D. (1999). Virus-encoded proteinases of the Togaviridae. *The Journal of general virology*, 80(Pt8), 1879-88, Epub 1999/08/31.

[10] Weaver, S. C., & Barrett, A. D. (2004). Transmission cycles, host range, evolution and emergence of arboviral disease. *Nature reviews Microbiology*, 2(10), 789-801, Epub 2004/09/21.

[11] Lindenbach, B. D., & Rice, C. M. (2003). Molecular biology of flaviviruses. *Advances in virus research*, 59, 23-61, Epub 2003/12/31.

[12] Elliott, R. M. (1990). Molecular biology of the Bunyaviridae. *The Journal of general virology*, 71(Pt 3), 501-22, Epub 1990/03/01.

[13] Elliott, R. M., Schmaljohn, C. S., & Collett, M. S. (1991). Bunyaviridae genome structure and gene expression. *Current topics in microbiology and immunology*, 169, 91-141, Epub 1991/01/01.

[14] Strauss, J. H., & Strauss, E. G. (1994). The alphaviruses: gene expression, replication, and evolution. *Microbiological reviews*, 58(3), 491-562, Epub 1994/09/01.

[15] Solomon, T. (2004). Flavivirus encephalitis. *The New England journal of medicine*, 351(4), 370-8, Epub 2004/07/23.

[16] Sips, G. J., Wilschut, J., & Smit, J. M. (2012). Neuroinvasive flavivirus infections. *Reviews in medical virology*, 22(2), 69-87, Epub 2011/11/17.

[17] Chen, W. J., Hwang, K. P., & Fang, A. H. (1991). Detection of IgM antibodies from cerebrospinal fluid and sera of dengue fever patients. *The Southeast Asian journal of tropical medicine and public health*, 22(4), 659-63, Epub 1991/12/01.

[18] Tournebize, P., Charlin, C., & Lagrange, M. (2009). Neurological manifestations in Chikungunya: about 23 cases collected in Reunion Island. *Revue neurologique*, 165(1), 48-51, Epub 2008/10/07.

[19] Varatharaj, A. (2010). Encephalitis in the clinical spectrum of dengue infection. *Neurology India*, 58(4), 585-91, Epub 2010/08/27.

[20] Hollidge, B. S., Gonzalez-Scarano, F., & Soldan, S. S. (2010). Arboviral encephalitides: transmission, emergence, and pathogenesis. *Journal of neuroimmune pharmacology : the official journal of the Society on NeuroImmune Pharmacology*, 5(3), 428-42, Epub 2010/07/24.

[21] Morris, C. D. (1988). Eastern equine encephalomyelitis. *In: Monath TP, editor. The Arboviruses: Epidemiology and Ecology. Boca Raton: CRC Press*, 2-13.

[22] Epidemiology and Ecology of Eastern Equine Encephalomyelitits [database on the Internet]. (2004). Available from: http://www.aphis.usda.gov/about_aphis/programs_offices/veterinary_services/ceah.shtml

[23] Takasaki, T. (2009). Flavivirus encephalitis. *Brain and nerve = Shinkei kenkyu no shinpo*, 61(2), 145-51, Epub 2009/02/25.

[24] Daniel, M., Benes, C., Danielova, V., & Kriz, B. (2011). Sixty years of research of tick-borne encephalitis--a basis of the current knowledge of the epidemiological situation in Central Europe. *Epidemiologie mikrobiologie, imunologie : casopis Spolecnosti pro epidemiologii a mikrobiologii Ceske lekarske spolecnosti JE Purkyne*, 60(4), 135-55, Epub 2012/02/14.

[25] Daniel, M., Kriz, B., Danielova, V., Valter, J., & Kott, I. (2008). Correlation between meteorological factors and tick-borne encephalitis incidence in the Czech Republic. *Parasitology research*, 103(suppl 1), S97-107, Epub 2008/11/23.

[26] Detels, R., Cates, M. D., Cross, J. H., Irving, G. S., & Watten, R. H. (1970). Ecology of Japanese encephalitis virus on Taiwan in 1968. *The American journal of tropical medicine and hygiene*, 19(4), 716-23, Epub 1970/07/01.

[27] Rosen, L. (1986). The natural history of Japanese encephalitis virus. *Annual review of microbiology*, 40, 395-414, Epub 1986/01/01.

[28] Mackenzie, J. S., Gubler, D. J., & Petersen, L. R. (2004). Emerging flaviviruses: the spread and resurgence of Japanese encephalitis, West Nile and dengue viruses. *Nature medicine*, 10(12), S98-109, Epub 2004/12/04.

[29] Mackenzie, J. S. (1999). Emerging viral diseases: an Australian perspective. *Emerging infectious diseases*, 5(1), 1-8, Epub 1999/03/19.

[30] Van-den-Hurk, A. F., Ritchie, S. A., Johansen, C. A., Mackenzie, J. S., & Smith, G. A. (2008). Domestic pigs and Japanese encephalitis virus infection, Australia. *Emerging infectious diseases*, 14(11), 1736-8, Epub 2008/11/04.

[31] Erlanger, T. E., Weiss, S., Keiser, J., Utzinger, J., & Wiedenmayer, K. (2009). Past, present, and future of Japanese encephalitis. *Emerging infectious diseases*, 15(1), 1-7, Epub 2009/01/01.

[32] Smithburn, K. C., Hughes, T. P., & Burke, A. W. (1940). A neurotropic virus isoalted from the blood of a native of Uganda. *Journal of tropical medicine & hygiene*, 20, 471-92.

[33] Komar, N. (2000). West Nile viral encephalitis. *Revue scientifique et technique*, 19(1), 166-76, Epub 2001/02/24.

[34] Petersen, L. R., & Hayes, E. B. (2004). Westward ho?--The spread of West Nile virus. *The New England journal of medicine*, 351(22), 257-9, Epub 2004/11/27.

[35] Calisher, C. H., Karabatsos, N., Dalrymple, J. M., Shope, R. E., Porterfield, J. S., Westaway, E. G., et al. (1989). Antigenic relationships between flaviviruses as determined by cross-neutralization tests with polyclonal antisera. *The Journal of general virology*, 70(Pt 1), 37-43, Epub 1989/01/01.

[36] Mc Lean, R. G., & Bowen, G. S. (1980). Vertebrate Hosts. *In: Monath TP, editor. St Louis Enecphalitis. Washington: American Public Health Association*, 381-450.

[37] Gubler, D. J. (2002). The global emergence/resurgence of arboviral diseases as public health problems. *Archives of medical research*, 33(4), 330-42, Epub 2002/09/18.

[38] La Crosse virus neuroinvasive disease-Missouri [database on the Internet]. (2010). Available from: http://www.cdc.gov/mmwr/preview/mmwrhtml/mm5928a2.htm

[39] Myint, K. S., Gibbons, R. V., Perng, G. C., & Solomon, T. (2007). Unravelling the neuropathogenesis of Japanese encephalitis. *Transactions of the Royal Society of Tropical Medicine and Hygiene*, 101(10), 955-6, Epub 2007/06/05.

[40] Solomon, T., Dung, N. M., Kneen, R., Gainsborough, M., Vaughn, D. W., & Khanh, V. T. (2000). Japanese encephalitis. *Journal of neurology, neurosurgery, and psychiatry*, 68(4), 405-15, Epub 2000/03/23.

[41] Johnston, L. J., Halliday, G. M., & King, N. J. (2000). Langerhans cells migrate to local lymph nodes following cutaneous infection with an arbovirus. *The Journal of investigative dermatology*, 114(3), 560-8, Epub 2000/02/26.

[42] Monath, T. P., Cropp, C. B., & Harrison, A. K. (1983). Mode of entry of a neurotropic arbovirus into the central nervous system. *Reinvestigation of an old controversy. Laboratory investigation; a journal of technical methods and pathology*, 48(4), 399-410, Epub 1983/04/01.

[43] Liou, M. L., & Hsu, C. Y. (1998). Japanese encephalitis virus is transported across the cerebral blood vessels by endocytosis in mouse brain. *Cell and tissue research*, 293(3), 389-94, Epub 1998/08/26.

[44] Mc Minn, P. C. (1997). The molecular basis of virulence of the encephalitogenic flaviviruses. *The Journal of general virology*, 78(11), 2711-22, Epub 1997/11/21.

[45] Mims, C. A. (1957). The invasion of the brain by yellow fever virus present in the blood of mice. *British journal of experimental pathology*, 38(3), 329-38, Epub 1957/06/01.

[46] Johnson, R. T., Burke, D. S., Elwell, M., Leake, C. J., Nisalak, A., Hoke, C. H., et al. (1985). Japanese encephalitis: immunocytochemical studies of viral antigen and inflammatory cells in fatal cases. *Annals of neurology*, 18(5), 567-73, Epub 1985/11/01.

[47] Kimura-Kuroda, J., Ichikawa, M., Ogata, A., Nagashima, K., & Yasui, K. (1993). Specific tropism of Japanese encephalitis virus for developing neurons in primary rat brain culture. *Archives of virology*, 130(3-4), 477-84, Epub 1993/01/01.

[48] Yamada, M., Nakamura, K., Yoshii, M., & Kaku, Y. (2004). Nonsuppurative encephalitis in piglets after experimental inoculation of Japanese encephalitis flavivirus isolated from pigs. *Veterinary pathology*, 41(1), 62-7, Epub 2004/01/13.

[49] Liu, T. H., Liang, L. C., Wang, C. C., Liu, H. C., & Chen, W. J. (2008). The blood-brain barrier in the cerebrum is the initial site for the Japanese encephalitis virus entering the central nervous system. *Journal of neurovirology*, 14(6), 514-21, Epub 2008/11/22.

[50] Silwedel, C., & Forster, C. (2006). Differential susceptibility of cerebral and cerebellar murine brain microvascular endothelial cells to loss of barrier properties in response to inflammatory stimuli. *Journal of neuroimmunology*, 179(1-2), 37-45, Epub 2006/08/04.

[51] Ballabh, P., Braun, A., & Nedergaard, M. (2004). The blood-brain barrier: an overview: structure, regulation, and clinical implications. *Neurobiology of disease*, 16(1), 1-13, Epub 2004/06/23.

[52] Bell, J. E., Busuttil, A., Ironside, J. W., Rebus, S., Donaldson, Y. K., Simmonds, P., et al. (1993). Human immunodeficiency virus and the brain: investigation of virus load and neuropathologic changes in pre-AIDS subjects. *The Journal of infectious diseases*, 168(4), 818-24, Epub 1993/10/01.

[53] Muller, D. M., Pender, M. P., & Greer, J. M. (2005). Blood-brain barrier disruption and lesion localisation in experimental autoimmune encephalomyelitis with predominant cerebellar and brainstem involvement. *Journal of neuroimmunology*, 160(1-2), 162-9, Epub 2005/02/16.

[54] Stephens, E. B., Singh, D. K., Kohler, M. E., Jackson, M., Pacyniak, E., & Berman, N. E. (2003). The primary phase of infection by pathogenic simian-human immunodeficiency virus results in disruption of the blood-brain barrier. *AIDS research and human retroviruses*, 19(10), 837-46, Epub 2003/10/31.

[55] Diamond, M. S., & Klein, R. S. (2004). West Nile virus: crossing the blood-brain barrier. *Nature medicine*, 10(12), 1294-5, Epub 2004/12/08.

[56] Hickey, W. F., Hsu, B. L., & Kimura, H. (1991). T-lymphocyte entry into the central nervous system. *Journal of neuroscience research*, 28(2), 254-60, Epub 1991/02/01.

[57] Griffin, D. E., Levine, B., Tyor, W. R., & Irani, D. N. (1992). The immune response in viral encephalitis. *Seminars in immunology*, 4(2), 111-9, Epub 1992/04/01.

[58] Chuang, C. K., Chiou, S. S., Liang, L. C., & Chen, W. J. (2003). Short report: detection of Japanese encephalitis virus in mouse peripheral blood mononuclear cells using an in situ reverse transcriptase-polymerase chain reaction. *The American journal of tropical medicine and hygiene*, 69(6), 648-51, Epub 2004/01/27.

[59] Mc Minn, P. C., Dalgarno, L., & Weir, R. C. (1996). A comparison of the spread of Murray Valley encephalitis viruses of high or low neuroinvasiveness in the tissues of Swiss mice after peripheral inoculation. *Virology*, 220(2), 414-23, Epub 1996/06/15.

[60] Campbell, G. L., Hills, S. L., Fischer, M., Jacobson, J. A., Hoke, C. H., Hombach, J. M., et al. (2011). Estimated global incidence of Japanese encephalitis: a systematic review. *Bulletin of the World Health Organization*, 89(10), 766-74, A-74E. Epub 2011/11/16.

[61] Gyure, K. A. (2009). West Nile virus infections. *Journal of neuropathology and experimental neurology*, 68(10), 1053-60, Epub 2009/11/18.

[62] Bargeron, Clark. K., Hsiao, H. M., Noisakran, S., Tsai, J. J., & Perng, G. C. (2012). Role of microparticles in dengue virus infection and its impact on medical intervention strategies. *The Yale journal of biology and medicine*, 85(1), 3-18, Epub 2012/03/31.

[63] Smith, D. R., Steele, K. E., Shamblin, J., Honko, A., Johnson, J., Reed, C., et al. (2010). The pathogenesis of Rift Valley fever virus in the mouse model. *Virology*, 407(2), 256-67, Epub 2010/09/21.

[64] Gordon, R. M., & Lumsden, W. H. R. (1939). A study of the behaviour of the mouthparts of mosquitoes when taking up blood from living tissues; together with some observations on the ingestion of microfilariae. *The Annals of tropical medicine & parasitology*, 33(3-4), 259-78.

[65] Griffiths, R. B., & Gordon, R. M. (1952). An apparatus which enables the process of feeding by mosquitoes to be observed in the tissues of a live rodent; together with an account of the ejection of saliva and its significance in Malaria. *The Annals of tropical medicine & parasitology*, 46(4), 311-9, Epub 1952/12/01.

[66] O'Rourke, F. (1956). Observations on pool and capillary feeding in *Aedes aegypti*. *Nature*, 177(4519), 1087-8.

[67] O'Neill, L. A. (2003). Therapeutic targeting of Toll-like receptors for inflammatory and infectious diseases. *Current opinion in pharmacology*, 3(4), 396-403, Epub 2003/08/07.

[68] Ramasubramanian, M. K., Barham, O. M., & Swaminathan, V. (2008). Mechanics of a mosquito bite with applications to microneedle design. *Bioinspiration & biomimetics*, 3(4), 046001, Epub 2008/09/10.

[69] Limon-Flores, A. Y., Perez-Tapia, M., Estrada-Garcia, I., Vaughan, G., Escobar-Gutierrez, A., Calderon-Amador, J., et al. (2005). Dengue virus inoculation to human skin explants: an effective approach to assess in situ the early infection and the effects on cutaneous dendritic cells. *International journal of experimental pathology*, 86(5), 323-34.

[70] Samuel, M. A., & Diamond, M. S. (2006). Pathogenesis of West Nile Virus infection: a balance between virulence, innate and adaptive immunity, and viral evasion. *Journal of virology*, 80(19), 9349-60, Epub 2006/09/16.

[71] Janssen, R., Gonzalez-Scarano, F., & Nathanson, N. (1984). Mechanisms of bunyavirus virulence. Comparative pathogenesis of a virulent strain of La Crosse and an avirulent strain of Tahyna virus. *Laboratory investigation; a journal of technical methods and pathology*, 50(4), 447-55, Epub 1984/04/01.

[72] Couderc, T., Chretien, F., Schilte, C., Disson, O., Brigitte, M., Guivel-Benhassine, F., et al. (2008). A mouse model for Chikungunya: young age and inefficient type-I interferon signaling are risk factors for severe disease. *PLoS pathogens*, e29, Epub 2008/02/20.

[73] Charles, P. C., Walters, E., Margolis, F., & Johnston, R. E. (1995). Mechanism of neuroinvasion of Venezuelan equine encephalitis virus in the mouse. *Virology*, 208(2), 662-71, Epub 1995/04/20.

[74] Vogel, P., Kell, W. M., Fritz, D. L., Parker, M. D., & Schoepp, R. J. (2005). Early events in the pathogenesis of eastern equine encephalitis virus in mice. *The American journal of pathology*, 166(1), 159-71, Epub 2005/01/06.

[75] Paessler, S., Aguilar, P., Anishchenko, M., Wang, H. Q., Aronson, J., Campbell, G., et al. (2004). The hamster as an animal model for eastern equine encephalitis--and its use in studies of virus entrance into the brain. *The Journal of infectious diseases*, 189(11), 2072-6, Epub 2004/05/15.

[76] Beasley, D. W., Davis, C. T., Whiteman, M., Granwehr, B., Kinney, R. M., & Barrett, A. D. (2004). Molecular determinants of virulence of West Nile virus in North America. *Archives of virology Supplementum* [18], 35-41, Epub 2004/05/04.

[77] Botha, E. M., Markotter, W., Wolfaardt, M., Paweska, J. T., Swanepoel, R., Palacios, G., et al. (2008). Genetic determinants of virulence in pathogenic lineage 2 West Nile virus strains. *Emerging infectious diseases*, 14(2), 222-30, Epub 2008/02/09.

[78] Labadie, K., Larcher, T., Joubert, C., Mannioui, A., Delache, B., Brochard, P., et al. (2010). Chikungunya disease in nonhuman primates involves long-term viral persistence in macrophages. *The Journal of clinical investigation*, 120(3), 894-906, Epub 2010/02/25.

[79] Miyake, M. (1964). The pathology of Japanese encephalitis. A review. *Bulletin of the World Health Organization*, 30, 153-60, Epub 1964/01/01.

[80] Rippy, M. K., Topper, M. J., Mebus, C. A., & Morrill, J. C. (1992). Rift Valley fever virus-induced encephalomyelitis and hepatitis in calves. *Veterinary pathology*, 29(6), 495-502, Epub 1992/11/01.

[81] Babu, G. N., Kalita, J., & Misra, U. K. (2006). Inflammatory markers in the patients of Japanese encephalitis. *Neurological research*, 28(2), 190-2, Epub 2006/03/23.

[82] Solomon, T., & Winter, P. M. (2004). Neurovirulence and host factors in flavivirus encephalitis--evidence from clinical epidemiology. *Archives of virology Supplementum*, 18, 161-70, Epub 2004/05/04.

[83] Sitati, E. M., & Diamond, M. S. (2006). CD4+ T-cell responses are required for clearance of West Nile virus from the central nervous system. *Journal of virology*, 80(24), 12060-9, Epub 2006/10/13.

[84] Mc Junkin, J. E., de los, Reyes. E. C., Irazuzta, J. E., Caceres, M. J., Khan, R. R., Minnich, L. L., et al. (2001). La Crosse encephalitis in children. *The New England journal of medicine*, 344(11), 801-7, Epub 2001/03/15.

[85] Rust, R. S., Thompson, W. H., Matthews, C. G., Beaty, B. J., & Chun, R. W. (1999). La Crosse and other forms of California encephalitis. *Journal of child neurology*, 14(1), 1-14, Epub 1999/02/20.

[86] Handique, S. K. (2011). Viral infections of the central nervous system. *Neuroimaging clinics of North America*, 21(4), 777-94, vii. Epub 2011/10/29.

[87] Dutta, K., Ghosh, D., & Basu, A. (2009). Curcumin protects neuronal cells from Japanese encephalitis virus-mediated cell death and also inhibits infective viral particle formation by dysregulation of ubiquitin-proteasome system. *Journal of neuroimmune pharmacology: the official journal of the Society on NeuroImmune Pharmacology*, 4(3), 328-37, Epub 2009/05/13.

[88] Mishra, M. K., & Basu, A. (2008). Minocycline neuroprotects, reduces microglial activation, inhibits caspase 3 induction, and viral replication following Japanese encephalitis. *Journal of neurochemistry*, 105(5), 1582-95, Epub 2008/01/23.

[89] Richardson-Burns, S. M., & Tyler, K. L. (2005). Minocycline delays disease onset and mortality in reovirus encephalitis. *Experimental neurology*, 192(2), 331-9, Epub 2005/03/10.

[90] Cassidy, L. F., & Patterson, J. L. (1989). Mechanism of La Crosse virus inhibition by ribavirin. *Antimicrobial agents and chemotherapy*, 33(11), 2009-11, Epub 1989/11/01.

[91] Thompson, B. S., Moesker, B., Smit, J. M., Wilschut, J., Diamond, M. S., & Fremont, D. H. (2009). A therapeutic antibody against west nile virus neutralizes infection by blocking fusion within endosomes. *PLoS pathogens*, 5(5), e1000453, Epub 2009/05/30.

[92] Levi, M. E., Quan, D., Ho, J. T., Kleinschmidt-Demasters, B. K., Tyler, K. L., & Grazia, T. J. (2010). Impact of rituximab-associated B-cell defects on West Nile virus meningoencephalitis in solid organ transplant recipients. *Clinical transplantation*, 24(2), 223-8, Epub 2009/08/08.

[93] Orlinger, K. K., Hofmeister, Y., Fritz, R., Holzer, G. W., Falkner, F. G., Unger, B., et al. (2011). A tick-borne encephalitis virus vaccine based on the European prototype strain induces broadly reactive cross-neutralizing antibodies in humans. *Journal of infectious diseases*, 203(11), 1556-64, Epub 2011/05/20.

[94] Rojanasuphot, S., Charoensuk, O., Kitprayura, D., Likityingvara, C., Limpisthien, S., Boonyindee, S., et al. (1989). A field trial of Japanese encephalitis vaccine produced in Thailand. *The Southeast Asian journal of tropical medicine and public health*, 20(4), 653-4, Epub 1989/12/01.

[95] Kurane, I., & Takasaki, T. (2000). Immunogenicity and protective efficacy of the current inactivated Japanese encephalitis vaccine against different Japanese encephalitis virus strains. *Vaccine*, 2, 33-5, Epub 2000/05/24.

[96] Duggan, S. T., & Plosker, G. L. (2009). Japanese encephalitis vaccine (inactivated, adsorbed) [IXIARO]. *Drugs*, 69(1), 115-22, Epub 2009/02/06.

[97] Fischer, M., Lindsey, N., Staples, J. E., & Hills, S. (2010). Japanese encephalitis vaccines: recommendations of the Advisory Committee on Immunization Practices (ACIP). *MMWR Recommendations and reports : Morbidity and mortality weekly report Recommendations and reports / Centers for Disease Control*, 59(RR-1), 1-27, Epub 2010/03/13.

[98] Halstead, S. B., & Thomas, S. J. (2011). New Japanese encephalitis vaccines: alternatives to production in mouse brain. *Expert review of vaccines*, 10(3), 355-64, Epub 2011/03/26.

[99] Reisen, W., & Brault, A. C. (2007). West Nile virus in North America: perspectives on epidemiology and intervention. *Pest management science*, 63(7), 641-6, Epub 2007/03/22.

[100] Heinz, F. X., & Stiasny, K. (2012). Flaviviruses and flavivirus vaccines. *Vaccine*, 30(29), 4301-6, Epub 2012/06/12.

Chapter 7

Genetic and Biological Properties of Original TBEV Strains Group Circulating in Eastern Siberia

I.V. Kozlova, M.M. Verkhozina, T.V. Demina, Yu.P. Dzhioev, S.E. Tkachev, L.S. Karan, E.K. Doroshchenko, O.V. Lisak, O.V. Suntsova, A.I. Paramonov, O.O. Fedulina, A.O. Revizor and V.I. Zlobin

Additional information is available at the end of the chapter

http://dx.doi.org/10.5772/54087

1. Introduction

In the XXI century tick-borne encephalitis (TBE) remains the most distributed severe natural foci infection transmitted by Ixodes ticks bite.

The causative agent of this infection is tick-borne encephalitis virus (TBEV). According to the modern classification it belongs to the group of mammal viruses transmitted by ticks, and is a member of the genus Flavivirus of the family Flaviviridae [23]. As a result of numerous studies devoted to TBEV genetic variability it was divided into three genotypes (subtypes): 1) genotype 1 (Far-Eastern (FE) subtype); 2) genotype 2 (European subtype); 3) genotype 3 (Siberian subtype). Each genotype is believed to distribute in its certain area where its absolute domination is observed [10, 20].

In Eastern Siberia the circulation of three TBE virus genotypes with the domination of genotype 3 was identified by the prior study. Moreover, the unique TBEV strains (886-84 and 178-79), which differed in genetic structure from all known TBEV genotypes, have been found on this territory [10].

Currently, with use of molecular hybridization of nucleic acids (MHNA) method with genotype-specific probes and sequencing of complete virus genome or its fragments we identified the group of 13 strains with high homology level to 886-84 strain that was conventionally defined as "group 886" [6]. The obtained results confirm the validity of "group 886" certification as possible separate TBEV genotype.

The unique genetic structure of "group 886" strains also manifests in original phenotype pattern that is quite significant from the scientific point of view. "Group 886" strains can be tested as prototype candidate strains for the design of universal vaccines effective against strains of different serotypes (genotypes) and TBEV test-systems.

The aim of the study was to investigate genetic and biological properties of TBEV "886 group" strains circulating in Eastern Siberia (territories of Irkutsk region, Buryat Republic, Transbaikalia) for estimation of their potential as candidates for test-systems and vaccine development.

2. Materials and methods

2.1. TBE virus

Thirteen TBEV strains from the collection of FSSFE "Scientific Centre of Family Health and Human Reproduction Problems, Institute of Epidemiology and Microbiology SB RAMS", Irkutsk were investigated in the study. By MHNA genotyping and full genome or fragments sequencing they were classified as "group 886" strains. Detailed information about strains is presented in Table 1.

Strain	The year of isolation	Isolation source	The location of sample collection
886-84	1984	*Myodes (Clethrionomys) rutilus*	Irkutsk region, Ekhirit-Bulagatskiy district
711-84	1984	*Myodes rufocanus*	Buryat Republic, Barguzinskiy district
740-84	1984	*Myodes rufocanus*	Buryat Republic, Bichurskiy district
712-89	1989	*I. persulcatus*	Transbaikalia, Krasnochikoyskiy district
780-89	1989	*I. persulcatus*	Buryat Republic, Bichurskiy district
617-90	1990	*I. persulcatus*	Buryat Republic, Bichurskiy district
636-90	1990	*I. persulcatus*	Buryat Republic, Bichurskiy district
608-90	1990	*I. persulcatus*	Buryat Republic, Bichurskiy district
606-90	1990	*I. persulcatus*	Buryat Republic, Bichurskiy district
691-90	1990	*I. persulcatus*	Buryat Republic, Bichurskiy district
418-90	1990	*I. persulcatus*	Transbaikalia, Krasnochikoyskiy district
733-90	1990	*I. persulcatus*	Transbaikalia, Krasnochikoyskiy district
742-90	1990	*I. persulcatus*	Transbaikalia, Krasnochikoyskiy district

Table 1. Information concerning "group 886" strains of TBE virus, isolated on the Eastern Siberia territory.

2.2. Strains genotyping

We used MHNA with three panels of 40 deoxyoligonucleic probes complemented to fragments of 10 genes of different TBEV genotypes. The probe description and their localization in TBEV genome was presented earlier by Demina *et al.* [6].

The total RNA extraction from infected mice brains or porcine embryo kidney cells, applying RNA onto kapron or cellulose nitrate filters and hybridization with probes were performed by the common methods [16].

The amplification was carried out with primers complemented to 5′- UTR fragment, to C-prM-E-NS1 genes, E gene or E-NS1 genes fragments, synthesized in the Institute of Chemical Biology and Fundamental Medicine SB RAS (Novosibirsk, Russia). RT-PCR was performed according to the "BioSan" company (Novosibirsk, Russia) protocol.

The sequence analysis of PCR products was carried out with BigDye Terminators Cycle Sequencing Kit v.3.1 (Applied Biosystems, USA) in DNA Sequencing Center SB RAS, Novosibirsk, Russia. The obtained data was analyzed by Mega 5.0 program [28]. The gene fragments sequences of TBEV strains belonging to the different genetic types from GenBank database were used as a material for comparison. BLAST program (http://www.ncbi.nlm.nih.gov/blast/) was used for homology search of obtained nucleotide sequences with already known fragments of TBEV genomes.

The genome fragments sequences of "group 866" strains obtained during the study have been deposited into GenBank database with access numbers EF469662, EU878281-EU878283, JN936341, JN936347, JN936349-JN936350, JN936353-JN936355.

The sequencing of full genome of 886-84 strain has been performed by Karan *et al.* in Central Research Institute of Epidemiology of Rospotrebnadzor RF, Moscow, Russia.

2.3. Strains immunotyping

The reaction of diffuse precipitation in agar (RDPA) was carried out by the method developed by Clark [12] with modifications by Rubin [27] and Bochkova [2]. We used immune sera against TBEV prototype strains of three serotypes (Sofjin – Far-Eastern serotype, 256 – Western serotype, Lesopark-11 and Aina/1448 – East-Siberian serotype) exposed to dosed adsorbtion with concentrated cultural antigens or cross-adsorbed sera against investigated strains [4].

The cytoplasmatic activity study was performed according to common methods. Virus titers were determined in tests on cell culture based on its cytopathic activity (CPA) by the full cumulative method (offered by Reed and Muench) and expressed as lg TCD_{50} [1]/ml [26].

2.4. Neuroinvasiveness

To estimate the neuroinvasiveness of TBEV strains we determined the index of invasiveness (II) – the difference between the virus titers after intracerebral (mNic) and subcutaneous

1 Tissue cytopathogenic dose

(mNsc) mice inoculation expressed as lg LD_{50}/ml [18]. Nonlinear mice (6-8 g in weight) were infected into brain with 0.03 ml or subcutaneously with 0.25 ml of inoculate. Animals infected intracerebrally were observed during 14 days while animals infected subcutaneously were observed during 21 days. Virus titers were detected by Reed and Muench method. The values of II 1-2.5 meant the high invasive activity of the virus, i.e. the ability of virus to overcome the blood-brain barrier to reach central nervous system (CNS) and propagate in it. The values of invasiveness index of equal or more than 3 indicated the lesser invasive activity of the virus strain.

2.5. Thermoresistance

Thermoresistance (T^{50}) of TBEV strains was tested by Ovchinnikova *et al.* method [17] using 24-hour cell culture grown in 96-hole plates at the presence of CO_2. The thermoresistance was determined by inactivation index – difference in lg of titers of virus samples heated at 50°C during 15 minutes or unheated (4°C). In case of titers difference equal or less than 2.0 lg the strain was characterized as T^{50+}, from 2.1 to 3.0 lg – as medium, equal or more than 3.1 lg – as T^{50-}.

2.6. Rct_{42}–feature

Rct_{42}-feature describes the ability of the virus to propagate at supraoptimal temperature. To determine rct_{42} the 24-hour cell culture grown in 96-hole plates was infected by different virus-containing suspensions (10^{-1} to 10^{-10}). One part of the cell cultures was infected with selected virus strain and incubated at 37°C, and other cells were infected with the same strain and incubated at 42°C at the presence of CO_2. Rct_{42} was determined on the sixth day after infection as a difference between lg of virus titers after the cultivation in cells at 37°C and 42°C. In case of titers difference equal or less than 2,0 lg the strain was characterized as $rct_{42}{}^{-}$, from 2.1 to 3.0 lg – as medium, equal or more than 3.1 lg – as $rct_{42}{}^{+}$.

2.7. S-feature

The cell culture was infected with TBEV strains undergone not more than 4 passages through the white mice brains and 3 cycles of cloning. The plaques appeared on the third or fourth day. The plaque size measuring was performed on the fifth day when they increased and become more sharp and transparent. S-feature was determined as S+ if plaque had the diameter (d)≥2.5 mm; S± at 2.5>d ≥2,0 mm; S– at 2.0>d ≥1,0 mm.

3. Results and discussion

For the first time the uniqueness of 886-84 strain was found during the investigation of its serological properties. Trukhina suggested that this strain takes the intermediate place between two TBEV serotypes – East-Siberian and Far-Eastern and shows the properties of both serotypes [21].

Then, 886-84 strain was described as a representative of the independent genotype according to criteria developed by our team after the comparing of difference level of 29 strains isolated on different territories of TBEV area [8]. In this study the fragment of E protein gene (positions 567-727 br) was used as a model. It was found that corresponding amino acid sequence of this fragment in 886-84 strain has Leu in position 206 as genotype 3 and Asp in position 234 as genotypes 1 and 2 [10]. At that time we did not find any homologous strains and isolates so the additional data were necessary to separate this TBEV strain into independent genotype.

Comparison of the strain 886-84 complete genome sequence (EF469662) with TBEV sequences available in GenBank has shown that it forms an independent branch and does not cluster with any strains of three main genotypes (Fig.1). It should be noted that nucleotide substitution level was close to the species separation border [11] (Table 2).

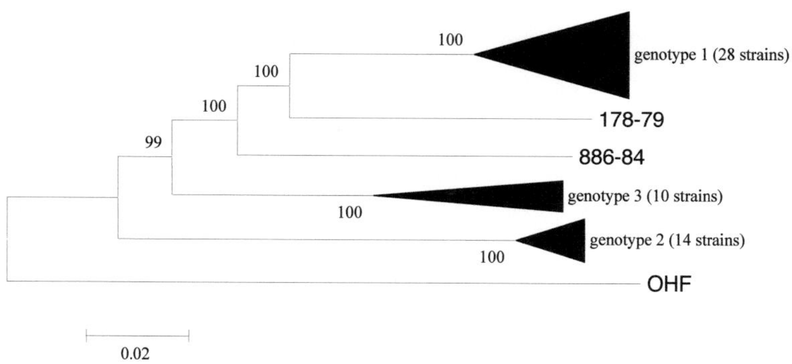

Figure 1. Phylogenetic tree demonstrating the genetic similarity level of 54 TBEV strains on the base of polyprotein coding region sequences (10242 nr). Genotype 1 cluster - Sofjin [25], AB022703, AB001026, DQ989336, AY182009, AY217093, JF316707, JF316708, FJ997899, EU816450-EU816455, AY169390, FJ906622, GQ228395, FJ402885, FJ402886, DQ862460, GU121642, HQ201303, HQ901367, HQ901366, HM859894, HM859895, JN003205; Genotype 2 cluster - TEU27495, TEU27491, TEU39292, AF091010, EU106868, DQ401140, GV266392, HM535610, HM535611, HM120875, GU183379-GU183381, GU183383; Genotype 3 cluster - L40361, AF527415, DQ486861, FJ968751, JN003206-JN003209, GU183382, GU183384. OHF – Omsk haemorrhagic fever virus.

	Nucleotide substitution level (%) (coding region of polyprotein, 10242 nr)		
	genotype 1	genotype 2	genotype 3
genotype 1	4,3		
genotype 2	16,4	2,3	
genotype 3	14,4	15,2	5,4
178-79	11,0	16,0	14,1
886-84	12,5	15,6	13,7
	Amino acid substitution level (%) (complete amino acid sequence of polyprotein, 3414 ar.)		
genotype 1	1,3		
genotype 2	6,9	0,9	
genotype 3	5,3	6,2	1,9
178-79	3,1	6,1	5,2
886-84	3,9	6,0	4,2

Comments: The level of nucleotide and amino acid substitutions within the genotype is marked with grey.

Table 2. Nucleotide and amino acid substitution level between different TBEV genotypes and strains 178-79 and 886-84.

The analysis of complete amino acid sequence of strain 886-84 polyprotein confirmed that it's the unique "mixture" of sequences common for genotypes 1, 2 and 3. For example, in the set of 22 positions which clearly differentiate all known TBEV strains into three genotypes the unique amino acids (alanine (A) in position C-108, serine (S) – NS2A-127 and glycine (G) – NS3-258) or interchange with amino acids typical for main TBEV genotypes were found in strain 886-84 polyprotein sequence [7] (Fig. 2).

protein	C		E		NS1			NS2A					NS3			NS4B			NS5			
Position number	3	108	206	317	54	141	285	100	127	174	175	225	126	258	376	21	28	96	18	297	671	832
Genotype 1	G	V/L/I	S	I/T	T	S/G	R	N	A	M/V	L	I/V	I	V	I/T	H	E	A/R	G	R	V/G	A/V/T
Genotype 2	K	I	V	A	S	Q	T	S	D/E	V	C	A	L/I	A	A	R/Q	S	T	N	E/A	L	M
Genotype 3	R	T	L	T	N	G	K	G/S	G	I/v	I/F	T	M/T	M/V/A	V	Q	G	S	S	G/R	I	T/A
178-79	R	V	S	T	T	S	K	N	G	M	L	T	I	V	V	Q	G	A	S	G	V	A
886-84	R	A	L	I	N	S	K	S	S	M	L	A	I	G	V	Q	G	A	S	G	V	A

Figure 2. The differences in 22 positions obtained by comparing of 54 TBEV strains polyprotein sequences; **Comments.** The cells marked with grey identify the amino acid residues corresponding to one of four TBEV genotypes. The unique amino acid for strain 886-84 is marked with black.

Thirty unique substitutions were detected in strain 886-84 polyprotein which could probably be the "genotype-specific" for "group 886" members. However, since studied polyprotein fragment for "group 886" strains was 1066 ar in length the "genotype-specific" uniqueness was confirmed only for 6 substitutions of 30 (Table. 3)

Protein	C		M	E		NS1
Position in polyprotein	98	108	270	688	735	898
Position in protein			158	408	455	122
genotype 1	A	V/L/I	V	K	L	S
genotype 2	A	I	V	K	L	S
genotype 3	T	T	V	K	L/M	S
178-79	A	V	V	K	L	S
"group 886"	V	A	A	R	I	A

Comments: genotype 1 is presented by translated nucleotide sequences X07755, AB022703, AB001026, DQ989336, AY182009, AY217093, JF316707, JF316708, FJ997899, EU816450-EU816455, AY169390, FJ906622, GQ228395, FJ402885, FJ402886, DQ862460, GU121642, HQ201303, HQ901367, HQ901366, HM859894, HM859895, JN003205; genotype 2 - TEU27495, TEU27491, TEU39292, AF091010, EU106868, DQ401140, GV266392, HM535610, HM535611, HM120875, GU183379- GU183381, GU183383; genotype 3 - L40361, AF527415, DQ486861, FJ968751, JN003206-JN003209, GU183382, GU183384. "Group 886" is presented by prototype strain sequence EF469662 (strain 886-84) and GenBank deposited (EU878281-EU878283) and non-deposited 617-90, 711-84 и 740-84 TBEV strains genome fragments.

Table 3. Unique substitutions in the polyprotein fragments (1066 ar) (proteins C, M, E and part of NS1) of TBEV "group 886" strains.

At present, using MHNA and sequencing methods we have found the group of 13 TBEV isolates with highly homologous genetic structure to the strain 886-84. For eight strains the genome fragments (1650 nr in length) coding proteins C, M, and E protein fragment were determined (GenBank accession numbers EF469662, EU878281-EU878283, JN936341, JN936347, JN936349-JN936350, JN936353-JN936355) (Fig.4). The homology level with the strain 886-84 genome sequence was 98.2-99.8% while the difference level with three main genotypes ranged from 13.1% (Sofjin) to 16.6% (Neudoerfl).

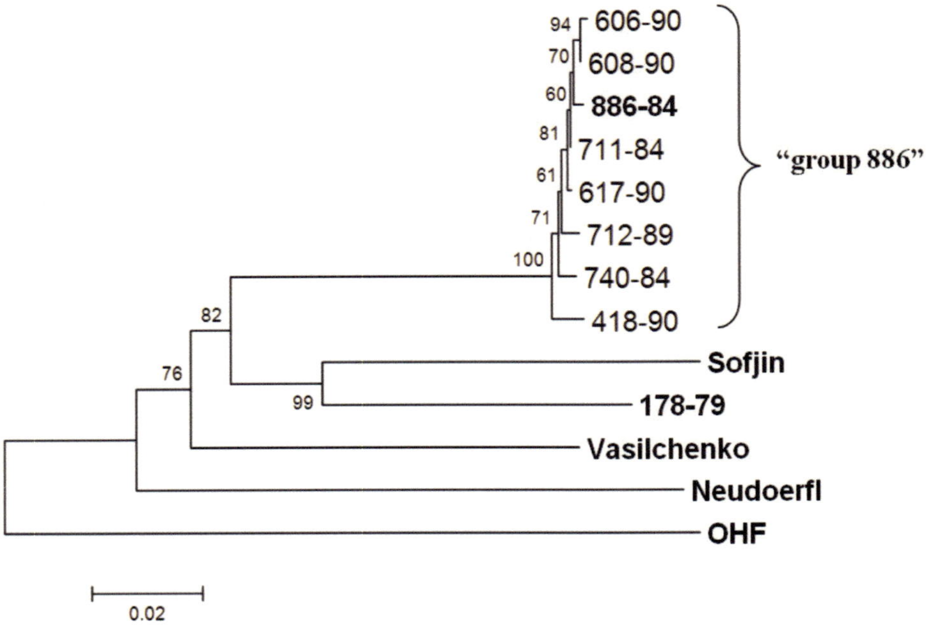

Figure 3. Phylogenetic tree (NJ, Kimura 2), based on TBEV genome fragments sequences (1650 nr in length) (proteins C, M, and E protein fragment).

Our study determined specific areas of habitat for TBEV "group 886" (Fig. 4).

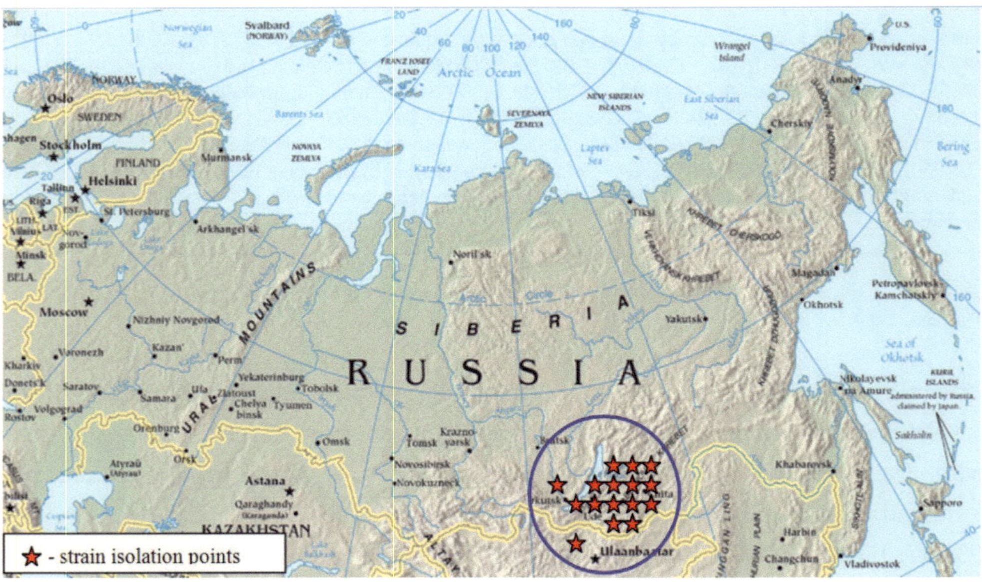

Figure 4. TBEV "group 886" area of habitat.

The strains forming this TBE virus variant were isolated from samples collected in Irkutsk region, Buryat Republic and Transbaikalia in 1984-1990. Also it was recently reported about two "group 886" strains isolated on the territory of National Park "Alkhanai" in Duldurginskiy district, Transbaikalia from *I. persulcatus* tick (in 1999) and one strain from *Myodes rutilus* (in 2010) [1]. Moreover, the case of meningoencephalitis with lethal outcome was described in Bulganskiy aimak in Mongolia caused by TBEV isolate with genome fragment sequence similar to strain 886-84 [24].

The common feature of above-listed territories is the presence of several landscape forms that could provide rich biodiversity of flora and fauna. The combination of forest landscapes with steppe areas is typical for Ekhirit-Bulagatskiy district of Irkutsk region. Bichurskiy district of Buryat Republic is presented by mountain forest ecosystems as well as submountain and mountain-valley areas including submountain landscapes with local pine woods and steppe-meadows. Barguzinskiy district is located from Barguzin river mouth along Barguzin river valley in mountain-forest zone. Its middle part corresponds an "island" of steppe and forest-steppe landscapes in isolated mountain valley surrounded by mountain-forest area. Krasnochikoiskiy district of Transbaikalia is the eastern frontier of South-Siberian mountain landscape territory. The basic components of foci territories are similar to ones from Irkutsk region and Buryat Republic south, where the combination of mountain-forest, forest-steppe and steppe landscapes could be observed. The landscape of National Park "Alkhanai" is also very diverse and includes steppes, meadows, forests and rocky mountains. The National Park location on the border of Eurasia boreal forests and Dauria steppes has the special biospheric importance and results in the significant biodiversity because of flora and fauna interpenetration. Bulganskiy aimak of Mongolia located in Selenga river basin is characterized by forest-steppe, steppe, dry steppe zones and river valleys landscapes.

Also for "group 886" strains we obtained the data concerning their ecological connections with all elements of transmissible chain. Thus, strains 712-89, 418-90, 606-90, 608-90, 617-90, 636-90, 691-90, 733-90 and 742-90 were isolated from *I. persulcatus* ticks, and 711-84 and 740-84 from gray-sided vole brain.

The case of meningoencephalitis with lethal outcome described in Bulganskiy aimak in Mongolia was caused by TBEV isolate highly homologous to strain 886-84. So it demonstrates that this TBEV variant may play the role in human infectious pathology. Also the strains isolation during the long period of time (since 1984 to 2010) confirms the stability of its circulation on Eastern Siberia territory.

Therefore, "group 886" strains seem to possess all necessary characteristics to separate them into the independent TBEV genotype. Earlier we suggested that two TBEV strains 178-79 and 886-84 are not the members of three known genotypes forming their own branch on phylogenetic tree and may be the representatives of genotypes 4 and 5 [8, 9]. The presented data confirm and develop this hypothesis and also allow to separate "group 886" strains into the new genotype 5 on the base of their properties described in our work.

Along with the original genome sequences of "group 886" strains we investigated their phenotypic characteristics which are the essential part of the virus nature and properties study and useful for practical virology.

The pathogenic properties of viruses are the most important biological characteristics. Taking into account that TBEV "group 886" strains play the role in human infectious pathology [24] it was extremely important to study their pathogenic potential.

We have estimated the virulence level of TBEV "group 886" strains according two parameters: the average infectious virus titers after intracerebral or subcutaneous inoculation of mice. Peripheral virus activity was characterized by index of invasiveness (II) (Table 4).

Strain	Isolaion source	mNic ($lgLD_{50}$/мл)	mNsc ($lgLD_{50}$/мл)	mNic-mNsc	II
691-90	*I. persulcatus*	7,02	5,1	1,92	+
418-90	*I. persulcatus*	9,72	7,8	1,52	+
886-84	*Myodes rutilus*	8,58	7,16	1,2	+
711-84	*Myodes rufocanus*	6,75	4,6	1,0	+
740-84	*Myodes rufocanus*	10,2	9,4	0,8	+
712-89	*I. persulcatus*	10,9	9,8	1,1	+
617-90	*I. persulcatus*	6,64	3,8	2,84	±
636-90	*I. persulcatus*	7,06	4,35	2,71	±
608-90	*I. persulcatus*	7,9	4,86	3,04	-
606-90	*I. persulcatus*	7,02	4,02	3,0	-

Table 4. The index of invasiveness (II) for TBEV "group 886" strains.

The virus titers after intracerebral inoculation of mice ranged from 6.64 to 10.9 lg LD_{50}/ml while after subcutaneous inoculation (peripheral activity) were found to be from 3.8 to 9.8 lg LD_{50}/ml. The determined virus indexes of invasiveness (II) had medium and high values (from 0.8 to 3.04 lg LD_{50}/ml). According to obtained results, six strains from "group 886" had high invasive properties that mean their ability to overcome the blood-brain barrier, penetrate into CNS and propagate in it. The highest invasive properties were observed in three strains isolated from rodents and in one strain isolated from tick collected in Krasnochikoiskiy district of Transbaikalia. Two strains (606-90 and 608-90) from Bichurskiy district, Buryat Republic had the lower neuroinvasive activity.

Additionally, to characterize the virulence of TBEV "group 886" strains we determined the average life time and lethality percent of infected mice (Table 5).

Strain №	Isolaion source	Life time (days ± m)	% of lethal cases (% ± m)
711-84	*Myodes rufocanus*	5,1±0,49	100
740-84	*Myodes rufocanus*	5,2±0,24	100
712-89	*I. persulcatus*	5,3±0,79	100
780-89	*I. persulcatus*	6,6±0,45	100
691-90	*I. persulcatus*	6,0±0,89	100
418-90	*I. persulcatus*	6,3±0,06	100
733-90	*I. persulcatus*	5,0±0,45	100
742-90	*I. persulcatus*	6,8±0,76	100
886-84	*Myodes rutilus*	6,1±0,35	93,8±1,91
606-90	*I. persulcatus*	5,9±0,27	93,3±1,98
636-90	*I. persulcatus*	5,3±0,44	88,9±2,5
608-90	*I. persulcatus*	6,4±0,89	77,8±3,3
617-90	*I. persulcatus*	5,3±1,03	70±3,65

Table 5. The average life time and lethality percent of mice infected with TBEV "group 886" strains.

The value of mice average life time after infection with different strains ranged from 5.0±0.45 to 6.8±0.76 days and lethality percent varied from 70±3.65 to 100%. It should be noted that the strains isolated from *I. persulcatus* ticks collected in Krasnochikoiskiy district caused the lethal outcome in laboratory animals in 100%.

Earlier, we have noted that registered and described severe clinical cases of TBE were found in the foci where "group 886" strains were isolated. The foci are located in Krasnochikoiskiy district of Transbaikalia and Bichurskiy district of Buryat Repblic [5, 15, 22].

Recently, the case of meningoencephalitis with lethal outcome was described in Mongolia caused by TBEV isolate possessed 98.5% homology level with strain 886-84 genome sequence. The infection of patient occurred after tick bite in Bulganskiy aimak bordering from south with four natural foci where TBEV "group 886" strains were isolated from collected samples. The patient was hospitalized on 11th day after the tick bite with diagnosis "meningoencephalitis" and died on 11th day of the disease. The presence of TBEV RNA in macromyelon samples, in core andmeninx vasculosa indicates the multilevel localization of lesions which are typical to the most severe forms of acute TBE resulting in lethal outcome or disability [19].

Taking into account the genetic and antigenic properties of 886-84 strain, the strain itself and the strains of the group could be considered as a candidates for development of universal vaccines and test-systems effective for different TBEV serotypes (genotypes). So we investigated "group 886" strains according the complex of criteria suggested by L.S. Vereta and M.S. Vorob'eva for the strains – candidates for vaccine prototypes [3].

The proteins of virus envelope are responsible for hemagglutination and antigenic activity, thermostability and some other properties. All TBEV "group 886" strains have shown the hemagglutination activity (titers in hemagglutination reaction 1:1280-1:10240) in the reaction with goose erythrocytes. In RDPA with cross-adsorbed strain-specific sera 886-84 strain demonstrated the same level of similarity with all TBEV subtypes. The high level of antigenic cross-reaction with East-Siberian and Far-Eastern subtypes was observed in RDPA and neutralization reaction (NR) tests for 886-84, 711-84 and 740-84 strains [4]. The results of antigenic typing are presented in Tables 6 and 7.

Strain antigen		Serum against strain							*antigenic typing results
		256, depleted by a/g Aina	Aina, depleted by a/g Sofjin	Leso-park11, depleted by a/g Sofjin	Sofjin, depleted by a/g 256	Aina, depleted by a/g 256	Sofjin, depleted by a/g Lesopark 11	Aina, depleted by a/g Lesopark 11	
Prototype Strains	Aina/1448	0	4	4	2	4	0	0	E-S
	Sofjin	0	0	0	4	0	4-8	0	F-E
	256	2-4	0	2	0	0	0	0	W
	Lesopark -11	2	4	2-4	0	2	0	0	E-S
"group 886" strains	*740-84*	0	4	4	0	0	0	0	E-S
	711-84	0	4-8	4	2-4	0	4	0	E-S F-E
	886-84	4	4	4	2	2	4-8	0	W, E-S, F-E

Comments: the reverse titers of precipitating antibodies are shown; 0-negative result at sera dilution 1:32; * marks: W – Western antigenic variant; E-S – East-Siberian; F-E – Far Eastern; a/g – antigen.

Table 6. Immunotyping of TBEV "group 886" strains by RDPA test.

	Strain	Immune sera				Antigenic typing results
		Sofjin	Lesopark	256	KFD	
Prototype TBEV strains and viruses of TBEV complex	Sofjin	**10240**	1280	1280	1280	F-E
	Lesopark-11	5120	**10240**	10240	1280	E-S
	256	10240	2560	**10240**	5120	W
	KFD	640	640	640	**5120**	KFD
TBEV "group 886" strains	740-84	**10240**	**10240**	2560	1280	F-E, E-S
	711-84	**5120**	**5120**	2560	1280	F-E, E-S
	886-84	**5120**	**10240**	2560	1280	E-S, F-E

Comments: reversed antibody titers are presented in the table; the significant values of neutralization marked with bold (the significant titers were corresponded to neutralization values of prototype strain with the same sera in homologous system). KFD – prototype strain of Kyasanur Forest disease virus. W – TBEV Western antigenic variant; E-S – East-Siberian; F-E – Far Eastern.

Table 7. TBEV "group 886" strains neutralization reaction test with antisera against prototype TBEV strains and viruses of tick-borne encephalitis virus complex.

http://dx.doi.org/10.5772/54087

Thermostability is one of the most important genetic features to which the attention should be paid during the selection of TBEV strains for inactivated vaccines production. The results of inactivation index determination for 13 TBEV "group 886" strains at temperature 50°C (T^{50}) are shown in Table 8.

Strain	Isolaion source	$lgTCD_{50}$/ml at 37°C	$lgTCD_{50}$/ml at 50°C	Difference 37-50°C	T^{50}
636-90	*I. persulcatus*	4,78	3,0	1,78	+
606-90	*I. persulcatus*	4,0	2,23	1,77	+
691-90	*I. persulcatus*	4,84	3,43	1,41	+
418-90	*I. persulcatus*	4,0	2,22	1,78	+
886-84	*Myodes rutilus*	7,08	6,9	0,18	+
711-84	*Myodes rufocanus*	8,26	7,07	1,2	+
712-89	*I. persulcatus*	4,0	2,23	1,77	+
733-90	*I. persulcatus*	4,25	2,5	1,75	+
742-90	*I. persulcatus*	3,5	2,23	1,27	+
608-90	*I. persulcatus*	4,5	2,0	2,5	±
287-83	*I. persulcatus*	5,33	2,5	2,83	±
740-84	*Myodes rufocanus*	7,18	4,78	2,4	±
617-90	*I. persulcatus*	8,0	3,67	4,33	-

Table 8. The results of thermal resistance determination for TBEV "group 886" strains.

The values of $lgTCD_{50}$/ml at 37ºC varied from 3.5 to 8.26. According to the thermoresistanse feature all tested strains were divided into three group: thermostable (T^{50+}) - nine strains; thermolabile (T^{50-}) – one strain; strains with medium thermoresistance – three strains. It should be noted that all strains isolated from *I. persulcatus* ticks collected in Krasnochikoiskiy district of Transbaikalia were thermostable.

The genetic features linked with intracellular TBEV proliferation are the cytopathic activity, plaque size and type in cells culture under agar layer (S-feature) and ability to proliferate at different temperatures (rct- or ts- feature).

All "group 886" strains caused the destruction of infected cells monolayer on 4th-6th day. The plaque size and type in cells culture under the agar layer differed depending on certain strain. Thus, strain 740-84 formed large plaques 3.0 mm in diameter (S+), strain 886-84 formed plaques of medium size (d=2.0 mm) (S±) and strain 711-84 formed small plaques with diameter 1-1.5 mm (S-).

The most of the viruses proliferate and form mature virus particles in sensitive cells in definite temperature limits. A number of authors investigating the proliferation of TBEV strains in cell cultures at different temperatures (rct-feature) came to the conclusion that this marker could be the important phenotypical characteristics of the virus and closely connected with its virulence [13, 14].

We investigated rct_{42} genetic marker for 12 TBEV "group 886" strains. The results are presented in Table 9.

Strain	Isolaion source	$lgTCD_{50}$/ml at 37°C	$lgTCD_{50}$/ml at 42°C	Difference 37-42°C	rct_{42}
636-90	*I. persulcatus*	4,78	5,78	-1,0	+
608-90	*I. persulcatus*	4,5	4,78	-0,28	+
606-90	*I. persulcatus*	4,0	6,83	-2,83	+
691-90	*I. persulcatus*	4,84	5,25	-0,41	+
418-90	*I. persulcatus*	4,0	3,0	1,0	+
740-84	*Myodes rufocanus*	7,18	6,95	0,23	+
712-89	*I. persulcatus*	4,0	2,23	1,77	+
733-90	*I. persulcatus*	4,25	5,57	- 1,32	+
742-90	*I. persulcatus*	3,5	3,0	0,5	+
711-84	*Myodes rufocanus*	8,26	5,90	2,36	±
617-90	*I. persulcatus*	8,0	5,67	2,33	±
886-84	*Myodes rutilus*	7,08	3,3	3,78	-

Table 9. Rct_{42} genetic marker for TBEV "group 886" strains.

"Group 886" strains demonstrated the high heterogeneity in proliferation ability at 42°C. Five strains propagated more effectively at supraoptimal temperature (42º). Moreover, eight of nine strains isolated from ticks had $rct_{42\pm}$ feature. The strains isolated from rodents were more heterogenic: strain 740-84 had rct_{42+} feature, strain 886-84 had rct_{42-} feature and strain 711-84 had $rct_{42\pm}$ feature. All TBEV "group 886" strains isolated from ticks collected in Krasnochikoiskiy district of Transbaikalia actively propagate at 42ºC.

4. Conclusions

1. The new data concerning original TBE virus variant circulating on the territory of Eastern Siberia have been obtained. We have demonstrated the unique genetic structure of

http://dx.doi.org/10.5772/54087

"group 886" strains that is the "mixture" of amino acid sequences typical for genotypes 1, 2 and 3.

2. This TBEV variant can be considered as an independent TBEV genotype 5 (high level of genetic difference compared to other genotypes – more than 12%, the existence of its own natural foci, the ecological connection with all elements of transmissive chain, the role in infectious pathology, stability and durational circulation in nature).

3. The ability to cause focal forms of tick-borne encephalitis with lethal outcome and laboratory results of virulence level evaluation testify the high pathogenic potential of TBEV "group 886" strains. During the study of the genetic markers connected with virus intracellular reproduction we have found that "group 886" strains have high adaptive ability and can easily accommodate to circulation in different biocenosises and in variety of landscape-geographical zones.

4. Some studied "group 886" strains possess the wide spectrum of antigenic properties, hemagglutination and neutralizing activity, high virulence and thermotolerance. They match the basic criteria of strains-candidates chosen for diagnostic and vaccine development.

Acknowledgements

The authors are greatly appreciated to all colleagues collected the field materials and to the staff of Natural-Foci Infection Department: E.V. Arbatskaya, I.V. Voronko, O.Z. Gorin, N.A. Gusarova, G.A. Danchinova, V.M. Kogan, S.I. Lipin, O.V. Melnikova, A.G. Trukhina. Also we acknowledge the partial financial support by Integration interdisciplinary project grant No. 135 from the Siberian Branch of the Russian Academy of Sciences.

Author details

I.V. Kozlova[1], M.M. Verkhozina[2], T.V. Demina[3], Yu.P. Dzhioev[1], S.E. Tkachev[4], L.S. Karan[5], E.K. Doroshchenko[1], O.V. Lisak[1], O.V. Suntsova[1], A.I. Paramonov[1], O.O. Fedulina[1], A.O. Revizor[3] and V.I. Zlobin[3]

1 FSSFE Scientific Centre of Family Health and Human Reproduction Problems SB RAMS, Irkutsk, Russia

2 Centre for Epidemiology and Hygiene in Irkutsk region, Irkutsk, Russia

3 Irkutsk State Medical University of Russian Ministry of Heath, Irkutsk, Russia

4 Institute of Chemical Biology and Fundamental Medicine SB RAS, Novosibirsk, Russia

5 Central Research Institute of Epidemiology of Rospotrebnadzor RF, Moscow, Russia

References

[1] Andaev, E.I., Sidorova, E.A., Borisova, T.I. et al. (2011). Tick-borne encephalitis in the Trans-Baikal region, and molecular-biological characteristics of the pathogen // "National priorities of Russia" (special issue). №2 (5), pp. 148-150 (Russian).

[2] Bochkova, N.G., Zhezmer, V.Y., Trukhina, A.G. et al. (1985) The study of Aina/1448 serotype of tick-borne encephalitis virus //Vopr. Virusol. № 5. pp. 572-575 (Russian).

[3] Vereta, L.A., Vorobyova, M.S. (1990). Natural heterogeneity and the purposeful selection of strains of tick-borne encephalitis virus. - M.: Medicine - 124 p. (Russian).

[4] Verkhozina, M.M. (2000). Molecular epidemiology and genetic characteristics of the regional population of tick-borne encephalitis virus in Eastern Siberia: PhD thesis. – Irkutsk. - 163 p. (Russian).

[5] Gorin, O.Z., Mungalova, N.P., Leonov, V.A. et al. (1992). The situation on tick-borne encephalitis in the west of the Chita region. In.: etiology, epidemiology and diagnosis of infectious diseases in East Siberia: comp. scientific works for the IEM RAMS 80th anniversary. - Irkutsk, pp. 44-53 (Russian).

[6] Demina, T.V., Dzioev, Yu.P., Verkhozina, M.M., Kozlova, I.V., Tkachev, S.E., Doroshchenko, E.K., Lisak, O.V., Zlobin, V.I. (2009). Genetic variability and genotyping of tick-borne encephalitis virus with desoxyoligonucleotide probes. Vopr. Virusol. №3. pp. 33-42 (Russian).

[7] Demina, T.V., Dzhioev, Yu.P., Kozlova, I.V. et al. (2012). Genotypes 4 and 5 of tick-borne encephalitis virus: structural features of genomes and a possible scenario for their formation. Vopr. Virusol. № 4. V. 57. P. 13-19 (Russian).

[8] Zlobin, V.I., Demina, T.V., Mamaev, L.V. et al. (2001). Analysis of genetic variability of TBEV strains on the primary structure of a cover protein's gene fragment. Vopr. Virusol. №1. pp. 12-16 (Russian).

[9] Zlobin, V.I., Demina, T.V., Belikov, S.I. et al. (2001). Genetic typing of TBEV strains in terms of homology analysis of an envelope protein's gene fragment. Vopr. Virusol. №1. pp. 17-22 (Russian).

[10] Zlobin, V.I,. Belikov, S.I., Dzioev, Yu.P. et al. (2003). Molecular epidemiology of tick-borne encephalitis. - Irkutsk: RRC ESSC SB RAMS, 2003. - 271 p. (Russian).

[11] Karan, LS, Malenko, G.V., Bochkova, N.G. et al. (2007). The use of molecular genetic techniques to study the structure of tick-borne encephalitis virus strains. Bull. RAMS. №4. pp. 34-40 (Russian).

[12] Clark, D. (1964). Further studies of antigenic relationships between group B arboviruses. Bull. WHO. T. 31. №1. pp. 50-67.

[13] Levkovich, E.N., Karpovich, L.G., Loginova, N.V. (1964). The study of tick-borne encephalitis virus strains grown in tissue culture at different temperatures // In.: Tick-

borne encephalitis, Kemerovo tick fever, hemorrhagic fever and other arboviral infections. - M., pp. 52-54 (Russian).

[14] Libikova, E., Stanchek, D. (1965). Characterization of three different variants of the same strain of tick-borne encephalitis // Acta Virol. V. 9. pp. 481-487 (Russian).

[15] Lochov, M.G., Blinnikova, I.A. (1986). To structural and functional characterization of foci of tick-borne encephalitis in the Bichursky area of Buryat Autonomous Republic. In.: Nidal infections in Eastern Siberia: comp. scientific works - Irkutsk: Irkut. Med. Inst, pp. 44-51 (Russian).

[16] Clinical Molecular Diagnostics: method / EdC. Herrington, J McGee. - Academic Press, 1999. 558 p.

[17] Ovchinnikov, E.A., Karpovich, LG., Levkovich, E.N. (1967). The study of thermal resistance of strains of tick-borne encephalitis complex having different neurovirulence for laboratory animals. Vopr. Virusol. №5. P. 607.

[18] Pogodina, V.V., Savinov, A.P. (1964). Variation in the pathogenicity of viruses of the tick-borne encephalitis complex for different animal species. I. Experimental infection of mice and hamsters. Acta virologica. №8. pp. 424-434.

[19] Pogodina, V.V., Levina, L.S,. Karan, L.S. et al. (2009). Fatal cases of tick-borne encephalitis caused by the Siberian subtype of the pathogen in the European part of Russia and in the Urals. Med. Virology. V. XXVI. pp. 121-122 (Russian).

[20] Pogodina, V.V., Bochkova, N.G., Karan, L.S. et al. (2004). Siberian and Far Eastern subtypes of tick-borne encephalitis in the European and Asian parts of Russia: genetic and antigenic characterization of strains. Vopr. Virusol. №3. pp. 20-25.

[21] Trukhina, A.G. Features of TBE pathogen circulation in the zone of the two serotypes distribution in the Baikal region: PhD thesis. - Irkutsk, 1989. – 176 p.

[22] Shasaitov, S.S., Domaev Yu.A. On the tick-borne encephalitis in the Chita region. In.: Zonal Conf. Ministry of Health of the Russian Federation "The influence of climatic factors on the functional state of the person." - Chita, 1980. pp. 97-99.

[23] Heinz, F.X., Collet, M.S., Purcell, R.H. et al. Family Flaviviridae // Virus taxonomy: classification and nomenclature of viruses: 7 report of the International committee of taxonomy of viruses. – San Diego, 2000. pp. 1217-1225.

[24] Khasnatinov, M.A., Danchinova, G.A., Unursaikhan, U. et al. (2009). Characterizaition of tick borne encephalitis virus that caused the lethal meningoencephalitis human in Mongolia. Inter. Conference Zoonotic infections desease and tourism. – Ulaanbaatar, pp. 88-93.

[25] Pletnev, A.G., Yamshikov, V.F., Blinov, V.M. (1990). Nucleotide sequence of the genome and complete amino acid sequence of the polyprotein of tick-borne encephalitis virus. Virology. V. 174. pp. 250–263.

[26] Reed, L., Muench, H.A. (1938). A Simple Method of Estimating Fifty Per Cent End-points. Am. J. Hyg.. № 27. pp. 493-497.

[27] Rubin, S.G., Chumakov, M.P. (1980). New data on the antigenic types of tick-borne encephalitis (TBE) virus. Arboviruses in the Mediterranen Countries. – Stutgart, New York, pp. 231-236.

[28] Tamura, K, Peterson, D, Peterson, N, Stecher, G., Nei, M, and Kumar S. MEGA5: Molecular Evolutionary Genetics Analysis using Maximum Likelihood, Evolutionary Distance, and Maximum Parsimony Methods. Molecular Biology and Evolution. 2011. V. 28. №10. pp. 2731-2739.

Chapter 8

The Pathomorphology of Far Eastern Tick-Borne Encephalitis

Larisa M. Somova, Galina N. Leonova, Natalia G. Plekhova, Yurii V. Kaminsky and Anna Y. Fisenko

Additional information is available at the end of the chapter

http://dx.doi.org/10.5772/53449

1. Introduction

In the 1990s, both in the Far East and other regions of Russia, has intensified the incidence of tick-borne encephalitis (TBE), which reached the 1940-1950s, with widespread worsening of clinical signs of infection (Mamunts, 1993, Zlobin & Gorin, 1996; Leonova, 1997; Erman et al., 1999, etc.). The Far Eastern version of the tick-borne encephalitis has long been known as a heavy neuroinfection clinically flows mainly in the focal paralytic forms with residual symptoms, high mortality rate reaching 30-35%, and sometimes a progressive transition to a chronic form.

Well-known in the literature, the classical data on the pathological anatomy and pathogenesis of human tick-borne encephalitis, date back to the early period of the study of this infection on Far East in 1940 - 1950's, given the generalized idea of the nature and location of the morphological changes in the central nervous system (Robinson & Sergeeva, 1939, 1940; Kastner, 1941; Panov, 1956; Shapoval, 1961; Belman, 1960).

In 1960 - 1990-s the study of pathology of tick-borne encephalitis occurred mainly in the experimental-morphological terms, and was aimed to clarify issues of pathogenesis and immunogenesis, the study of viral neurovirulence strains, and their differentiation to find high-performance candidates for the preparation of vaccine against tick-borne encephalitis (Rozina, 1972; Frolova, 1965, 1967, 1973, 1975; Konev, 1982, 1995; Kvetkova, 1984; Erman et al., 1999, etc.).

The experience 75- years of the study showed that the tick-borne encephalitis is not monolithic and heterogeneous infection, including several subspecies: the Far-Eastern, the Siberian and other variants, which differ in the clinic, the severity and outcome of disease, as well as antigenic and genetic structure of pathogens, habitats and mechanisms of transmission (V.I. Votyakov et al., 1978; A.A. Smorodintsev, A. Dubov, 1986; V.I. Zlobin et al., 1996; M.P. Isaeva, 1998; Y.P.Dzhioev, 2000, G.N. Leonova, 2009; H. Holzmann et al., 1991; G.N. Leonova et al, 1999).

It is shown that the disease is characterized by polymorphism of clinical manifestations from inapparent to severe fever and focal forms, from the acute to progressive chronic course, from the complete recovery to the serious residual effects and death.

Characteristic features of the pathogenesis of tick-borne encephalitis are: the presence of two phases of infection - visceral and neural; hematogenous, lymphogenous, and neural pathes the generalization of infection and penetration of the pathogen in the central nervous system (CNS); the marked tropism of the virus to lymphoid tissue, an early and active involvement of the immune system in the process of reproduction of the virus and the patholigical process; the pronounced neurotropizm and the diffuse spread of the virus in the CNS. The incubation period for TBE is an average of 7-14 days.

The well-known in the literature, the classical description of the pathomorphology of acute TBE in human is mainly characterized by the stage of maximum expression of the pathological process in the CNS. The evaluation of encephalitic changes carried out in accordance with general pathological knowledge that existed in the mid-twentieth century and up until the last decade (Erman et al, 1999; Ierusalimsky, 2001) did not undergo correction in terms of immunopathogenesis.

On examination of the dead peoples they often have a strong constitution and good physical development (Shapoval, 1980). Macroscopic changes appear only hyperemia and edema of the meninges and brain substance. There are a small subarachnoid and subpial hemorrhages. The figure matter of the spinal cord is blurred, especially in the neck and shoulder level. In the anterior horns of the spinal cord revealed small foci of hemorrhage, and softening. In the internal organs is determined the congestive hyperemia and degenerative changes. The serous and mucous membranes often have pinpoint hemorrhages. The spleen is usually hyperplasive. Some of the dead people have the thinning of the cortical layer of the adrenal glands.

The histopathological picture of acute tick-borne encephalitis is characterized by diffusely distributed in the central nervous system inflammatory changes that are made up of alterative, exudative and proliferative effects. The most severe changes with necrosis and massive deposition of motor nerve cells observed in the indicator areas (Nathanson et al., 1966): in anterior horns of the cervical and thoracic spinal cord, the nucleus of the hypoglossal and the vagus nerves, the reticular formation and inferior olive of the medulla oblongata as well as its own nucleus Varoliy pons, red nucleus and substantia nigra of the brain legs and in the cortex and nuclei of cerebellum (Robinson & Sergeeva, 1940). The pathological process with necrobiosis of nerve cells is also observed in the thalamus, caudate and lenticular nuclei, and diffusely in the cerebral cortex of the brain. The degree of severity of the process decreases in the oral direction of CNS. Alterative changes in the nerve cells are combined with severe exudative phenomena with the formation of perivascular infiltrates consisting of lymphocytes, monocytes, plasma cells, histiocytes, as well as with diffuse proliferative glial response. As pointed out by Kestner (1941), the pathological process can be described as an acute non-purulent meningo-polioencephalomyelitis involving all sections of the central and peripheral nervous system. Pathological changes are found in sensory and vegetative nodes, as well as in peripheral nerves (Semenov-Tien Shansky & Shapoval, 1949; Dekonenko et al., 1994).

In the pia mater and vascular plexuses of brain ventricles observed redness, swelling, and stratificatione, perivascular infiltrates of lymphocytes and histiocytes, to a lesser extent – leukocytes and plasma cells. Revealed the destruction and proliferation of ependyma cells of the ventricles, subependimar glia cells, as well as the central gray matter of the Sylvius aqueduct.

The permanent feature of TBE pathomorphology are the vasomotor disturbances. There has been a dramatic expansion and vascular hyperemia until capillary stasis, diapedetic hemorrhages, coagulation thrombi, sometimes fibrinoid necrosis of vessel walls.

Nerve cells in the affected area are in a state of acute swelling, vacuolization, the perinuclear or the total chromatolysis, kariocytolisis, cytolisis elting, neuronophagia. It is characteristic of the TBE the piknomorfic (hyperchromic) changes of nerve cells.

The destructive changes occur in hematogenous cells of inflammatory infiltrates and in proliferating glial cells with the expressed klasmatodendrosis. In the subsequent formation of multiple foci of softening, localized in the varoliav pons, medulla oblongata, bain legs, hypothalamic area, basal ganglia and spinal cord. The deep destructive changes also occur in the vascular wall and in the white matter of the brain with signs of myelin and axons disintegration.

The most mobile part of the pathological process are inflammatory changes that already in the acute stage are not always identical. In most cases, there is an abundant infiltration of vessels wall, perivascular infiltration of lymphocytes and histiocytes with an admixture of polymorphonuclear leukocytes and a small amount of plasma cells. With the prolongation of infection the infiltration of lymphocytes and plasma cells increases, the massive perivascular infiltrates as a muffs appeared.

There is the focal and diffuse proliferation of microglia, astrocytes and oligodendroglia (Shapoval, 1961; Zlotnik, 1968; Zlotnik et al., 1976). There are formed numerous glial nodules, granulomas in place the dead nerve cells and around capillaries.

Thus, the preferential injury of Varoliy pons, medulla oblongata nuclei and the motor neurons of the anterior horn of the cervical spinal cord is the main feature of the topography of the histo-pathological changes typical for TBE.

Sometimes the inflammation in the brain at TBE passes in atypical with little or no productive and exudative changes. The perivascular infiltration is isinsignificant, the inflammatory response is expressed in the form of microglial nodules. In these cases, you should emphasize the discrepancy between the severity of the clinical course and low severity of inflammation in the presence of the intensive dystrophic and destructive changes in neurons (Robinson & Sergeeva, 1939; Kastner, 1941; Belman, 1960; Somova, 2010). In the early occurrence of deep disturbances of consciousness (coma) in the cerebral cortex and other parts of the brain observed the common hyperchromatosis of neurons with a peculiar dark staining and wrinkling their (Shapoval, 1980).

The lack of etiotropic treatment of TBE dictated the need to further develop the issues on pathogenesis and morphogenesis of infection with the calculation of the especial feature of regional TBE strains, in order to support more efficient methods of pathogenetic therapy.

In the 1980-1990-s there is evidence of the involvement of lymphoid organs (thymus, spleen, lymph nodes) in the TBE virus reproduction, which greatly complement the information on the pathogenesis of acute and chronic processes during this infection (Pogodina et al., 1986; Rychkov et al., 1989, 1990; Karmysheva & Pogodina, 1990, 1991; Leonova &. Isachkova, 1995; Malkova & Frankova, 1959; Malkova & Smetana, 1966; Kopecky, 1987).

Using highly specific method of molecular hybridization of nucleic acids in cryostat sections of lymph nodes, spleen and brain of experimental animals (Zinoviev et al., 1990; Konev et al., 1991; Rychkov, 1992) it is found that on acute and chronic TBE is resettlement and virus replication in cells of the sinuses and T-dependent areas of lymphoid organs at the same time with the development of these reactions, reflecting the formation of an immune response. In the dynamics of the incubation period the TBE virus is accumulated in the lymphoid organs, especially the regional to the site of infection lymph nodes, and subsequently recorded in the area of vascular lesions of the brain, where the beginning of clinical manifestations of the disease the virus is detected by IFA and electron microscopy.

It is determined that the damage of the lymphoid organs with subsequent development of the immune deficiency leads to the development of inflammation in the brain with a quick invasion of his virus, and the degree of damage of lymphoid organs is an important criterion for prediction of viral infection (Konev, 1994, 1995). According to the author, in an experiment on animals the dependence of TBE morphogenesis and relationships in the "brain - lymphoid organs" from the degree of susceptibility of the host to the virus, the causative agent, take a place. In a susceptible animal the necrotic reaction develops in the lymphoid organs with subsequent formation of encephalitis in the background of secondary immunodeficiency, and in insensitive animal the damage of lymphoid organs and, accordingly, the immunodeficiency are absent, and encephalomyelitis does not develop.

Karmysheva and Pogodina (1991) in experiments on hamsters received the evidence about the active involvement of the thymus in the infectious process in the tick-borne encephalitis, with nature and extent of lesions of the thymus is heavier under the introduction of highly virulent strains than for infection caused fainly virulent strains. Immunological methods is shown that a severe course of TBE is associated with the expressive delay hypersensitivity (DH) under a weak antibody production, and asymptomatic infection – with a weak sensitization, an early and strong reaction of antibody-forming cells and increased nonspecific resistance (Perehodova et al., 1976; Pogodina et al., 1984). A more favorable prognosis when infected by fainly virulent strains, apparently, to a large extent dependent on the less affected of immune system organs and the development in these proliferative processes. A number of authors (Spindles, 1969; Vargin & Semenov, 1980; Konev, 1982; Alexandrov & Kislitsyna, 1982; Kvetkova & Shmatko, 1983; Webb & Smith, 1966) suggest that the failure of the immune system is an important factor in the pathogenesis of TBE.

For tick-borne encephalitis has been shown experimentally that the virus from the primary foci of multiplication in the skin and subcutaneous fat is distributed in the body with lymphogenous and hematogenous routes (Pogodina et al., 1986; Albrecht, 1968). The penetration of the virus in the brain associated with overcoming the blood-brain barrier through the wall of blood capillaries located in the parenchyma of the nervous tissue. This barrier is a complex system of defense mechanisms, including vascular plexus, the meninges, the wall of blood vessels and glial elements.

Pogodina et al. (1986), summarizing data on the immunopathogenesis of the disease, indicates that the TBE holds a pronounced immune response, characterized by a deficiency of T-lymphocytes, B-lymphocyte proliferation, macrophage reaction, the appearance of antibodies in the blood and cerebrospinal fluid, cellular immune responses in brain tissue, which in general have both protective and pathologic effects.

Thus, by the early 2000s, the accumulated extensive experimental material has prepared the basis for the specification of views on the nature of the pathological process in the CNS in human tick-borne encephalitis. On the basis of modern ideas that the inflammatory response, which is realized hematogenous elements, provides a basal level of immunity, we saw fit to approach the study of the pathology of tick-borne encephalitis in terms of immunopathological nature of central nervous system damage.

The main goal of our research was focused on an integrated assessment of the nature of the pathological process in the central nervous system in tick-borne encephalitis and identification of clinical and morphological variants of the disease caused her immunopathogenetic mechanisms. An important aspect of the study, in our opinion, was the distinction, on the one hand, the primary damage to tissue-structural elements of the CNS, directly related to the cytopathic effect and intracellular reproduction of the TBE virus, on the other hand, reactive and immunopathological changes with the definition of pathogenetic importance of the last in the development of various clinical and morphological forms of encephalitis. The study was based on the autopsy material from 35 patients aged 4 to 68 years old, ill tick-borne encephalitis in different parts of the Primorye Territory in the 1990s and died in different periods from the onset.

Date of death from the disease ranged from 3 to 28 days. The duration of hospital stay ranged from 1 hour to 25 days. The incubation period from the time of tick suction on bite before the first symptoms of the disease lasted from 7 to 23 days, an average of 15 days. In 6 cases there were multiple bites of ticks, so specify the duration of the incubation period was impossible. In two cases, infection occurred in the crushing ticks with the aid of arms.

For pathohistological study samples from different parts of the central nervous system were dissected: the anterior central gyrus, stem sections at the levels of the brain legs, Varolii pons and medulla, as well as the cortex and the vermis of cerebellum, cervical spinal cord.

2. The overall clinical and anatomical characteristics of tick-borne encephalitis

For the duration of the disease, all patients were divided into four groups in which the death occurred respectively in the first, second, third and fourth week of the onset of clinical symptoms. In all cases there was an acute onset of temperature increase to high numbers 38 º - 39 º C, quickly joined the general brain symptoms as headache, nausea, vomiting, stupor, and disorders of consciousness and sometimes convulsions. In the early days of the onset of the disease appeared meningeal syndrome and focal symptoms of central nervous system involvement: paresis and paralysis of the limbs, neck, bulbar disorders, due to which almost all patients at different times transferred to a ventilator.

From the brain of all died patients was isolated tick-borne encephalitis virus, and sera were determined by specific antibodies in diagnostic titers. At autopsy, macroscopic changes in the CNS manifested by edema and vascular injection of the meninges and brain substance, sometimes point hemorrhages scattered in different parts of the brain. The boundary of gray and white matter was somewhat effaced, especially in the cervical spinal cord and parts of the brain stem. There were congestion and degenerative changes in parenchymal organs (heart, kidney, liver), hyperemia of spleen. According to our observations, pathoanatomical diagnosis of tick-borne encephalitis should continue to be based on microscopic examination of brain and spinal cord. At the same time the crucial importance to the diagnosis has an analysis of pathological changes in the so-called indicator areas of the brain.

3. Morphogenesis of changes in the central nervous system

In the study of morphogenesis of tick-borne encephalitis in humans the main attention was paid to the sequence of the individual components of the inflammatory process, an assessment of their importance in the formation of various clinical manifestations of disease. In the first week of the disease (*the first group* - 5 cases) all deaths revealed an acute microvascular response in the central nervous system - congestion of vessels up to the capillaries, stasis, endothelial vacuolation. There were plasma soaking, stratification and focal fibrinoid necrosis of vessel walls. Frequently observed diapedetic hemorrhages, pronounced the virhov expansion space around the vessels due to edema (Fig. 1a).

In the pia mater were observed the stratification, the mucoid and fibrinoid swelling, the proliferation arahnoidendoteliya places, some parts of it were infiltrated with lymphocytes and histiocytes, to a lesser extent, erythrocytes and polimorphonuclear leukocytes. In the matter of the brain and spinal cord were determined the severe dystrophic and destructive changes of neurons - perinuclear and diffuse chromatolysis, in the part of neurons - the ectopic nucleus and kariolizis with the formation of cell-shading. There were also hyperchromatic cells. Alterative changes in the increasingly covered the neurons of the indicator brain areas: pyramidal cells of the motor cortex, nuclei of the substantia nigra, red and vestibular nuclei, inferior olive, nuclei of the caudal cranial nerves, cortex and nuclei of cerebellum, the anterior horn of the spinal cord, mainly in the cervical region (Fig. 1b, d). In the cerebellar cortex is constantly met the degeneration and loss of Purkinje cells. At the nucleus of Semmering black substance the part of neurons was reduced the content of the pigment melanin.

The attention is drawn to the distinct focal reaction of microglia and oligodendroglia with neuronophagia and the formation of glial nodules on the site of dead nerve cells. In areas of inflammation was observed a significant admixture of polymorphonuclear leukocytes. There was also a diffuse infiltration of the brain substance by lymphocytes, polymorphonuclear leukocytes and glial cells. In the white matter of the brain and spinal cord was detected fragmentation of nerve fibers, were seen clusters of large, basophilic-stained cells. The inflammation around blood vessels of the brain substance were not common, however, in some places were found loose histiocytic and lymphocytic perivascular infiltrates, in which there was an admixture of neutrophils (Fig. 1 c).

In general, the pathological process in the CNS of patients with the first group can be characterized as meningo-polioencephalomielitis with a predominance of exudative phenomena and alterative changes in the nerve cells. The severe damage to the wall of blood vessels, edematous hemorrhagic component of inflammation with exudation of polymorphonuclear leukocytes showed marked sensitization of the organism in response to the introduction of the virus in the CNS with the presence of morphological reactions of immediate hypersensitivity (IH).

The second group of deaths was the most numerous (17 cases) and was 48.5% of cases. All died patients in the second week of the disease were observed in the brain the pronounced breach of hemocirclulation: eritrostasis, the presence of fibrin in the lumen of blood vessels, the expressive swelling of the brain tissue of spongy type. Vascular endothelium was in a state of proliferation, there was damage to the endothelial layer, porosity of the wall of blood vessels, often identified microhemorragii in different parts of the brain (Fig. 2 a). The elastic membrane of blood vessels had the irregular thickness, stratification, and sometimes not detected. There were the mucoid and fibrinoid swelling, the fibrinoid necrosis and aneurysmal expansion of vessels wall.

In the meninges, in addition to plethora, revealed swelling, stratification, proliferation of arahnoidendotelium, loose perivascular infiltrates of lymphocytes, histiocytes, with a small admixture of plasma cells.

In the vascular plexus of the brain ventricles were observed the rough swelling of the villi, the plethora and the homogenization of capillary wall, the degeneration, and in some places proliferation of the epithelium lining the villi. Ependyma cells were able to hyperplasia with areas of proliferation.

As in the previous period, the neuronal pathology was significantly expressed at different stages of damage. There were the diffuse chromatolysis, cell death and neuronophagia, focal loss of neurons with microglial reaction in these areas (Fig. 2b). Processes of nerve cells are often not reviewed, observed their destruction - klazmatodendrosis. Often hyperchromic cells were seen.

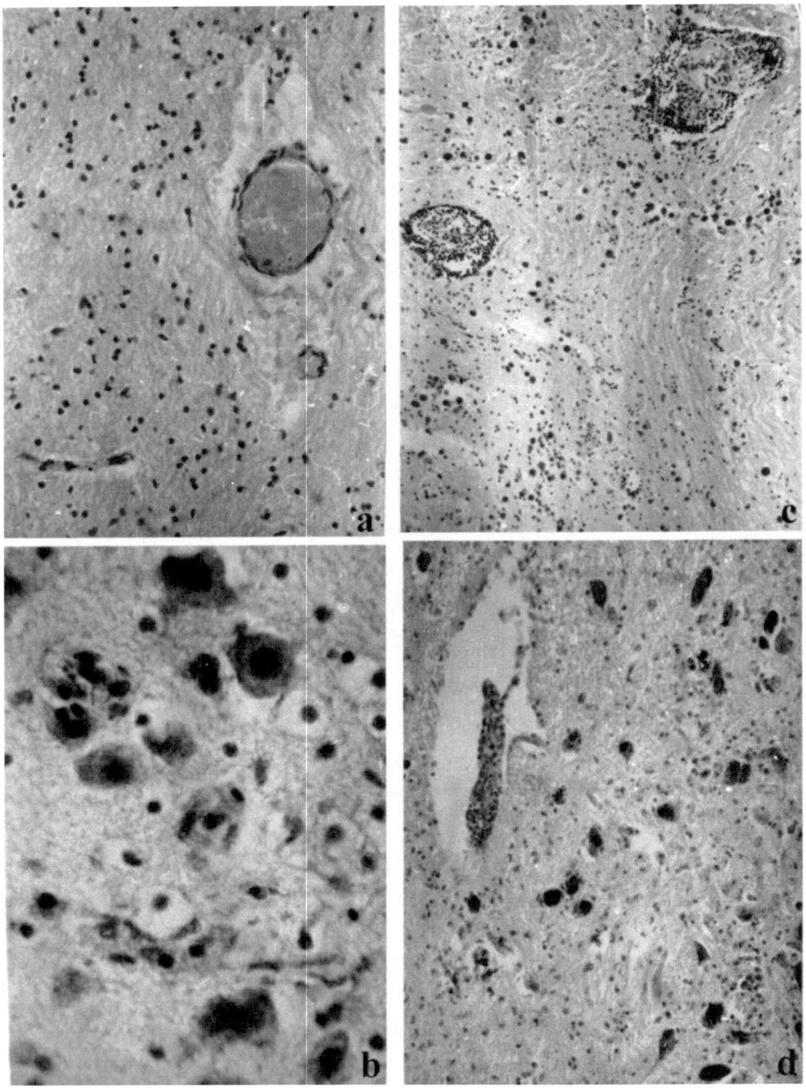

Figure 1. Pathological changes in the human brain with tick-borne encephalitis, 1st week of illness. a - hyperemia of blood vessels, diapedetic hemorrhage, intensive perivascular edema, diffuse glial reaction in the subcortical regions, x 100, b - alterative changes of neurons in the nucleus of the pons: chromatolysis, ectopia, hyperhromatosis, kariolisis, nodular glial reaction, x 200; c - plethora of vessels, leukocytosis and loose perivascular infiltration, accumulation of basophilic cells in the subcortical region, x 80, d - dystrophic changes in neurons of the black substance in the midbrain, small glial nodules, vasculitis, a dramatic expansion of perivascular spaces, x 125. Stained with hematoxylin and eosin (a, c, d) and cresyl violet by Nissl (b).

The most severe damage of neurons were located in the III-V layers of the cortex of the anterior central gyrus, brain legs, Varolii pons and medulla oblongata, and especially significant - in the anterior horns of the cervical spinal cord (Fig. 2 b, d). In the pathological process are constantly involved neurons of red nuclei, substantia nigra, vestibular nuclei, nuclei of the bulbar cranial nerves and the cerebellar vermis. In the cerebellum, in all cases revealed common areas of loss of Purkinje cells, swelling and lysis of surviving ganglion cells, focal thinning of the granular layer cells (Fig. 2 c). In the field of loss of Purkinje cells was observed the expressive proliferation of Bergman glia in the spread of the molecular layer. Nerve fibers of the white matter of the brain and spinal cord were able to disorganization, fragmentation, and in some places granular disintegration.

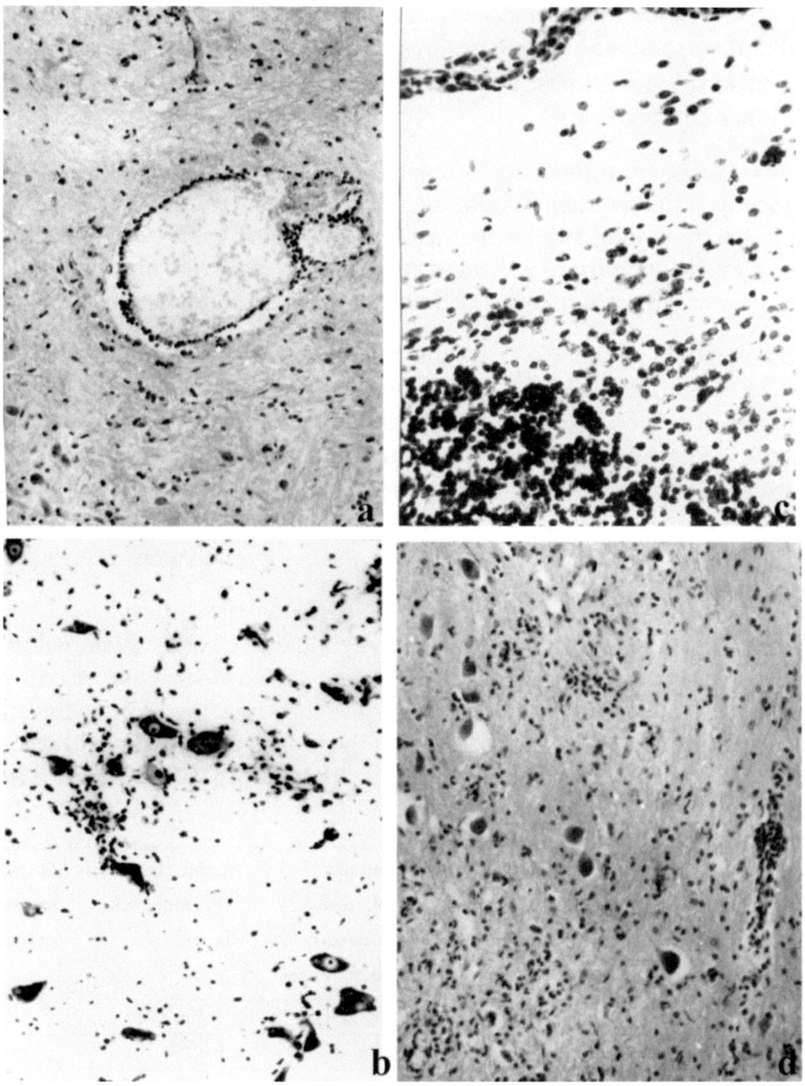

Figure 2. Pathological changes in the brain of human with tick-borne encephalitis, 2nd week of illness. a-porosity of the vascular wall, eritrodiapedesis, damage to neurons in the type of lysis in the medulla, x 125, b - diffuse chromatolysis and loss of neurons, kariolisis, neuronophagia, x 200; c - loss of Purkinje cells in the ganglionic layer of cerebellar cortex, the proliferation of Bergman glia, inflammatory infiltration of the pia mater, x 200; d - heavy damage and loss of neurons in the medulla, diffuse and nodular glial reaction, productive vasculitis, x 125. Stained with hematoxylin and eosin (a, d) and by Nissl (b, c).

Inflammatory - infiltrative changes in the second week of the disease were different in intensity at different dead patients. In 23.5% of cases the marked perivascular infiltration mainly by lymphocytes and histiocytes with an admixture of plasma cells were detected. The response of polymorphonuclear leukocytes in this period was negligible. Perivascular infiltrates were located in the meninges, and very often in the gray matter of the brain in the indicator areas. In the vessels the leukocytosis was observed, met perivascular "muffs."

Thus, in the second week of tick-borne encephalitis in the pathological picture in the background of alterative-proliferative changes in some of the dead patients, compared with the first group, detected the increased infiltrative reaction with the predominance of mononuclear cells in inflammatory foci.

In the next two weeks from the start of tick-borne encephalitis died 37.2% of patients.The pathological study of the central nervous system revealed that during this period changed the ratio of expression of various components of the inflammatory process. This is manifested by the increased intensity of infiltrative changes around the vessel in the meninges, and especially in the brain matter with a predominance of them in the indicator areas of the CNS.

In the third group of died patients (4 cases) the moderate hemo- and moderate liquorodynamic disorders were determined. In the brain, the stasis, sludge, diapedetic hemorrhages were found. In the lumen of blood vessels fibrinopurulent leukocyte thrombi often revealed. Perivascular spaces were greatly widened, areas by dilution (lysis) of the brain substance near the vessels were determined. On the background of the diffuse glial proliferation, glial nodules were also seen on the site of dead neurons. Along with the progressive (hyperplasia) changes in glial cells, the regressive (dystrophic-destructive) changes are found related to microglia and astrocytes.

For the objectification of the expression of alterative component of the inflammatory process in the dynamics of tick-borne encephalitis, the calculation of glial index was carried out, ie ratio of total number of glial cells to the number of neurons in the same area of brain tissue. It is established that the destruction and loss of neurons in the most damaged structural formations of the central nervous system were accompanied by an increase of glial index (Table 1).

The term bark disease	**Anterior central gyrus**	**Midbrain (substantia nigra nucleus)**	**Medulla oblongata (nucleus of the vagus nerve)**	**Cerebellum (Purkinje cell layer)**	**Spinal cord (anterior horn motor neurons)**
Control	7.26±0.06	2.82±0.03	2.67±0.04	3.45±0.06	3.12±0.04
The first week	8.15±0.04*	3.15±0.04*	5.13±0.03*	6.38±0.05*	7.26±0.04*
The second week	9.36±0.04*	3.85±0.03*	6.26±0.03*	10.26±0.04*	11.15±0.02*
The third week	10.28±0.06*	4.05±0.02*	6.36±0.03*	10.87±0.06*	12.05±0.03*
The fourth week	10.15±0.03*	4.17±0.04*	6.27±0.05*	11.25±0.04*	12.54±0.05*

Note: * - P <0.05 compared with control

Table 1. The glial index in the indicator areas of the brain at different times of acute tick-borne encephalitis (M ± m)

http://dx.doi.org/10.5772/53449

As the table shows, the significant increase in glial index occurred in the first - the second week of illness, and further significant change in performance was not found. This indicates that from the third week of tick-borne encephalitis is not going the increase in severity of alterative component of the inflammatory process, with the deepening of neuronal damage in the indicator areas of the central nervous system.

In the third group of died patients the mesenchymal inflammatory reaction around the blood vessels was greater than in the previous period, with the significant ($p < 0.05$) increase in the number and density of perivascular infiltrates (Table 2).

The evidence of inflammation intensity	Ratios of inflammation per unit area (M ± m)			
	The first week	The second week	The third week	The fourth week
The number of perivascular infiltrates (in sight)	1.8±0.01	2.8±0.01	4.6±0.02	4.8±0.02
The density of perivascular infiltrates (mm^2)	6.7±2.1	12.2±4.3	18.7±5.4	19.1±6.1

Table 2. The intensity of infiltrative changes in the brain at different times of acute tick-borne encephalitis

The perivascular infiltration with the formation of "muffs", consisting of mononuclear cells, was detected in various parts of the brain, the gray matter of spinal cord, mainly in the anterior horns of the cervical spine and a moderate degree in some areas of the meninges (Fig. 3 a, b). By the third week of the disease, compared with the initial period, in the inflammatory infiltrates the percentage of lymphocytes and plasma cells significantly increased. Using the method of fluorescent antibody (IFA), the specific emission of immunoglobulins is detected in the inflammatory infiltrates, which is consistent with the reaction of plasmocytes. For histochemical study in the foci of inflammatory cells, giving a positive reaction for acid phosphatase and α-naftilatsetatesterase, were observed, indicating that they belong to the T-lymphocytes (Fig. 3 c, d).

The attention is drawn to the expressive damage of blood vessels wall: thinning, vacuolization, blurring the structures of the vascular wall, breaking-stost endothelium, the deformation of the vessels lumen with the formation of aneurysmal extension, damage to elastic fibers. It should be noted that the penetration of cells of perivascular infiltrates into the surrounding brain tissue observed in the initial stages of the disease (first - second weeks), was limited in the third week of increasing the density of infiltrates, suggesting a decrease in diffuse lesions of the brain during the development of local (tissue) immune.

Thus, in dead patients on the third week of tick-borne encephalitis in the histopathological picture of the central nervous system the perivascular infiltrative changes were predominant, characterizing immunopathological process with expressive cell reactions of the immediate hypersensitivity type.

In the group who died on *the fourth week* of tick-borne encephalitis on *in the fourth group* of died patients (9 cases) revealed the pathological picture in general analogous to that in the third group. All patients of the fourth group in a long time (25 days) were unconscious, with severe focal disorders of the central nervous system, disorders of vital functions and connection to a ventilator.

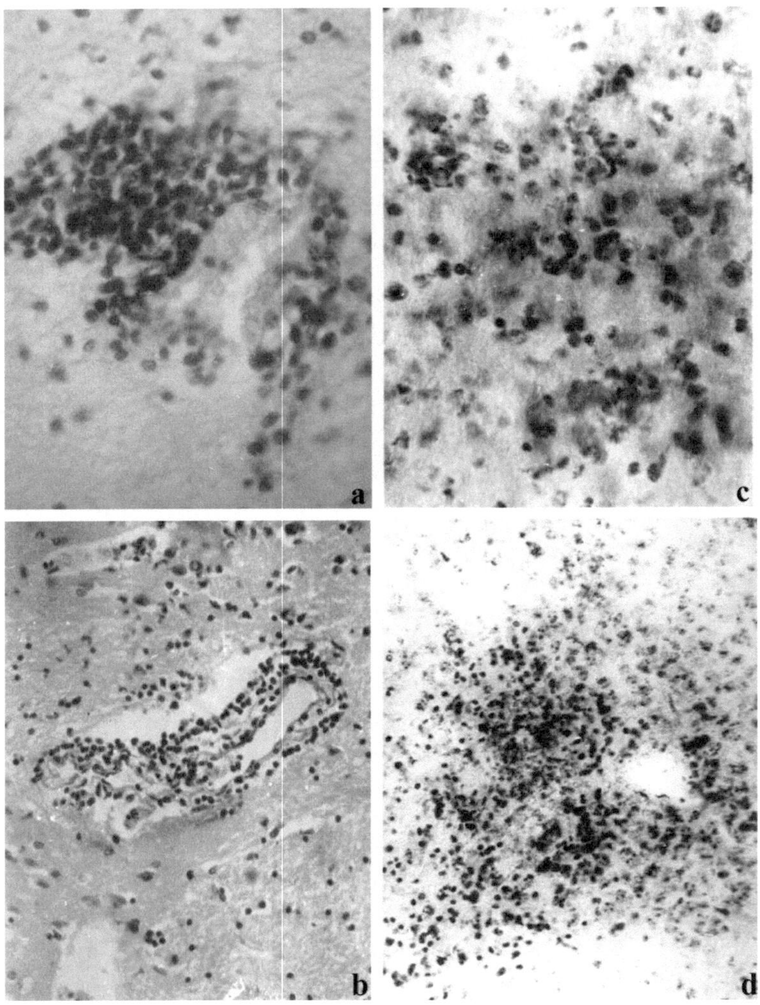

Figure 3. Pathological changes in the brain of human with tick-borne encephalitis. 3-d week of illness. a – destructive-productive vasculitis with the formation of perivascular "muff" in the pons, x 400, b - the venule with thinned wall and deformation of lumen, perivascular infiltration of lymphocytes, hystiosytes and plasma cells in the caudal brain stem, x 200; Stained with hematoxylin and eosin (a, b); a positive reaction to acid phosphatase in the cells of the perivascular infiltrate by Gomori (c), × 200, d-α-naftilatsetatesterase in cells of the inflammatory foci, the color by Pigarevsky - Zeltser, x 400.

In the indicator areas of the brain, in areas with destructive changes of nerve cells, the focal proliferation of microglial, oligodendroglial and astrocytic cells was observed with the formation of large glial nodes (Fig. 4 a). The surviving neurons were generally able to diffuse chromatolysis with the conversion of some of them in a cell-shade. In the cerebellar cortex of all the dead patients the total and subtotal loss of Purkinje cells, the focal thinning of the granular layer cells were discovered (Fig. 4 c). In the anterior horns of the cervical spinal cord single hyperchromic neurons were retained. In the brain stem marked neuronal lipofuscinosis of large neurons were observed.

There were the abrupt disruption of the gray and white matter of the brain through the spongy edema, widespread dystrophic and destructive changes of vessels with thinning and loosening of theirs wall, the mucoid and fibrinoid swelling, vacuolation of it. The lumen of many vessels contained fibrin threads, a few blood cells, in small vessels - hyaline thrombi. In some vessels were found clusters of white blood cells, in which there was a distinct part of the fragmentation of the nucleus with the location of its fragments on the periphery of the cytoplasm, which was similar to apoptosis (Fig. 4 b). Quite often diapedetic hemorrhages met around the vessels.

The expression of the infiltrative component of inflammation in the brain varied in different cases and manifested in the presence of vasculitis, and perivascular infiltrates, and in some cases the formation of "muffs" (Fig. 4). Inflammatory infiltrates composed of lymphocytes, histiocytes and plasma cells, they were detected histochemically cells with positive reaction to acid phosphatase (T-lymphocytes).

In general, in the fourth group of died patients, compared with the third group, the significant increase of the severity of infiltrative and proliferative changes in the brain and spinal cord, as well as significant changes in the percentage of cells of inflammatory infiltrates were not observed.

Thus, in died pations in the fourth week of tick-borne encephalitis the pathological process in the central nervous system should be characterized as meningoencephalomielitis, which clearly expressed alterative component of inflammation with widespread heavy damage and loss of nerve cells in the indicator areas of the brain, as well as the effects of spongiosis and focal gliosis of cerebral matter with the increase in morphological manifestations of immunodeficiency. In our observations, the absence of the clear increase of the severity of inflammation in the CNS of died patients in the later stages of the disease may be associated with significant virus-induced suppression of the immune system and profound disturbances of metabolic processes in the body.

Summary of results of morphological studies our observed fatal encephalitis cases in humans gives an idea of the features of the morphogenesis of the Far Eastern varient of this neuroinfection flowing with focal lesions of the nervous system, as well as to determine the value of the main components of the inflammatory process at different stages of the disease. The obtained data showed that the focal forms of tick-borne encephalitis in the initiation stage the leading importance belongs to the primary damage of the structures of the blood-brain barrier and neurons of the brain and spinal cord. There is the rapid development of

CNS pathology, morphological manifestations of which indicate the nature of hyperergic inflammation. A change in the morphogenesis of the CNS in tick-borne encephalitis reflects the basic laws of development of the inflammation in the immune basis with the presence of tissue-specific features of its various components.

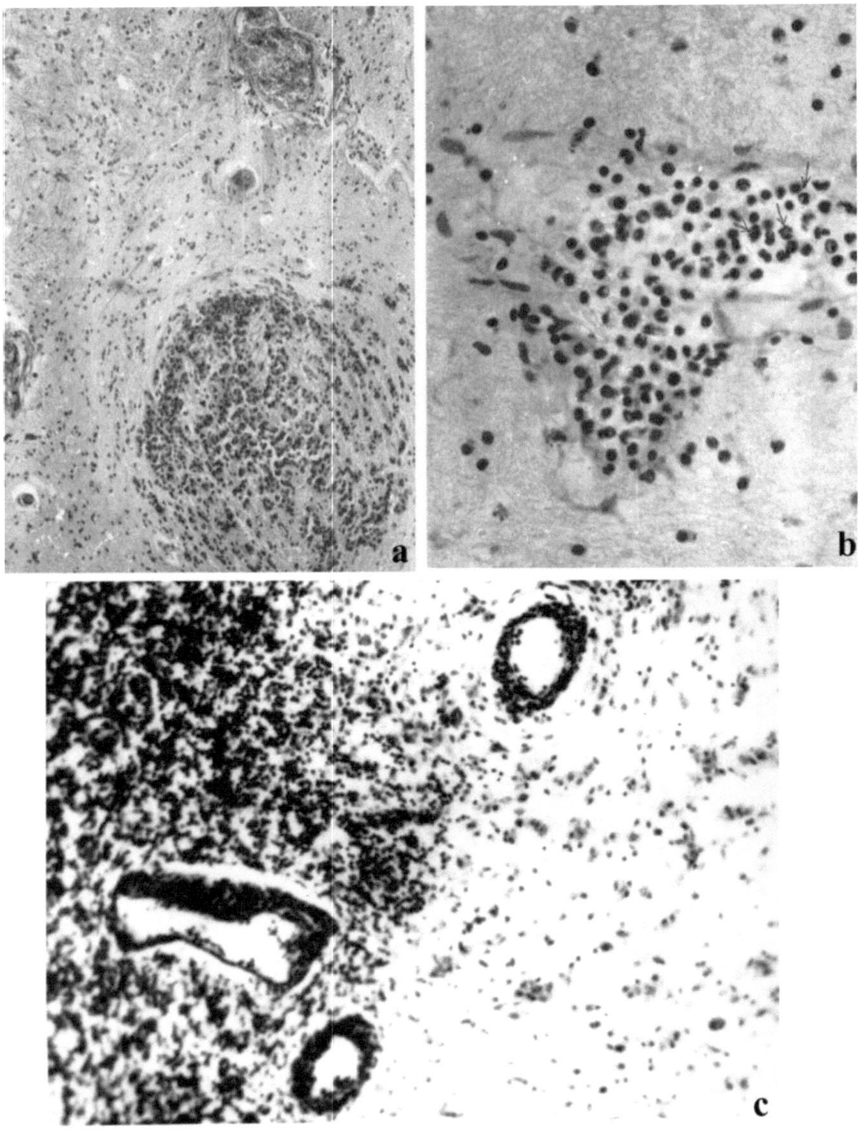

Figure 4. Pathological changes in the brain of human with tick-borne encephalitis. 4th week of illness. a - a major inflammatory infiltrate around the central canal in the spinal cord, to the right - a vessel with the wall stratification and eritrostasis, x 80, b - a destructive vasculitis, fibrin and leucocytes in the lumen of the vessel, fragments of the nucleus in some cells (arrows), x 320; c - numerous perivaskular "muffs", pronounced glial reaction in the area adjacent to the cerebellar cortex, x 100. Stained with hematoxylin and eosin (a,b) and by Nissl (c).

http://dx.doi.org/10.5772/53449

Thus, the histopathological study of material taken from patients who died during the first, second, third and fourth weeks of the first clinical manifestation of symptoms, possible to trace the morphogenesis of tick-borne encephalitis, and select the individual components of the pathological process. The feature of the pathological process in the first week of the disease is the low intensity of inflammatory changes around the vessels of the meninges and matter brain in the presence of infiltrates of neutrophils, lymphocytes and histiocytes.

The profound degenerative changes of the brain vascular lesions with accumulation of mucopolysaccharides, as well as neurons in conjunction with the exudation of polymorphonuclear leukocytes into the brain, on the background to identify with the IAF-specific antigen in the brain cells, suggest that these changes are due to a direct damaging effect of tick-borne encephalitis virus, over-coming the blood-brain barrier in the pathogenesis of neural phase of infection.

In addition, the proof of this fact is the data on the distribution of viral RNA in the brain and blood cells of died patients, as well as white mice infected subcutaneously with a prototype Sofjin strain of TBE virus (Demenev et al., 1990; Konev et al., 1990; Konev, 1996). Using a highly specific method of nucleic acid hybridization in situ were identified by the authors RFID viral RNA during the first week of the disease over the cytoplasm of morphologically intact and exposed to destruction of neurons, over the endothelial cells of capillaries and choroid plexus. Polischuk (1999) in experiments on white mice found that the RFID virus RNA appear in the vascular structures of the brain and spinal cord in the incubation period from 12 to 48 hours after infection.

In addition to the direct damaging effects of tick-borne encephalitis virus in the mechanism of pathological changes in neurons and other cells of the brain, apparently, to consider the possibility of cytolytic activities of specific antibodies determined already in the early acute stage of the disease, Semenov & Gavrilov (1976) suggested that the reaction of antibodies with virus-induced antigens (autoantigens - in Kanchurin, 1964), lead to the immunolisis of cells and are one of the launchers mechanisms of inflammation in viral infections, as well as the autoimmune process. The latter is known to regard the cells of the central nervous system (Strukov et al., 1982). This is consistent with the data Nathanson & Panitch (1978), Morishima et al. (1984).

The expressed alterative and exudative components of inflammation in the first or second week of illness, in our opinion, points to the hyperergic nature of the initial changes in tick-borne encephalitis, with symptoms of immediate hypersensitivity (ITH). Such changes in the weak expression of the cellular reactions in the most severe cases of TBE previously attributed to the atypical (Robinzon & Sergeeva, 1940; Robinzon, 1975).

If we consider that in endemic foci of the Far East, people often have the multiple, repeated sucking ticks, it is logical to assume the sensitization, previous the acute symptomatic infection of tick-borne encephalitis. Here the analogy with hemorrhagic dengue fever are reviewed (Halstead, 1973; Russell et al., 1969; Barnes & Rosen, 1974), in which the immunopathological mechanism of acute vascular reaction was determined, occurring in response to the release of histamine from cells under the influence of excessive amounts of specific immune complexes in the presence of C3A, C5a complement components.

Along with the deep alterative and proliferative changes, the characteristic of pathological changes found in the died patients in the second week of tick-borne encephalitis should be considered more pronounced, than in the previous period, the cellular infiltration in the pia mater, choroidal plexus and around the cerebral vessels with the appearance of perivascular "muffs". In the composition of inflammatory infiltrates dominated by lymphocytes and histiocytes with the admixture of plasma cells. Neutrophil response in this period was minimal. In the 1/3 cases histiocytic and lymphocytic infiltration was significant.

The identification in cells of the inflammatory infiltrate as a specific antigen, and antitick-borne immunoglobulins, as well as the intense reaction to ribonucleoproteins, acid phosphatase (EC) and α-naftilatsetatesterase indicate the strengthening of immunopathological component of inflammation with a predominance of delayed-type hypersensitivity (DTH).

In recent years, began to pay attention to the value of immunological reactions in the pathogenesis of viral infections, including tick-borne encephalitis (Erman et al., 1996; Konev, 1989; Kvetkova, 1984; Pogodina et al., 1984; Barnshteyn, 1989.). Based mainly on experimental data, the pathology of central nervous system was seen in the close relationship with virus-induced damage of the immune system, coming back in the visceral phase of the TBE pathogenesis (Karmysheva & Pogodina, 1991; Rychkov, 1992; Tulakina et al., 1994). In the analysis of relationships in the "brain - lymphoid organs"system was found the strong direct correlation between the vascular and inflammatory changes and the state of the T-dependent areas of lymphoid organs (Konev et al., 1991; Polischuk et al., 1990).

Our studies with human tick-borne encephalitis confirm that the infiltrative component of inflammation in the form of a perivascular "muffs", local and diffuse cellular infiltrates, consisting mainly of T-lymphocytes, histiocytes and macrophages, should be seen as manifestations of the reactions of the cell (tissue) immunity. To this phenomenon it is also concerned the neuronophagia actively carried out mainly of microgliacytes related to the macrophage system. Using the MFA we found in the brain tissue the components of specific immune complexes (antibody-containing and antigen-containing cells) are yet another confirmation of the immune basis of inflammation in tick-borne encephalitis.

It should be noted that during the first - the second week of the onset of clinical symptoms of tick-borne encephalitis died most of the patients - 22 of 35 people, representing 62.9% of cases, in spite of all the patients carried out by the intensive therapy with the mechanical ventilation. This is the indirect proof of the predominant importance of destructive changes in the structure of the pathological process with the irreversible damage to cells of the vital areas central nervous system.

On the third or fourth week of the disease in inflammatory infiltrates increased the content of acid-phosphate-positive cells, indicating that they belong to the T-lymphocytes and macrophages, and plasma (antibody-containing) cells. In the indicator areas of the brain and spinal cord revealed extensive glial foci and nodules on the site of dead nerve cells. The expression of inflammatory cellular changes differed in each case, but generally on the third

- the fourth week of the disease in the brain infiltrative and proliferative components of inflammation dominated.

Thus, the study of morphogenesis of focal forms of tick-borne encephalitis, observed in the Primorye Territory, found that the pathological process in the central nervous system is a multi-component and, in all morphological characters, from the very beginning of its development is immunopathological in nature. In this case there is a consistent deployment of cell-tissue reactions immediate and delayed types. The trigger of the encephalitic process is certainly damage to mesenchymal structures of blood-brain barrier and nerve cells caused by the direct action of tick-borne encephalitis virus in its penetration and intracellular replication in the CNS, which immediately leads to the sensitization of immunologically isolated brain tissue. The immunological basis of inflammation in the brain at the tick-borne encephalitis, and assumed Robinzon and Frolova (1964), Girs (1976), Yaroslavsky et al. (1977).

On our data, the observed variations of the intensity of alterative-exudative and infiltrative-proliferative changes in the brain at tick-borne encephalitis depend, on the one hand, from the stage of inflammation, but on the other hand, from the type of immune responses in individual patients. This data confirms that high levels of specific antibodies in the blood and cerebrospinal fluid, and a more pronounced imbalance of immune responses observed in patients with severe focal forms of TBE than in patients with fever, meningeal, and blurred forms (Kvetkova et al., 1981; Leonova, 1989, 1997; Vereta et al., 1990; Sysolyatin et al., 1990; Shien et al., 1996).

To emphasize the importance of immunoreactivity in the development of inflammatory cell response in the brain at tick-borne encephalitis, it is necessary to refer to the work Pogodina and Frolova(1962, 1965, 1984), performed on a large number of monkeys. These data show that intracerebral infection of animal by neurovirulent TBE virus strains, when the infection was reproduced, bypassing the visceral stage of the pathogenesis without the severe damage to the lymphoid organs, morphological changes in the central nervous system are more pronounced the infiltrative-proliferative component of inflammation, with the domination of DTH reactions than in cases of fatal encephalitis in humans.

One of the factors, the lack of the full symptom- complex of inflammation in viral infections can be the possibility of virus to suppress the inflammatory cell reaction (Avtsyn, 1983). Our morphological data confirm that the tick-borne encephalitis is associated with the known immunosuppressive action of the virus and the resulting state of immunodeficiency (Ryabov et al., 1990; Konev, 1995; Leonova, 1997).

It is known that the severity of the inflammatory process depends not only on the immunological reactivity of the organism, but also on the degree of virulence of the pathogen. The data on the comparative pathology of tick-borne encephalitis, caused by virus strains of high and reduced neurovirulence, based almost solely on the experimental data using to infect animals with different sensitivity to TBE virus (Robinzon & Popova, 1949; Levkovich et al., 1967; Rozina, 1972; Frolova, 1964, 1967; Zinovev et al., 1978a, 1978b, etc.). It should be noted that these studies were mainly focused on characterization of pathogenicity of attenuated tick-borne encephalitis virus strains and the clarification of the pathogenesis of infection in order to find variants of the virus that are suitable for the development of an effective vaccine for the prevention of TBE.

Our experimental studies have focused on the establishment of the morphological basis of different clinical manifestations of the Far Eastern tick-borne encephalitis, referred Shapoval (1980) to the main nozogeografic version of tick-borne encephalitis (Somova et al, 2001). To address this issue we have studied the morphology of experimental encephalitis on the model of golden hamsters induced by subcutaneous (analogical flowing natural infection process) infection of the virus strains isolated from patients with different clinical forms of infection. This model allows us to differentiate between virulent and attenuated strains of TBE virus (Pogodina et al., 1984). Morphological changes were compared in four groups of animals, ranging from the first up to 21 days after infection.

The histopathological study of animals in Group 1, infected with TBE virus strain 582, isolated from human white blood cells with the inapparent form infection, showed that this strain has a reduced neurovirulence and cause minor inflammatory changes in the brain (Fig. 5 a) and reversible changes in neurons in the form of the swelling and the perinuclear chromatolysis. The appearance of the brain to the 11-14th days after infection the lymphocytic-histiocytic infiltrates with the presence of plasma cells indicating the nature of the immune inflammatory response in the CNS (Fig. 5 b, c). The inflammatory changes concerned mainly the pia mater and the choroid plexus of the brain ventricles. We can assume that the asymptomatic form of the infectious process is limited to the visceral phase of the pathogenesis of TBE, when an adequate immune response flowing spread of the virus in the CNS is limited due to the development of protective immunomorphological changes in the structures of the blood-brain barrier. It is assumed that the asymptomatic form of tick-borne encephalitis is quite common in endemic areas (Shapoval, 1961; Levkovich et al., 1967). In the seropositive cases of TBE the low levels of specific antibodies are determined (Leonova, 1997).

The animals in Group 2, infected with TBE virus strain 208, isolated from a patient's white blood cells with the febrile form infection, the pathological process in the central nervous system characterized by a predominance of infiltrative and proliferative changes (Fig. 6 a, b). Distinct vascular and inflammatory reactions in the pia mater and substance of the brain were detected at an earlier date than the animals in Group 1. Perivascular infiltrates were distributed along the vessels from the pia mater to the deep brain substance. The response of nerve cells to viral infection manifested degenerative changes, the vacuolation of nuclei of individual neurons, the loss of small groups of Purkinje cells in the ganglionic layer of the cerebellum. In general, pathological changes in the central nervous system caused by the TBE virus strain 208, were identified as meningoencephalitis, and in some cases animals with paresis of the extremities and eyelids were observed a more widespread phenomenon of inflammation.

The conduct clinical and morphological parallels in experimental animals and humans can suggest that the absence of neurologic symptoms in patients with febrile form of tick-borne encephalitis does not exclude the involvement of the CNS in the pathological process. Most likely, reactive cellular changes in the arahnoidendotelium, choroidal plexus and ependyma of ventricles inhibit the penetration of the virus in nerve cells during infection of strains with reduced neurovirulence. In this regard, the data from V.P. Konev (1995) are of interest, which in inapparent infection in hamsters infected subcutaneously with TBE virus, through MGNA in situ, detected the virus components in the structures of the microvasculature, although the alteration and signs of inflammation in the brain is almost absent. At the same reactions in the lymphoid organs reflect the active formation of cellular and humoral immune response.

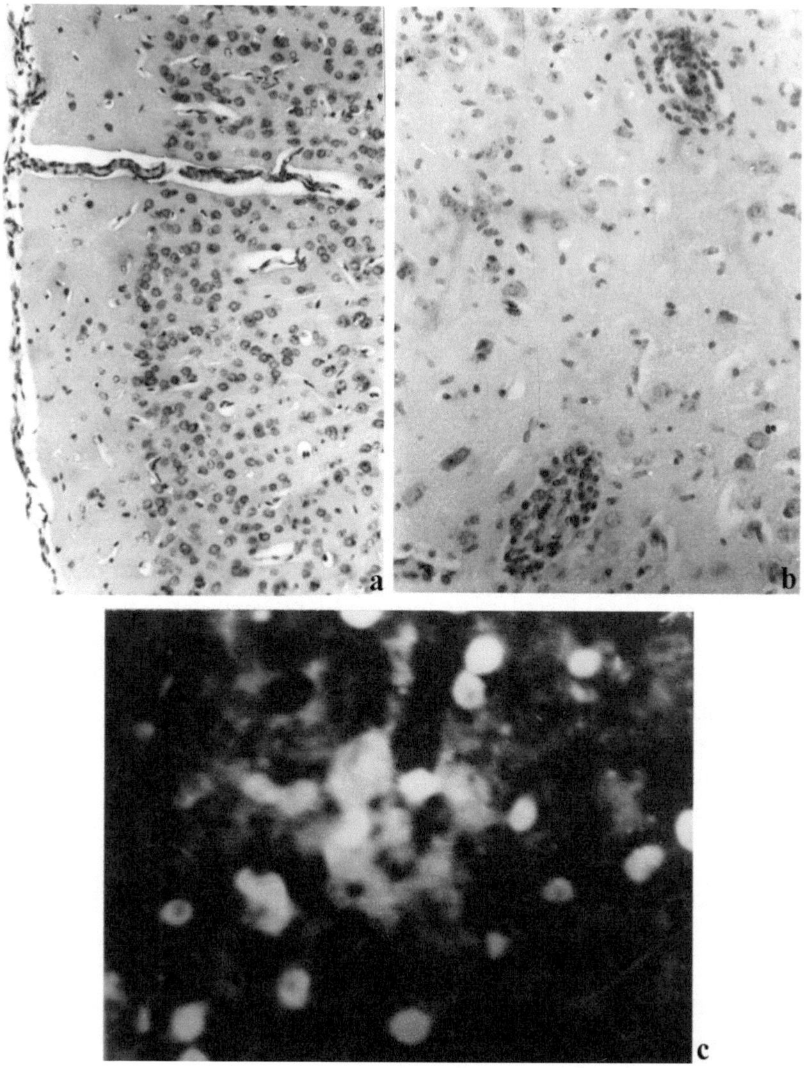

Figure 5. Pathological changes in the brain of hamsters infected with 582 strain of tick-borne encephalitis virus, isolated from human blood with inapparent form of infection, 11 days postinfection. a – the slight lymphocytic- histiocytic infiltration of pia mater in the spread of the brain substance, x 80, b – perivascular mononuclear infiltration in subcortex, x 200, stained with hematoxylin and eosin (a, b); c - specific immunoglobulin in the cells of perivascular infiltrate, x 200, the indirect IFA (c).

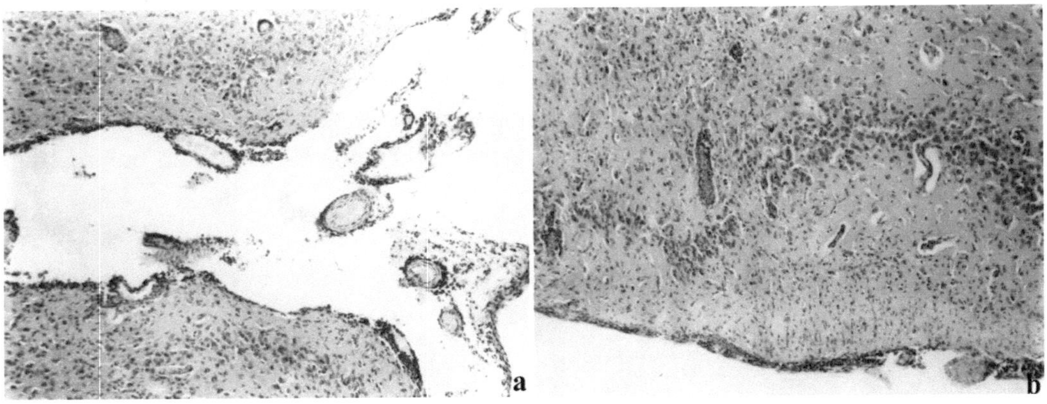

Figure 6. Pathological changes in the brains of hamsters infected with 208 strain of tick-borne encephalitis virus, isolated from the blood of patients with febrile form of infection, 11 days postinfection. a-plethora, edema and inflammation of pia mater in the sagittal sulcus of the brain, perivascular infiltration, x 80; b – the infiltrative and proliferative changes in the pia mater and the cerebral cortex, x 80. Stained with hematoxylin and eosin.

On the basis of morphological data can be assumed that the clinical differentiation of feverish, worn and meningeal forms of encephalitis, apparently, is conditional. In this regard, it should also pay attention to the experimental data (Frolova, 1967; Rozina, 1972) that even the attenuated and vaccine strains of tick-borne encephalitis virus can cause meningoencephalitis asymptomatic lesions without large foci neurons damage, with the formation of perivascular "muffs", glial reaction, as well as events of ependimitis and horioplexitis as indicators of immunomorphological reactions.

The experimental infection in animals infected with tick-borne encephalitis virus strains, isolated from patients with focal forms of the disease, manifested in the brain the development of the microscopic changes characteristic of a typical meningoencephalomielitis. Some animals were observed limb paresis, weakness. Thus, in the third group of animals, infected with strain 336, isolated from a patient's white blood cells with non-fatal, focal form TBE, the exudative and alterative component of the pathological process was pronounced (Fig. 7 a, b). Dystrophic and destructive changes in the nerve cells predominated in the brain areas adjacent to the ventricular system - Ammon's horn, subcortical layer of the cortex, around the Sylvius aqueduct. In hamsters, in addition to acute swelling of nerve cells in the cortical layer of the hippocampus is often observed oxyphilic foci of degeneration of neurons with their nuclei hyperchromatosis.

The infiltrative and proliferative component of the inflammation has been clearly expressed in the period from the 7th to the 14th days after infection, and manifested the moderate lymphocytic-histiocytic infiltration of the meninges, the choroidal plexus, the formation of glial "pillows" in the subependimal layer of the lateral ventricles. By 21 days the intensity of inflammatory changes decreases.

In the 4th group of animals infected with the "Walecki" strain of tick-borne encephalitis virus, isolated from the brain of the died patient with the focal form of the disease, the phenomenon meningoencephalomielis determined at an earlier date and were more expressive pronounced in comparison with the animals of group 3 (Fig. 8). The dynamics of the pathological process was similar among patients who died of the tick-borne encephalitis.

There were severe degenerative and destructive changes in the nerve cells in the indicator areas of the brain, which combined with severe exudative and infiltrative changes around the pial vessels and in the brain substance with the formation of perivascular "muffs". As in patients with tick-borne encephalitis in the animals of the fourth group in the morphogenesis of inflammation discernible the change in the cellular composition of infiltrates with an increase in the percentage of lymphocytes and plasma cells with the growth of the duration of the infection.

The poor demarcation of inflammatory lesions with the penetration of hematogenous elements into the surrounding brain tissue, the expressed neuronal damage with loss of cell groups, as well as the active glial proliferation indicated on the high neurovirulence of the "Walecki" strain and on the severity of encephalitic process with immunopathological in nature.

In the study, from 5-th to 21-th day after infection in sera of animals antibodies to tick-borne encephalitis were determined in the HAI with an increase in their titers. However, in animals of group 4 showed the inhibition of the immunogenesis. This is consistent with the data of morphological studies of lymphoid organs, showed a significant degree of depletion of cellular responses in the spleen (delimphatization) and the accidental transformation of the thymus in animals infected with the "Walecki" strain. The phenomenon of the virus-induced immunodeficiency is also confirmed the redaction in the thymic index in animals of all four groups in proportion to the degree of neurovirulence of tick-borne encephalitis virus strains, taken for infection.

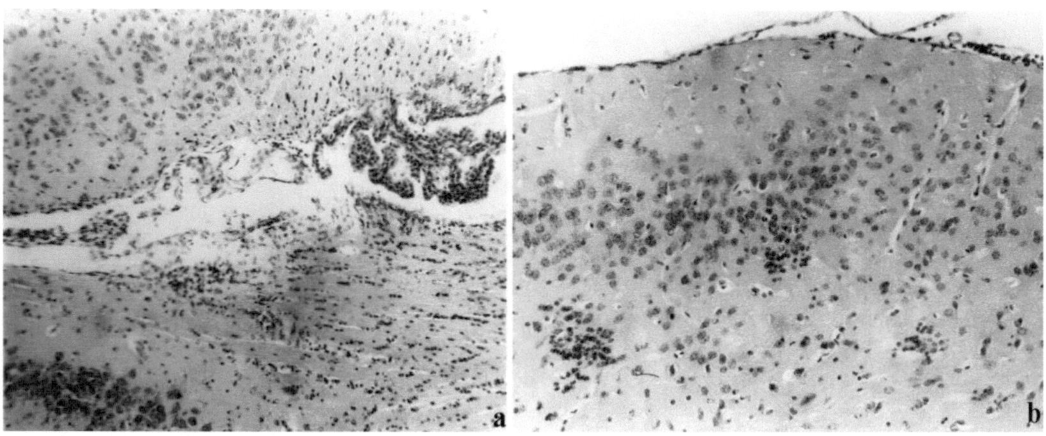

Figure 7. Pathological changes in the brain of hamsters infected with 336 strain of tick-borne encephalitis virus, isolated from the blood of patients with focal form of infection, 1 day postinfection. a – a part of the hippocampus, adjacent to the lateral ventricle of brain, inflammatory changes of the choroidal plexus, the focus of destruction under the ependyma with glial reaction, x 80; b - glial nodules in the cortical layers of the cerebral hemispheres, lymphoid infiltration of the pia mater, x 125. Stained with hematoxylin and eosin.

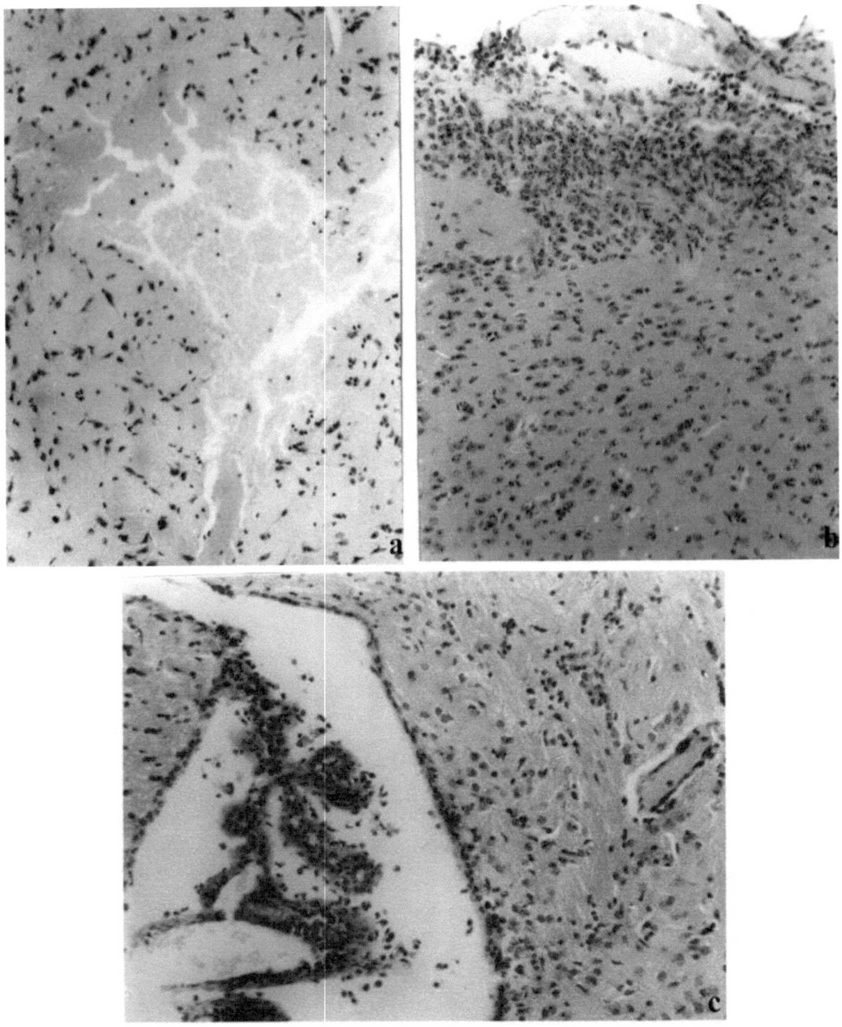

Figure 8. Pathological changes in the brain of hamsters infected with the "Walecki" strain of tick-borne encephalitis virus isolated from brain the died patient with the focal form of infection, 5 days postinfection. a – a hemorrhage around the necrotic vessel in the brain stem, glial reaction, x 125; b – the abundant infiltration of the pia mater and cortical brain regions by hematogenous elements, x 125; c –the expressive proliferation of ependyma of lateral ventricle, infiltrative-proliferative changes in the brain substance, x 125. Stained with hematoxylin and eosin.

Thus, our experimental studies were evidence the dependence of morphogenesis of tick-borne encephalitis from the characterictic of infecting virus strains. The direct evidences for virus-induced immunodeficiency in TBE received Konev (1995), who showed in experiments using in situ MGNK the selective accumulation of the virus in lymphoid organs from the first day of infection in macrophages and lymphocytes of the T-dependent zones. According to the author, who used to infect animals Sofjin Far East neurovirulence strain, the nature of brain damage, the dynamics of the immune response with the morphological equivalents in the lymphoid organs also depend on the specific susceptibility of animal models (mice, hamsters).

Our materials are allowed to evaluate the pathology of tick-borne encephalitis, caused by a heterogeneous viral population, in terms of a common mechanism underlying the protective and damaging effects of immunomorphological reactions. Based on the analysis of own and literature data were divided into three clinical-morphological variants of tick-borne encephalitis (table 3).

The first variant of the acute TBE is characterized by pronounced cerebral disorders, the high mortality during the first week of the disease, the prevalence of exudative and alterative components of inflammation and haemocirculating disorders in the CNS. The heavy damage to neurons has the direct connection to the intracellular reproduction of the virus. The development of this version of the tick-borne encephalitis is caused by highly virulent strains of TBE virus, as well as the specific sensitization of the organism dominated by immediate hypersensitivity reactions.

The second variant, the most typical of the acute TBE, is characterized by a slow rate in the development of changes in the CNS, focal symptoms, fatalities on 2 - 4th week of the disease. In the pathological pattern prevails the infiltrative-proliferative component of the inflammation with the presence of perivascular "muffs" as well as the severe nodular and diffuse glial reaction. These changes are the consequence of immunopathological process inherent in delayed-type hypersensitivity.

The third variant is characterized feverish, worn and inapparent forms of tick-borne encephalitis. The selecting this variant was possible on the basis of experimental elaboration during infection caused by attenuated strains of TBE virus, including those in the literature (Rozina, 1972), with the vaccination and the passive immunization of specific gamma globulin. In the pathological picture there are reactive changes in the structures of the blood-brain barrier in the form of the productive arachnoiditis, horioplexitis and ependimitis that protect nerve cells from the virus.

In parallel with our research, a lot of attention to the modern pathomorphosis of tick-borne encephalitis drew scientists of the Ural region (Erman et al, 1999), where by the end of the 1990s saw the significant increase in the incidence of tick-borne encephalitis, weighting the clinical course and outcome of disease. Based on analysis of 32 fatal cases of acute encephalitis authors, along with the general features characteristic of the disease, identified three types of pathological changes in the nature of the inflammatory response: the alterative-productive inflammation, the alterative-exudative inflammation and the alterative inflammation. The differences of these types of inflammation, according to the authors, was relative.

Based on our own research results of the Far Eastern tick-borne encephalitis cases, we believe that the differentiation of the pathological process, carried out by Yerman et al. (1999) without delay the onset of fatal diseases, caused by the morphogenesis of changes in the central nervous system during development of infection and in general similar to that described by us pathological picture of tick-borne encephalitis. In our opinion, the authors made a logical conclusion that the unstable cellular inflammatory response, from the intense diffuse and focal perivascular infiltrates and proliferates to a small or virtually absent cellular inflammation is associated with the virulence of the virus strains and to a large extent with the immunological reactivity of the organism to infection. In assessing the nature of the pathological process, we stand in solidarity with Yerman, concluding that the immunopathology of tick-borne encephalitis includes both immediate type hypersevsitivity, and delayed-type hypersevsitivity, a different combination of which creates the impression of different types of inflammatory reaction.

Indexes	**Clinical and morphological variants of the disease**		
	The first	**The second**	**The third**
The clinical picture			
Cerebral symptoms	+++	+/++	-
Focal neurological symptoms	++	+++	-
The current of disease	heavy	heavy / moderate	light, with or without clinical picture
The during the onset of death, week	the first week	2-3-4 weeks	Till one week
Mortality	100 %	2 weeks. -56.6% 3 weeks. - 13.4% 4 weeks. - 30%	no
The morphological picture			
Alteration of neurons	+++	++/+++	+/±
Gemocirculating disorders	+++	++/+++	±/-
Infiltration due to:			
neutrophils	++	+	±/-
lymphocytes/ histiocytes	+/++	++/+++	++
Proliferation of glia:			
focal	++	++/+++	+/±
diffuse	++	++/+++	-
Reactions of ITH	+++	±/+	-
Reactions of DTH	±/+	++/+++	+/±

Note: + + + pronounced, + + moderate severity, + weak expression, ± low intensity, - the lack of symptom/sign.

Table 3. Clinical and morphological variants of tick-borne encephalitis

http://dx.doi.org/10.5772/53449

4. Conclusion

On the basis of their own and literature data is given the modern interpretation of the pathomorphology of tick-borne encephalitis (TBE) in terms of immunopathological nature of the inflammation. It is shown that the pathological picture of central nervous system reflects the hyperergic nature of inflammation with TBE. In the morphogenesis of the pathological process traced the consistent development of immediate type hypersensitivity reactions, initiated by the damaging effect of the virus in brain tissue, and delayed type hypersensitivity reactions to ensure the formation of local (tissue) immunity. For a comprehensive assessment of pathology of tick-borne encephalitis in humans and experimental animals set the variability of its manifestations, this depends on the properties of the infecting virus strain, such as the virus-induced immune response and the stage of disease morphogenesis. On this basis, divided into three clinical and morphological variant manifestations of infection with TBEV.

Acknowledgment

This investigation was supported by the International Science and Technology Center a grant N^0 4006.

Author details

Larisa M. Somova[1], Galina N. Leonova[1], Natalia G. Plekhova[1], Yurii V. Kaminsky[2] and Anna Y. Fisenko[2]

1 Lab. Pathomorphlogy and Electron Microscopy, Lab. Tick-Borne Encephalitis, Institute of Epidemiology and Microbiology, Siberian Branch of the Russian Academy of Medical Sciences, Vladivostok, Russia

2 Vladivostok State Medical University, Vladivostok, Russia

References

[1] Albrecht, P. 1968. Pathogenesis of neurotropic arbovirus infection, Current Topics in Microbiol and Immunol. Vol. 43. pp. 247-259.

[2] Alexandrova, N.N., Kislitsyna, I.L. 1982. The study of the immune status of children with tick-borne encephalitis. In.: Children viral infection. Sverdlovsk, pp. 81-84.

[3] Avtsyn, A.P., Shroyt, I.G., Erman, B.A. 1983. The originality of inflammatory processes in viral infections J. of Med. Sciences of the USSR. Vol. 11. pp. 3-10.

[4] Barnes, W., Rosen, L. 1974. Fatal hemorrhagic disease and shock associated with primary dengue infection. Amer. J. Trop. Med. Vol. 23. pp. 495-501.

[5] Halstead, S.B., Shotwell, H., Casals, J. 1973. Studies on the pathogenesis of dengue infection in monkeys. II. Clinical laboratory responses to heterologous infection. J. Infect Dis. Vol. 128(1). Pp. 15-22.

[6] Barnshteyn, Y.A. 1989. Immunodeficiency and infectious process. VIII All-Union Congress of Pathologists: Proc. Reports. Moscow. pp. 152-154.

[7] Belman, H.L. 1960. Tick-borne encephalitis. Leningrad, 198 p.

[8] Gears, B.K. 1976.Changes in the vessels of the brain and spinal cord of monkeys with experimental acute and subacute infections caused by strains of tick-borne encephalitis virus with different biological properties. Proceedings of the inter-institutional Scientific conference. Join. devoted. 70th anniversary of the opening of the Tomsk NIIVS. Tomsk. pp. 56-58.

[9] Dekonenko, E.P., Umansky, K.G., Frolova, M.P., Skurda, M.P. 1994. Clinic and pathogenesis of poliradikuloneuropatia with tick-borne encephalitis. J. Neuropathol. Psychiatr. Them. S.S. Korsakov. № 4. pp. 27-31.

[10] Demenev, V.A., Schikova, M.A., Artemenko, N.L., Nebaykina, Y.V. 1990. Methodological features of electron-microscopic indication of tick-borne encephalitis virus in immunocompetent cells of the peripheral blood of patients. All-Union Symposium "Current problems of epidemiology, diagnosis and prevention of tick-borne encephalitis": Proc. Reports. Irkutsk. pp. 95-96.

[11] Dzhioev, Yu.P. 2000. Molecular- epidemiological and phylogenetic analysis of the genetic heterogenecity of populations of tick-borne encephalitis virus in the Asian territory of Russia: Abstract. thesis. ... Candidate. of Biological. Sciences, Irkutsk. p. 22.

[12] Erman, B.A., Konev, V.P., Royhel, Y.V. 1996. Viral infections of the central nervous system (pathological anatomy, pathogenesis, diagnosis). Ekaterinburg. 72 p.

[13] Erman, B.A., Zaitseva, L.N., Volkova, L.I., Obraztsova, R.G. 1999. The pathological anatomy of modern tick-borne encephalitis in the Ural. Ekaterinburg. 80 p.

[14] Frolova, M.P. 1964. The pathology of experimental monkey encephalitis caused by virus strains isolated in the eastern regions of the USSR. Tick-borne encephalitis. Moscow. pp. 40-43.

[15] Frolova, M.P. 1965. Characteristic properties of neurotropic strains of the spring-summer encephalitis, isolated from healthy individuals of virus, on the monkeys model. In.: Tick-borne encephalitis. Minsk. pp. 80-87.

[16] Frolova, M.P. 1967. Morphological study of the central nervous system of monkeys infected with virulent strains and attenuated variants of tick-borne encephalitis virus and Langat (strain TR-21). Proceedings of the XIII session of the Institute of Poliomyelitis and Viral Encephalitis of Medical Sciences of the USSR. Moscow. p. 114.

[17] Frolova, M.P., Karpovich, L.G., Levkovich, E.N., Ralph, N.M. 1973. The study of residual pathogenicity of attenuated variant of the TR-21-237 virus Langat in monkeys. II. Pathological indicators of residual neurovirulence. Medical Virology. Moscow. T. 21, Vol. 1. pp. 150-160.

[18] Frolova, M.P., Pogodina, V.V. 1984. Persistence of tick-borne encephalitis virus infection in monkeys. VI. Pathology of chronic process in the central nervous system. Acta virologica. T. 28. pp. 232-239.

[19] Frolova, M.P., Tikhomirova, T.I., , Shestopalova, N.M. 1975. Some questions in the pathogenesis of tick-borne encephalitis. Problems of medical virology. Moscow. S. 82-83.

[20] Holzmann, H., Heins, F.X., Mandel, Ch.W. et al. 1991.Molecular studies on the virulence of tick-borne encephalitis virus. J. Cell Biochem. Suppl. 15 E. p. 86.

[21] Isaeva, M.P. 1998. Molecular and genetic characterization of tick-borne encephalitis virus population of the South Sikhote-Alin focal region: Abstract. thesis. ... Candidate of Medical Sciences, Vladivostok. 22 p.

[22] Jerusalemsky, A.P. 2001. Tick-borne encephalitis. Novosibirsk. 360 p.

[23] Kanchurin, A.H. 1964. By the pathogenesis of allergic (demyelinating) lesions of the central nervous system: Abstract. thesis. ... Candidate of Medical Sciences, Moscow. 24 p.

[24] Karmysheva, V.J., Pogodina, V.V. 1990. The lesion of the thymus in the pathogenesis of experimental tick-borne encephalitis. Problems of virology. № 2. pp. 144-146.

[25] Karmysheva, V.J., Pogodina, V.V. 1991. The lesion of the immune system as a factor in the pathogenesis of tick-borne encephalitis. Microscopic aspects of the pathogenesis of viral infections: Proc. Reports. Novosibirsk. p. 16.

[26] Kastner, A.G. 1941. Pathological anatomy and histology of the spring-summer (taiga) encephalitis in human and experimental animals. In.: Tick-borne encephalitis. Khabarovsk. pp. 116-121.

[27] Kvetkova, E.A. 1984. Virological and immunological aspects of the pathogenesis of tick-borne encephalitis: Abstract. thesis. … Doctor of Medical Sciences, Leningrad. 35 p.

[28] Kvetkova, E.A., Konev, V.P. 1996. Immunopathogenesis of infection and the vaccination process in the tick-borne encephalitis. Viral, rickettsial and bacterial infections carried by ticks: Proc. Reports of the International conference, Irkutsk. pp. 146-147.

[29] Kvetkova, E.A., Shmatko, V.G. 1983. Immunopathology of Nervous and Mental Diseases. Moscow. pp. 83-83.

[30] Konev, V.P. 1982. The morphogenesis of tick-borne encephalitis in the strain variations in the pathogen and passive immunization: Author. thesis. ... Candidate of Medocal Sciences. Novosibirsk. 22 p.

[31] Konev, V.P. 1994. Interorganal relationships in morphogenesis of acute tick-borne encephalitis. Actual problems of medical virology. Ekaterinburg. pp. 123-127.

[32] Konev, V.P. 1995. The natural morphogenesis and induced pathomorphosis of tick-borne encephalitis: Author. thesis. ... Doctor of Medical Sciences, Omsk. 39 p.

[33] Konev, V.P., Kosterina, L.D., Kvetkova, E.A., Rychkov ,A.A., Polishchuk, T. I. 1989. Immunodeficiencies in morphogenesis of neuroviral infections. VIII All-Union Congress of Pathologists: Proc. Reports. Moscow. pp. 208-209.

[34] Konev, V.P., Kvetkova, E.A., Polishchuk, T.I., Tulakina, LG, Rychkov, A.A., Ilyushenko, L.P. 1991. The correlation relationship of brain damage and lymphoid organs in acute tick-borne encephalitis. Nature-focal diseases in human, Omsk, pp. 74-78.

[35] Kopecky, J., Tomkova, E., Grubhoffer, L., Krivance, K. 1987. Immune Response of host to the tick-borne encephalitis virus infection // III Intern. Symposium on Ecology of Arboviruses: Abstracts, Smolenice. pp. 44.

[36] Leonova, G.N. 1989. The effectiveness of vaccination and serotherapy in tick-borne encephalitis in the Primorsky Territory. J. of Microbiology. № 10. pp. 59-64.

[37] Leonova, G.N., Isachkova, L.M., Kruglyak, S.P. 1995. Pathogenic criteria for evaluating the virulence of tick-borne encephalitis virus strains isolated in the south of Far East. Problems of Virology. № 4. pp. 165-169.

[38] Leonova, G.N. 1997. Tick-borne encephalitis in the Primorsky Krai. Vladivostok: Dal'nauka. 187 p.

[39] Leonova, G.N., Kozhemyako, V.B., Borisevich, V.G. 1999. Molicular-genetic basis of heterogenicity of the Far East population of tick-borne virus. 3rd Intern Conference "Ticks and tick-borne Pathogens": Into the 21st Century, Slovakia. p. 25.

[40] Leonova, G.N. 2009. Tick-borne encephalitis: current aspects. Vladivostok. 168 p.

[41] Levkovich, E.N., Pogodina, V.V., Zasukhina, G.D., Karpovich, L.G. 1967.Viruses of the tick-borne encephalitis complex. Leningrad.: Medicine. 245 p.

[42] Malkova, D., Frankova, V. 1959. The role of the lymphatic system in the development of encephalitis in mice Acta virologica. Vol. 3. pp. 210-215.

[43] Malkova, D., Smetana, A. 1966. The role of the lymphatic system for direct introduction of tick-borne encephalitis virus in the blood of white mice susceptible Acta virologica. Vol. 10. pp. 471-474.

[44] Mamunts, A.Z. 1993. Tick-borne encephalitis in children. Pediatrics. Vol. 6. pp. 81-85.

[45] Morishima, T., Hanada, N., Nishikawa, K. 1984. Kinetics of antibody production in central nervous system and the damage of blood-borne in virus infection. 6th Intern. Congress of Virology, Sendai, pp. 79.

[46] Nathanson, N., Davis, M., Thind, I.S., Price, W.H. 1966. Histological Studies of the monkey neurovirulence of group B arboviruses. II. Selection of indicator centers. Amer. J. Epidem. Vol. 84. pp. 524-540.

[47] Nathanson, N., Panitch, H. 1978. Immunological aspects of viral infections. Handbook of Clinical Neurology, Amsterdam-New York-Oxford. Vol. 34. pp. 39-62.

[48] Panov, A.G. 1956. Tick-borne encephalitis. Leningrad: Medgiz. 282 p.

[49] Perehodova, S.K., Semenov, B.F., Kvetkova, E.A., Konev, V.P. 1976. The study of delayed-type hypersensitivity in experimental tick-borne encephalitis. J. of Microbiol. Vol. 10. pp. 120-124.

[50] Pogodina, V.V., Larina, G.I., Frolova, M.P., Bochkova, N. G. 1984. Variants of host immune response to the tick-borne encephalitis virus. Problems of Virology. Vol. 6. pp. 708-715.

[51] Pogodina, V.V., Frolova, M.P., Erman, B.A. 1986. Chronic tick-borne encephalitis. Novosibirsk: Nauka. 232 p.

[52] Polishchuk, T.I. 1999. Morphogenetic evaluation of the migration of the virus in the incubation period of acute tick-borne encephalitis. 2nd Congress of the International Union of Pathologists: Proc. Reports. Moscow. pp. 239-241.

[53] Polishchuk, T.I., Shamanin, V.A., Rychkov, A.A., Konev, V.P. 1990. The relationship of morphological changes in the brain and lymphoid organs in the tick-borne encephalitis Human Health in Siberia. Abstracts of the 5th scientific and practical conference "Young scientists - practical health care." Krasnoyarsk. pp. 104-105.

[54] Robinson, I.A. 1975. General questions of pathogenesis and pathologic anatomy of the nervous system infections. In. M.B. Zucker: Meningitis and encephalitis in children. Moscow. pp. 5-72.

[55] Robinson, I.A., Popova, L.M. 1949. Histopathological characteristics of experimental tick-borne encephalitis. IV Scientific session of the Institute of Neurology, Academy of Medical Sciences: Proc. Reports., Moscow, pp. 8-17.

[56] Robinson, I.A., Sergeeva, Y.S. 1939. Pathological changes in the nervous system during the spring-summer (taiga) encephalitis Archives of Biological Sciences. Vol. 5. pp. 71-82.

[57] Robinson, I.A., Sergeeva, Y.S. 1940. On the localization of inflammatory changes in the spring-summer meningoencephalomyelitis J. of neuropathology and psychiatry. T. 9,Vol. 1-2. pp. 31-37.

[58] Robinson, I.A., Frolova, M.P. 1964. Some questions of pathology and pathogenesis of tick-borne encephalitis. Proceedings of the 11th Scientific Sessions of the Institute of Poliomyelitis and Viral Encephalitis AMS USSR, Moscow. pp. 36-38.

[59] Russell, P.X., Intavivat, A., Kachenapilant, S. 1969.Anti-dengue immunoglobulins and serum globulin levels in dengue shock syndrome. J. Immunol. Vol. 102. pp. 412-420.

[60] Rozina, E.E. 1972. Experimental viral infections. Moscow: Meditsina. 262 p.

[61] Ryabov, V.I., Motyreva, A.I., Olenev, O.G. 1990. The state of immune reactivity and natural resistance in patients with tick-borne encephalitis. Nature-focal diseases in human. Omsk. pp. 43-47.

[62] Rychkov, A.A. 1992. Structural equivalents of tick-borne encephalitis virus infection in lymphoid organs: Author. thesis. ... Candidate of Medical Sciences, Chelyabinsk. 23 p.

[63] Rychkov, A.A., Konev, V.P., Kvetkova, E.A., Shamanin, V.A. 1990. Lymphoid organs in acute and chronic tick-borne encephalitis: detection of viral RNS, morphofunctional assessment. Problems of the Epidemiology, Immunology and Diagnosis of viral infections, Sverdlovsk. pp. 42-46.

[64] Rychkov, A.A., Zinoviev, A.S., Kvetkova, E.A., Pletnev, A.G., Konev, V.P., Polischuk, T. I. 1989. Pathology of lymph nodes in humans with acute tick-borne encephalitis. Nature-focal diseases in human, Omsk. pp. 79-83.

[65] Semenov, B.F., Gavrilov, V.I. 1976. Immunopathology in viral infections. Moscow: Medicine. 173 p.

[66] Semenova-Tienshanskaya, V.V., Shapoval, A.N. 1949. The pathology of tick-borne encephalitis. Experience of medicine in the Great Patriotic War of 1941-1945. Vol. 26. pp. 146-161.

[67] Smorodintsev, A.A., Dubov, A.V. 1986. Tick-borne encephalitis and its vaccination. Leningrad.: Medicine. 232 p.

[68] Shien, W.J., Ksaizek, T., Bethke, F.R. et al. 1996. Immunochistochemical Diagnosis of flavivirus Infection in paraffin-embedded human tissues. Lab. Invest. Vol. 74., N 1. pp. 764.

[69] Somova (Isachkova), L.M., Leonova, G.N., Frolova, M.P., Fisenko, A.Y. 2001. Experimental study of variability of clinical and morphological manifestations of tick-borne encephalitis. The Pacific Med. J. № 2. pp. 88-91.

[70] Somova, L.M, Leonova, G.N., Fisenko, A.J., Plekhova, N.G., Kaminsky, Y.V. 2010. Morphogenesis of the Far Eastern tick-borne encephalitis. Archives of Pathology. № 5. pp. 47-52.

[71] Strukov, A.I. 1982. Inflammation. In: General human pathology (ed. A.I. Strukov, V. Serov V.V., Sarkisov D.S.), Moscow: Medicine. pp. 271-328.

[72] Sysolyatin, V.A., Selyutina, I.A., Caravanov, A.S. 1990. Features of the immune response in patients with tick-borne encephalitis. All-Union Symposium "Modern

problems of Epidemiology, Diagnosis and Prevention of tick-borne encephalitis": Proc. Reports, Irkutsk. pp. 125-126.

[73] Shapoval, A.N. 1961. Tick-borne encephalitis (encephalomyelitis). Moscow: Medgizh. 317 p.

[74] Shapoval, A.N. 1976. Chronic forms of tick-borne encephalitis. Leningrad: Medicine. 176 p.

[75] Shapoval, A.N. 1980. Tick-borne encephalomyelitis. Leningrad: Medicine. 256 p.

[76] Tulakina, L.G., Konev, V.P., Polischuk, T.I. 1994. The ultrastructural pathology of the lymph nodes in the tick-borne encephalitis. Actual problems of Medical Virology, Ekaterinburg. pp. 132-135.

[77] Vargin, V.V., Semenov, B.F. 1980. Characterization of autoreactive T cells, detected by experimental infection of mice infected with Langat virus. Immunology, Moscow. № 2. pp. 74-76.

[78] Vereta, L.A . 1969. Immunology of tick-borne encephalitis based on clinical, experimental and epidemiological studies in areas of Amur Region: Abstract. thesis. ... Doctor of Medical Sciences, Moscow. 30 p.

[79] Vereta, L.A., Nikolaeva, S.P., Zaharycheva, T.A. et al. 1990. Virological and immunological analysis of meningoencephalitic and meningoencephalomyelitic forms tick-borne encephalitis. Proc. Symposium "Current problems of epidemiology, diagnosis and prevention of tick-borne encephalitis": Proc. Reports, Irkutsk. pp. 111-112.

[80] Votyakov, V.I., Protas, I.I., Zhdanov, V.M. 1978. Western tick-borne encephalitis. Minsk: "Belarus". 256 p.

[81] Webb, H.E., Smith, C. E. 1966. Relation of immune response to development of central nervous system lesions in virus infection of man. Brit. Med. J. N 2. pp. 1179-1181.

[82] Yaroslavsky, V.E., Dubov, A. V, Gears, B.K. 1977. Questions of the pathogenesis of experimental infections caused by tick-borne encephalitis virus strains with different biological properties. In: The pathogenesis of chronic and latent neuroviral and coxsackie-viral infections. Tomsk. pp. 33-36.

[83] Zinoviev, A.S. , Konev, V.P., Kvetkova, E.A., Perehodova, S.K. 1978a. The role of morphological changes in microvascular of brain in the pathogenesis of experimental tick-borne encephalitis. Questions of immunity and disease diagnosis of natural-focal diseases, Leningrad. pp. 59-65.

[84] Zinoviev, A.S., Konev, V.P., Kvetkova, E.A., Perehodova, S.K. 1978b.The morphological manifestations of experimental tick-borne encephalitis, caused by a group of West Siberian virus strains. Mixed infections with natural foci, Omsk. pp. 49-55.

[85] Zlobin, V.I., Gorin, O.Z. 1996. Tick-borne encephalitis. The etiology, epidemiology and prevention. Novosibirsk: Nauka. 177 p.

[86] Zlotnik, I. 1968. The reaction of astrocytes to acute virus infections of central nervous system. Brit. J. Exper. Path. Vol. 49, N 6. pp. 555-564.

[87] Zlotnik, I., Grant, D.P., Carter, G.B. 1976. Experimental infection of monkeys with virus of tick-borne encephalitis complex. Degenerative cerebellar lesions following inapparent form of the disease of recovery from clinical encephalitis. Bri. J. Exper. Path. Vol. 57. pp. 200-210.

Chapter 9

Active Natural Foci of Tick-Borne Neuroinfection in the North-West Region of Ukraine

I. Lozynski, H. Biletska, O. Semenyshyn, V. Fedoruk, O. Drul, I. Ben, A. Shulgan and R. Morochkovski

Additional information is available at the end of the chapter

http://dx.doi.org/10.5772/54912

1. Introduction

The formation natural foci of tick-borne infections is closely connected to three physically–geographical zones in Ukraine: Ukrainian Polissya (mixed forest zone - (woodlands), Forest–Steppe zone, Steppe zone and two extra-zonal natural areas – Carpathian and Crimean mountains.

On the territory of Ukrainian Polissya there are favourable conditions for the formation of natural foci of mainly those types of arboviruses and bacterial infections, which are transmitted by ticks – tick-borne viral encephalitis, Tribec, Uukuniemi, ixodid tick-borne borreliosis, human granulocytic anaplasmosis (HGA), others.

Tick-borne viral encephalitis (TBVE), ixodid tick-borne borreliosis (ITBB) and mixed-infection (TBVE and ITBB) are the most prevalent feral herd transmissible infections in Ukraine. Numerous aspects of these infections require to be better looked into or need more accurate definitions. First of all, this refers to the regional peculiarities of epidemiology and clinical manifestations, diagnostics, treatment and also the efficiency of preventive measures taken. There is an urgent need in studies of special clinical features of late manifestations and chronic course of these neuroinfections, as well as their better timely diagnostics and etio-pathogenetic therapy.

2. Abiotic and biotic peculiarities of Volyn oblast

Volyn oblast is located on far north-west part of Ukraine and occupies the western part of plain territories of two geographic zones of Ukraine – Ukrainian Polissya and Forest-Steppe. On the south it borders with Lviv oblast, on the east with Rivne oblast, on the north with the Republic of Belarus, on the west (along the Western Bug) with Poland.

Climate of Volyn oblast is mild-continental, with mild winters, short periods of freezing, frequent thaws, mild summers, without significant heat waves, heavy percipitation, long springs and autumns. Average January temperature is +4,5 ^{0}C, for July it is +18,6 ^{0}C. Vegetation period lasts for about 200 days. The sums of the temperatures for the periods with stabile temperatures above +10, make 2495-2580 ^{0}C. Percipitation makes 550-600 mm a year. Relative humidity of the air is in the reverse proportion to its temperature: in the winter it exceeds 80 %, in the summer it reaches 65-70 % [1].

Territory of Volyn oblast is the part of Eastern-European province of broadleaf forests of the European Broadleaf Zone. The landscapes of the zone are of two types: Polissya, with high prevalence of swamps, meadows, oak-pine and narrow-leaf forests and Forest-Steppe type zone, with prevalence of meadow steppes and oak-hornbeam forests in prehistoric times, which are mainly farming lands nowadays.

Due to its zoo-geographic parameters, Volyn oblast is a borreal-forest zoo-geographic type of zone. Its territory hosts 301 vertebral species, among them 183 species of nesting and non-migrating birds, 64 species of mammals. Among small mammals, which are within the range of parasitory system of tick-borne infections, there are *Sorex araneus, Castor fiber, Apodemus agrarius, Arvicolla terrestris* (*amphibious*), *Microtus oeconomus*. To woods species belong *Sciurus vulgaris, Microtus subterraneus, Meles meles*. In zoocenozes also are distributed *Dryomys nitedula, Glis glis, Muscardinus avellanarius, Myodes Clethrionomys glareolus, Sylvaemus sylvaticus, Sylvaemus tauricus, Talpa europaea, Erinaceus europaeus* [2]. All territory of the oblast is within the area of *I. ricinus* ticks - main vector of tick-borne pathogenes in Europe.

The findings of the complex studies and surveillance, conducted in the period of 1990-2011, showed the presence of active natural foci of TBVE and ITBB on the considerable part of the territory of the oblast.

Aims of study: to look at the incidence rates of tick-borne infectious diseases and analyse the range of their clinical manifestations in north-west region of Ukraine taking Volyn oblast as a sample territory during the period of 1990-2011.

3. Tikc-borne viral encephalitis

3.1. TBVE Epidemiology

Virological surveillance, that has been conducted by scientists of the laboratory of Transmissible Viral Infections (TVI) of State Institution "Lviv Research Institute of Epidemiology and Hygiene Ministry of Health of Ukraine" (LRIEH), enabled detection of 38 strains of TBVE virus. Most of them (26 strains) were isolated from *I. ricinus* ticks, whose rates of TBVE infection in active natural foci are 19,5 %, from mouse-like rodents (*Apodemus agrarius, A. sylvaticus*) – 2 strains, from birds (*Fulica atra*) – 1 strain and from TBVE patients – 9 strains.

Due to their antigen characteristics, strains of TBE virus isolated in Ukraine belong to ricinus-serotype (genotype 2) and have almost same biological characteristics as causative agent of Central-European encephalitis of countries of Eastern and Western Europe [3, 4].

For 2011 enzootic as to TBVE territories, distinguished according to one or combination of such characteristics as natural infection (presence of antigen) of ixodid ticks and small mammals (potential carriers and reservoirs of pathogen) with causative agent, diagnosed cases of the disease with local infection, high degrees of population immunity, were registered in 33 settlements of 9 districts of Volyn oblast [5] (fig.1).

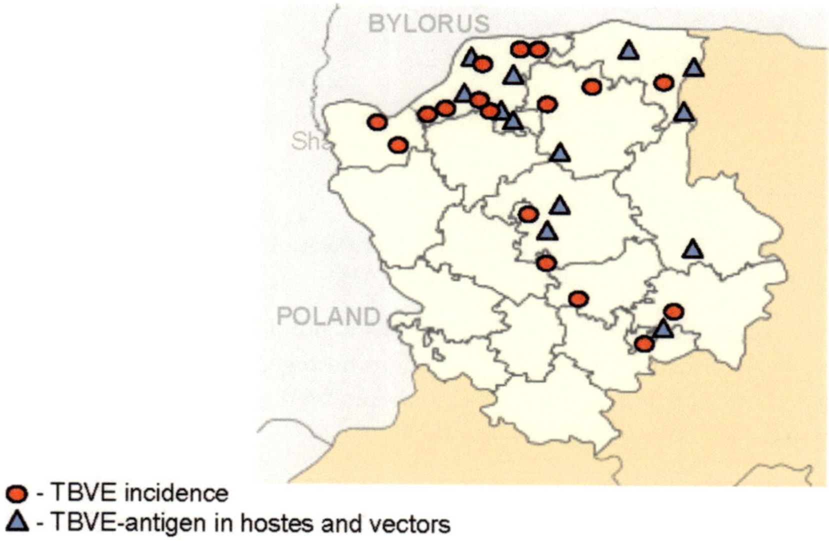

Figure 1. Shematic map of TBVE enzootic territories in Volyn oblast

The main reservoirs of TBVE virus in nature are *Microtus arvalis, Myodes glareolus,* and *Apodemus agrarius,* where the part of *M. arvalis* makes more than 50 %.

Among ixodid ticks, the species which are more often infected with TBE virus are *Dermacentor reticulatus* (64,3 %), while among the *Ixodes ricinus* this number is 35,7% [6].

3.2. TBVE incidence rates

Tick-borne viral encephalitis is one of the most prevalent arboviral infections in Ukraine. People get infected with it through the tick bite or by consuming raw, mainly goat milk.

For present moment local cases of TBVE among people are registered yearly in 16 out of 25 oblasts of Ukraine, in cities Kyiv and Sevastopol. However the official data don't reflect the real state of things with the morbidity in Ukraine [7].

During the period of 1955 to 2010 there were only 580 TBVE cases registered, while 132 of them were registered in the period of 2000–2011 (fig. 2). And correspondingly, the indices of morbidity in Ukraine during the decade varied in the range 0,001 – 0,03/100 000 population, including per oblast from 0–1,5 [8].

During the period of 2003-2010 we observed 223 cases of seroconversion in diagnostic titers of people from 14 oblasts of Ukraine. Among them in Volyn oblast - 77 cases [9].

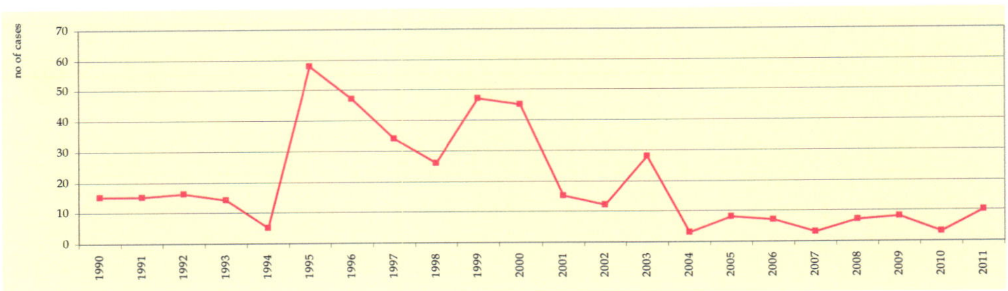

Figure 2. Cases of TBVE in Ukraine (1990-2011)

On the territory of Volyn oblast on the whole, there were 187 cases of TBVE reported. This is almost third of all reported cases for Ukraine (32,5 %).

Within the range of natural foci described, the TBVE morbidity is characterized by a sporadic occurance, its clinical course is similar to western noso-geographic form of the disease. The considerable part of foci forms of TBVE was reported from Ukrainian Polissya (Volyn, Zhytomyr and Kyiv oblasts) [10].

The most active natural TBVE foci, which manifested itself with group morbidity, was detected in Ratne district of Volyn oblast. It was confirmed by isolation of TBVE virus strains from *I. ricinus* ticks and results of antigen screening in *D. reticulatus*, *I. ricinus* and body organs of *Apodemus agrarius*.

During the period of April-October 1995, there were more than 80 patients hospitalized, with fever, and the air-ways and central nervous system lesions. The largest part of cases was reported during the period of June-September, which is related to the berries-mushrooms season.

The largest part of cases appeared in residential areas that are in the close proximity to the forests and is caused by tick bites.

The disease was registered in spring-autumn period, starting in May and ending in November, with the peak in July-August. The main means of infection was transmitting (68,0 %). The cases of alimentary infection with TBVE (32,0 %) were due to a consumption of raw goat and cow's milk and its products. The development of a severe and complicated clinical forms of a disease was more common in terms of the transmitting way of infection ($P<0,05$).

In general TBVE in Volyn is characterized by one-wave feverous period, with predomination of feverous (60 %) and meningeal (24 %) forms of a disease with only 16 % of focal form (fig. 3), coordination disorders, insignificant quantity of paralytic forms and cases of a development of a chronic disease.

http://dx.doi.org/10.5772/54912

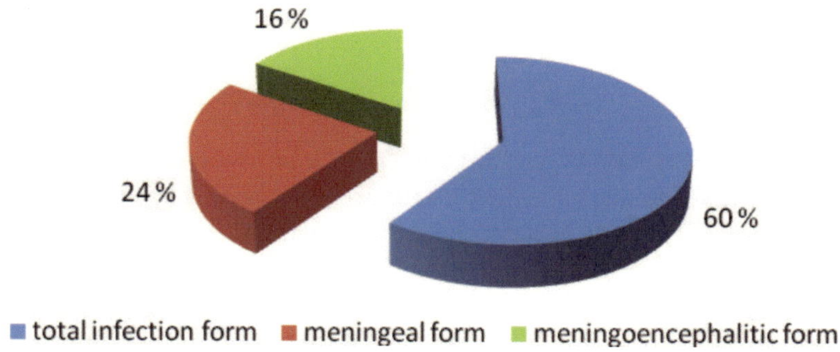

Figure 3. The main clinical forms of TBVE in Volyn oblast

Clinical manifestations are similar to the western type of this infection, but there predominated one-wave character of thermal curve, while two-wave type of fever and changes in hemogram were observed in half frequency. The temperature curve of part of the patients had three waves.

In terms of neurological complaints there predominated the vertigo, walk unsteadiness, bones and lips tremor. Sensitivity disorders in forms of paresthesia were common as well. From the side of vegetative nervous system during the acute period the leading symptoms were the following: bradycardia, growth of blood pressure, clearly manifested hyperhidrosis, stable diffuse dermographism. In the acute period of the disease some patients developed thyroid enlargement, asymmetry of skin temperature. Highly notable were various "pseudonevrasthenic" complaints which followed the course of the disease: memory decrease, irritability, obsessive fears and thoughts, emotional lability. The before-mentioned clinical form was called by author as"attenuate TBVE" [12].

Almost half of patients (48,2 %) – the initial stage of the disease was characterized by some prodromal indications, manifestation of which wasn't pathognomonic for the given disease. As a result of a transmissible form of infection ($P<0,05$), there were more complicated manifestations of it, when in terms of clearly manifested intoxication and general-cerebral syndrome, changes from the side of a nervous system there developed a disfunction of a vegetative nervous system which prevailed in different parts of it ($P<0,05$), there were observed pathologic indications in cardio-vascular system ($P<0,05$), liver enlargement ($P<0,001$). All disorders of a vegetative nervous system were of central genesis as a rule, and developed mainly as a result of more considerable lesions of a central nervous system. As a common indication there was observed a skin hyperhidrosis, especially of a local character, which developed in all patients with poliomyelitic –like form of a disease.

It has to be mentioned that the rates of TBVE forms with the lesions of a central nervous system which followed the tick bites and those which followed the alimentary way of infection didn't differ significantly ($P>0,05$).

We found that TBVE area includes Ratne and some more districts, which is confirmed by new cases reported, positive results of TBVE antigen screening in *Ixodid* ticks and rodents, and positive immune layer among healthy population in Kivertsi, Kovel, Rozhysche, Lyuboml, and Lutsk districts [13].

4. Ixodid tick-borne borreliosis (Lyme Borreliosis)

4.1. Natural foci of ITBB

In the course of our investigation of *I. ricinus* and *D. reticulatus* ticks collected in Kivertsi, Ratne and Turiysk districts of Polissya in 1998-2011, natural infectioning with *Borrelia burgdorferi s. l.* was identified in 19,8 % of *I. ricinus* and 3,8 % of *D. reticulatus* on the average. The highest prevalence of infected *I. ricinus* – 25,0 % - was identified in Kivertsi, Ratne (19,3 %) and Manevychi (16,7 %) districts, while the lowest rates were reported from Turiysk - 6,7 %. Sixty-two population units in all 16 districts of the oblast were found ITBB enzootic.

4.2. Population immunity

The evidence of the endemic status of ITBB natural foci on the territory of the oblast were collected in terms of serologic screening of 2122 persons among healthy population of five districts of Ukrainian Polissya (Kivertsi, Kovel, Manevychi, Ratne and Rozhysche) and three districts of a Forest-Steppe zone (Volodymyr-Volynskyi, Ivanychi and Lutsk) (table 1).

Seropositive layer of screened persons was within the range of 18,6-45,6 % (the mean value for oblast was 28,6 %), thus exceeding 10 % threshold - the estimated level of active natural foci of Lyme-borreliosis in other districts [14]. More than 20 % of population in 5 out of 12 screened districts of Volyn oblast (Volodymyr-Volynskyi, Gorohiv, Kovel, Lutsk and Ratne were found to have higher titres of Ig G antibodies (1:400-1:1600).

№	Districts	Total of observed patients	Found positive:			
			n	%	incl. in titres 1:400-1:1600	
					n	%
1	Volodymyr-Volynskyi	114	52	45,6	49	43,0
2	Gorokhiv	99	30	30,3	30	30,3
3	Ivanychi	20	5	25,0	0	0
4	Kamin-Kashyrs	59	11	18,6	10	16,9
5	Kivertsi	452	124	27,4	80	16,9
6	Kovel	206	80	38,8	37	18,0
7	Liubeshiv	111	31	27,9	31	27,9
8	Lutsk	194	64	33,0	57	29,4
9	Manevychi	347	80	23,0	64	18,4
10	Ratne	418	108	25,8	96	23,0
11	Rozhysche	49	12	24,5	11	22,4
12	Staro-Vyzhva	53	14	26,4	6	11,3
	Total	2122	609	28,6	471	22,2

Table 1. Seroprevalence of ITBB in human probands from different areas of Volyn oblast

http://dx.doi.org/10.5772/54912

The same districts had on the average 1,6 times higher level of the specific antibodies among the group of high professional risk (forestry workers), which was anticipated. This can be expained by the permanent being in natural foci, they contact with infected ticks more often (table 2). The antibodies were detected in 129 out of 281 (45,9 %) of the screened persons.

№	Districts	Total of observed patients	Found positive:	
			n	%
1	Kivertsi	46	29	63,0
2	Kovel skyi	74	25	33,8
3	Manevychi	21	9	42,8
4	Ratne	39	24	61,5
5	Rozhyshche	65	26	40,0
6	Staro-Vyzhva	36	16	44,4
	Total	281	129	45,9

Table 2. Seroprevalence of ITBB in human risk groups from different areas of Volyn oblast

4.3. Epidemiology

Upon observation of 1117 patients from 15 administrative districts of Volyn oblast, who were suspected of having ITBB or diagnosis which don' t exclude it (primarily with the preliminary diagnosis of TBVE), the antibodies to *B. burgdorferi s. l.* in diagnostic titres (1:100-1:1600) were detected in 267 (23,9 %) (table 3).

№	Districts	Number of patients*	Antibodies found:		Range of morbidity**
			n	%	
1	Volodymyr-Volynskyi	34	5	14,7	3,9
2	Gorokhiv	20	3	15,0	1,9
3	Ivanychi	76	11	14,5	3,7
4	Kamin-Kashyrsk	18	2	11,1	2,7
5	Kivertsi	150	21	19,0	3,6
6	Kovel	127	28	22,0	3,5
7	Lokachi	19	3	21,4	4,4
8	Lutsk yi (incl. Lutsk city)	262	92	35,1	5,3
9	Liubeshiv	18	3	16,7	8,3
10	Liuboml	14	3	21,4	7,5
11	Manevychi	31	5	16,1	2,3
12	Ratne	225	72	32,0	12,6
13	Rozhysche	62	7	11,3	4,3
14	Staro-Vyzhva	14	2	14,3	3,2
15	Shatsk	47	7	14,9	5,9
Total		1117	267	23,9	2,1

* - number of patients observed with the fever and a tick bite

** - range of morbidity (mean for 2000-2011 year, per 100 000 population)

Table 3. Results of serologic revealtion of ITBB patients in Volyn oblast

According to the data of clinically-epidemiological survey of 267 laboratory-confirmed cases, we determined the main clinical manifestations and epidemiologic peculiarities of ITBB.

Almost 80 % (77,9 %) of the patients experienced the tick bite or "unknown insect's bite", which preceded the development of the disease. The incubative period in the course of tick borrelioses lasted 10 days on the average-from 3 to 45 days.

Seasonal character of tick borrelioses - spring-summer, which responds to the period of seasonal activity of *I. ricinus* ticks. First cases are reported in April, peak of prevalence (45,0 %) is observed in June, July and August, the latest new cases come out in November. Thus the season of the highest risk of infectioning lasts for 6-8 months - from April to November. If we compare encephalitis and tick-brome borreliosis, we can see that the cases of ITBB (up to 14-15 %), are reported in winter and early spring, but this is related to the clinical manifestations of 2-3 stages of the disease (fig. 4).

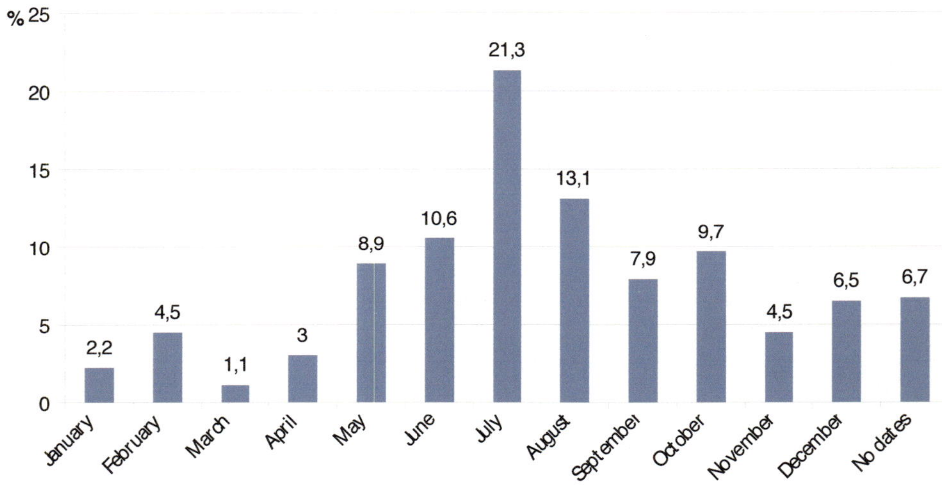

Figure 4. Seasonal distribution of ITBB cases in Volyn oblast, 2000-2011 (n= 267)

Within the structure of patients with the laboratory confirmed diagnosis of ITBB there prevailed the residents of big and small towns of the region - 58,1 % (154), rural population's part made 41,9 % (111). The zones of major infectioning were forest zones and forest-park zones attached to them. Seventy cases of infectioning occurred within the rural/countryside areas (26,2 %). There was a new phenomena in the science of epidemiology observed - a considerable urbanization of natural foci: 13,1 % of patients were infected on the territory of recreation zones (parks, natural relax zones, gardens, etc) of oblast's center - Lutsk city as well as districts' centers. In fact, we have ample evidence to claim that there are not natural foci, but anthropurgic and transient foci of ITBB and other TBI on the territory of Volyn oblast.

Within the gender structure of patients male made 40,2 %, female - 59,8 %.

All age groups were found vulnerable to ITBB - from the age of 1,2 to 80 years old people. Children below 10 and senior citizens (above 60) get sick less often - 9,0 % and 9,8 % (5 persons) respectively (fig. 5). Age risk group is the one of adult working age, 31-60 years old (52,7 % of cases, 141 persons).

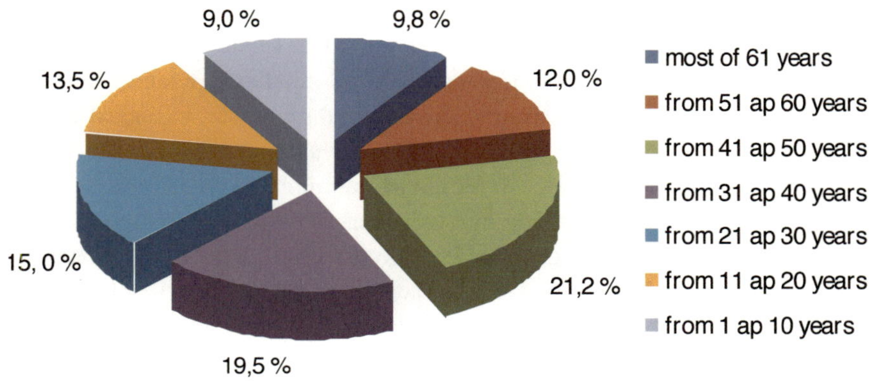

Figure 5. ITBB cases by age in Volyn oblast, 2000-2011 (n= 267)

Concerning the socially-professional structure of the disease, the highest risk of infectioning (62,2 %) was detected among office and labour workers, pensioners and unemployed.

4.4. Clinical manifestations

The spectrum of the main clinical manifestations was analysed according to the reported cases and was found typical for ITBB (table 4).

Clinical manifestations	Detection rates:		
	Volyn oblast		Ukraine
	n	%	%
ME	156	58,4	64,9
Syndrome of total infectioning	182	68,2	43,3
Nervous system lesions	86	37,0	21,4
Locomotor system lesions	56	21,0	24,1
Heart lesions	23	8,6	8,3

Table 4. Frequency and spectrum of ITBB clinical manifestations

The initial clinical manifestation of the disease was erythema migrans (58,4 %) and a syndrome of total infectioning (68,2 %).

A heart pathology was observed in 8,6 % of patients. Ischemic disease, myocarditis and pericarditis etc were diagnosed in regard to the cardio-vascular lesions.

On the other hand, in more than 20 % of the patients the course of the disease was characterised by the manifestations of locomotor system, the lesions of joints (arthritis, arthralgia) and periarticular tissues (bursitis, synovitis, plexitis).

Neurologic lesions, which are considered to be as prevalent lesions in the course of ITBB as erythema migrans in Europe [4], were observed in 37,0 % of patients, which is 16 % more than in Ukraine on the whole. Thus, according to the accumulative data, in regard to the clinical manifestations in the country on the whole, locomotor system lesions take the second place, after erythema migrans, and make 24,1 %. While in Volyn oblast the second most prevalent manifestation is neuroborreliosis. Taking into consideration the known fact, that there is an ethiologic mutual dependence between some genotypes of a causative agent and nozologic types of ITBB [15, 16], it can be assumed that the considerable prevalence of the patients with nervous system lesions can be caused by the prevalence of *B. garinii* within the spectrum of *B. burgdorferi s. l.*, which is believed to be the cause of neuroborreliosis.

On the acute stage of the disease, among the main manifestations of neuroborreliosis there were lesions of both peripheric nervous system (migrating pains, mono- and polyneuritis of scull nerves, polyradiculoneuritis, lack of skin sensitivity of a local character, paresthesia, relapsing neuritis of a facial nerve), which appeared mostly on the acute stage of the disease, and of central nervous system - manifested by meningitis, encephalitis, meningoencyphalitis, arachnoiditis, rigidity of neck muscles, nausea, headache, which manifested on the second stage of ITBB development. It has to be noted that in Ukraine, the major part of complicated lesions of the central nervous system in the course of ITBB is mainly observed in three oblasts – Volyn, Kherson and Zaporizzya.

On the second stage of Lyme Borreliosis the lesions of a cerebral cortex were manifested by different encephalopathia (9,5 %), such as speech problems, coordination, sleep, sight, memory, short-term black-outs. In a part of the patients (3,43 %) we were observing the signs of astheno-neurotic syndrome, such as often headaches, fatiguability, migrains, nervousness etc, some patients (1,47 %) had torpid paresis of facial muscles, in some rare case (0,49 %) the epileptic syndrome developed.

Cerebrospinal fluid has lymphocitaric pleocitosis, number of cells - dozens and hundreds in 1 mkl; lymphocitis make 70-100 % of total amount of cells, quite often, especially in the course of meningoradiculitis, there is an increase in protein amount - sometimes more than 1-2 mmol/l.

4.5. Neurologic manifestations with or without a erythema migrans

The peculiar feature of neuroborreliosis in Volyn oblast is the lack of the migratory erythema at the initial stage of the disease in 81,4 % of patients, which approximately equals the number for Ukraine - 80,9 %, and also the manifestations of total infectioning syndrome - hyperthermia, fatigness, dizzyness in 21,4% (for Ukraine on the whole - 24,1 %).

Overall, the analysis of the clinical course of non-erythemic forms of ITBB and comparing it to erythemic forms, shows that the course of the former was more complicated with the involvement of infectioning of other organs and systems, than that of the latter (fig. 6.)

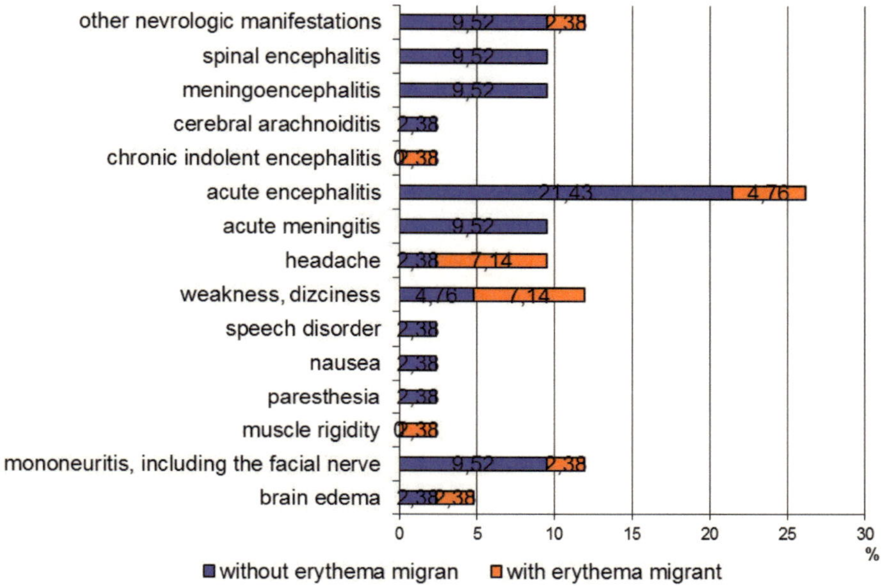

Figure 6. Spectrum of neurological manifestation in patient of erythemic and non-erythemic forms.

There were observed certain differences such as the syndrome of total infectioning with higher and continuous fever, which needs to be confirmed by a larger studies. The symptoms as the headache and dizcyness were observed 1,5 times more often, syndrome asthenovegetative-1,3 times more often.

As for the gender structure, male prevailed and made 53,5 %, while the part of female was 46,5 %. The age of patients was fluctuating of 1,2 up to 80 years, but neurology pathology was observed in children under 10 (18,6 %), teenagers (16,3 %) more often, while the largest group (40,7 %) was made of the persons of working age: 31-40 (25,6 %) and 41-50 (15,1 %) years old.

Up to 50 % of the patients with the borreliosis lesions of the nervous system were sick in the period June-October after the incubatory period, that lasted from few days to few weeks.

Taking into consideration the neuroborreliosis manifestations (neurologic lesions) observed in one third of the patients, we conducted a target serologic examination for ITBB of the patients of out-hospital departments of Volyn oblast. In the course of the examination of 107 patients with the neurologic lesions (hemyparesis, paresthesia, myalgia), the antibodies to Borrelias were detected in 20 (28,9 %), among them 10 cases (27,9 %) - had it in higher titres.

In some patients (6,86 %), the course of the disease and the character of neurologic manifestations (acute outset, temperature reaction, rigidity of neck muscles, fading of reflexes, inflammation of CLS, etc), Lyme Borreliosis was very similar to TBVE, especially in its encephalopoliomyelitic manifestations, which lead to the preliminary diagnosis of TBVE, which was not confirmed by the further serologic tests. Similar indicators of the disease are observed in some regions of Russia [17], but are manifested very rarely in patients from other countries.

4.6. Mixed infections of TBVE-ITBB

The presence of causative agents of different diseases (TBVE, ITBB, HGA) in parazyte systems, common vectors (*I. ricinus* and *D. reticulatus* ticks) and host-reservoirs (*Myodes glareolus* and *Sorex araneus* etc) with certain residing areas of each, predetermine similarities in epidemiologic structure of these infections. It is proved that one ixodid tick can contain 5-7 pathogenes at the same time [18]. The main social factors, predetermining the main features of TBVE, ITTB and HGA are also similar. Given all these facts, it may cause regular simultaneous infectioning of people with several causative agents.

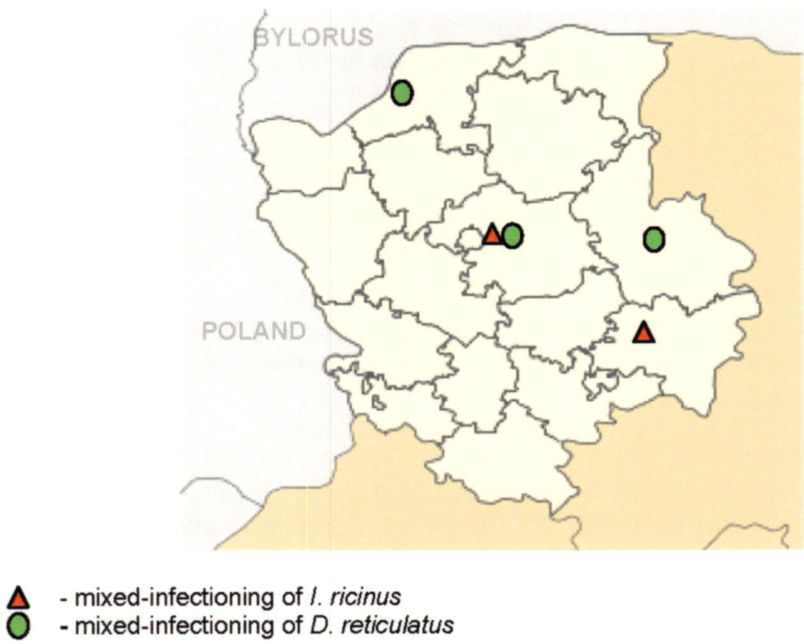

Figure 7. Connected natural foci of ITBB and TBVE in Volyn oblast

Retrospective analysis showed that the considerable part of cases with the preliminary diagnosis of TBVE, was, in fact, the cases of neuroborreliosis, including mixed infections of TBVE and neuroborreliosis.

http://dx.doi.org/10.5772/54912

In Volyn oblast, we got the evidence of the existance of territory-connected natural foci of ITBB and TBVE for 6 districts (fig. 7). The existance of population-connected foci of these two zoonoses is proven by cases of mixed-infectioning of *I. ricinus* ticks with TBE virus and *Borrelia burgdorferi s. l.*, which we detected in Kovel and Kivertzi districts, and *D. reticulatus* ticks - in Manevychi, Ratne and Kovel districts.

On the territory of oblast out of 267 cases of ITBB 29 (10,9 %) appeared to be TBVE mixed infection: the majority of them were found in Ratne (18) and Lutsk (8) rayons, few of them in Kivertzi (2), Kovel (1), Lyubeshiv (1) and Shatsk (1) districts [19].

5. Conclusions

1. North-West region of Ukraine is one of the regions with high prevalence of TBVE and ITBB.

2. There are an active natural foci of TBVE and ITBB in Ratne district of Volyn oblast. High epidemic potential is confirmed by isolation of TBE virus strains, detection of the antigen of a causative agent in vectors and reservoirs, as well as by a population morbidity.

3. We found the evidence to confirm the previously made hypothesis as for the existance of polivector (binar) TBVE and ITBB foci in Ukraine, where the circulation of the causative agent is done by two dominating species of *ixodids* - *Ixodes ricinus* and *D. reticulatus*, which makes the risk of a population infectioning higher. The range of vertebral-reservoirs of causative agents of Lyme Borreliosis and TBVE, includes not only those known in Europe, but also other species of small mammals.

4. The TBVE incidence manifests itself by regular sporadic cases of the disease and outbreaks. In terms of clinical manifestations, there dominate forms with total-infectioning with the non-malignant course of the disease (60 %). Meningeal forms make 24 %, meningo-encephalitic -16 %.

5. ITBB is an endemic disease for Volyn oblast, caused by the presence of *I. ricinus* and *D. reticulatus* ticks there. High prevalence rates are reported in Kivertsi, Lutsk, Manevychi, Ratne, Rozhysche districts, were 16,7 % up to 25 % of ticks are infected with the ITBB causative agent, the rates of population contact with ticks is within 30-40 %, risk group makes 40-60 %, mean indicator of the incidence (based on many years of surveillance) is 0,39-4,33 per 100 000 population.

6. The range of clinical manifestations of ITBB includes most of symptoms, which are described in scientific literature: starting from the erythema migrans, and syndrome of total infectioning to nervous system lesions, as well as lesions of locomotor and cardiovascular system. The distinctive feature of the manifestations of the acute form of the disease is high prevalence of non-erythemic forms (41,6 %) as well as high percentage of cases with nervous system involvement (37,0 %).

7. There were numerous combined natural tick-borne mixed infections foci detected: TBVE, ITBB, HGA. First time in Ukraine, there were cases of all possible combinations of mixed infections of these nosologic forms found.

8. The findings of our study serve as a theoretic base for the surveillance over the extremely dangerous natural foci infections in the country, implementation of anti-epidemic and preventive measures into the practice of a health care system, search for the new approach to diagnostic, prevention and treatment of these infectious diseases.

Author details

I. Lozynski[1], H. Biletska[1], O. Semenyshyn[1], V. Fedoruk[1], O. Drul[1], I. Ben[1], A. Shulgan[1] and R. Morochkovski[2]

1 State Institution "Lviv Research Institute of Epidemiology and Hygiene Ministry of Health of Ukraine", Lviv, Ukraine

2 Infections Hospital of Volyn oblast, Lutsk, Ukraine

References

[1] Gerenchuk, K. Nature of Volyn oblast. Lviv: Vyscha shkola; (1975).

[2] Tatarinov KVertebrate Fauna of the Western Ukraine. Lviv: Lviv University, (1973).

[3] Vynograd, I, Biletska, H, & Lozynski, I. Tick-borne encephalitis and other arboviruses infections in Ukraine. Infectious Diseases (1996). , 1996(4), 9-13.

[4] Gratz, N. (2005). Vector-borne infectious diseases in Europe, *WHO Regional Office for Europe*. Retrieved from: http://www.euro.who.int/pubrequest.

[5] Enzootics territories with especially dangerous natural-focal infectious diseases in Ukraine and measures of their preventionInformation letter of the Ministry of Health of Ukraine, Kyiv. (2011).

[6] Fedoruk, V. I, Pidoprygora, R. I, Shman, M. Y, & Valovenko, G. Hondoga A.I., Lozynskyi I.M. Features ecology of the virus of tick-borne encephalitis in the Polissya region: proceedings of the Materials of scientific practical conference "Actual problems of control of especially dangerous and guided infections in Ukraine", May 2004, Lviv, Ukraine. Lviv: Kolir Pro Servis; (2004).

[7] Lozynskiy, I. Arbovirusses and arboviral infections in forest-step zone inUkraine. Microbiology Journal (1998). , 60

[8] Pavlikovska, T. Sytuation of TBE in Ukraine since 1955 to 2010 years: proceedings of the Materials of ukrainian seminar on the current issues of surveillance of viral and especially dangeruos infections, (2011). Sumy, Ukraine.

[9] Biletska, H. V, Semenyshyn, O. B, Ben, I. I, Fedoruk, V. I, Drul, S, Shulgan, A. M, Sholomey, V, Rogochiy, E. G, & Lozynskiy, I. M. Actual tick-borne natural focal infections in Ukraine // National Scientific Conference "Natural focal infections", May 2012, Uzhgorod, Ukraine. Ternopil:Ukrmedknyha; (2012).

[10] Lozynskyi IBiletska H.V., Semenyshyn O.B., Fedoruk V.I., Drul O.S., Maretc' L.I., Sholomey M.V. Features of epidemiology and clinival manifestations of arboviral infections in Western oblasts of Ukraine: proceedings of the Materials of scientific practical conference "Modern problems of epidemiology, microbiologe and hygiene". May 2008, Lviv, Ukraine. Lviv: Kolir Pro Servis; (2008).

[11] Vynograd, I. A, Berezovskiy, S, & Biletska, H. V. Lozynskyi I.M. Outbreak of tick-borne encephalitis in Volyn oblast: proceedings of XIII Congress of the Ukrainian Society of microbiologists, epidemiologists and parasitologists named D.K.Zabolotnyi "Actual problems of microbiology, epidemiology, parasitology and prevention of infection disease", (1996). Vinnica, Ukraine.

[12] Morochkovski, R. Clinical characteristics of tick-borne encephalitis in Volyn' and optimization of treatment: PhD thesis, State establishment "Lev Gromashevsky Institute of Epidemiology and Infectious diseases of Academy of Medical Sciences of Ukraine", Kyiv, (2003).

[13] Biletska, H, Lozynskiy, I, Drul, O, Semenyshyn, O, Ben, I, Shulgan, A, & Fedoruk, V. Natural focal transmissible infections with neurological manifestations in Ukraine. Flavivirus Encephalitis. Dr. Daniel Ruzek (Ed.), 978-9-53307-669-0InTech, Avialable from:http://www.intechopen.com/books/flavivirus-encephalitis/natural-focal-transmissible- infections-with-neurological-manifestations-in-ukraine.

[14] Biletska, H. V. Lozynskyi I.M., Semenyshyn O.B., Morochkovska H.V., Morochkovski R.S.,Kozlovskiy M.M., Drul O.S., Rogochiy E.G., Sholomey M.V., Bon' O.S., Kinah A.A., Berezovskiy S.O. Identification and study of Lyme disease in Volyn' oblast. Infectious Diseases (2003). , 2003(4), 53-56.

[15] Lindgren, E. T, & Jaenson, G. Lyme borreliosis in Europe: influences of climate and climate change, epidemiology, ecology and adaptation measures:- Copenhagen: World Health Organization, (2006). http://www.euro.who.int.

[16] Ornstein, K, Berglund, J, Bergstrom, S, et al. Three major Lyme Borrelia genospecies (Borrelia burgdorferi s.s., B. afzelii and B.garinii) identified by PCR in cerebrospinal fluid from patients with neuroborreliosis in Sweden. Scand. J. Infect. Dis. (2002). , 5-341.

[17] Lobzin, Y. V, Uskov, A. N, & Kozlov, S. S. Lyme borreliosis (Ixodic tick-borne borreliosis). St-Peterburg. Foliant; (2000).

[18] Danielová, V, Rudenko, N, Daniel, M, et al. Extension of Ixodes ricinus ticks and agents of tick-borne diseases to mountain areas in the Czech Republic. Int. J. Med. Microbiol. (2006). , 48-53.

[19] Biletska, H. V. Lozynskyi I.M., Semenyshyn O.B., Fedoruk V.I., Rogochiy E.G., Drul O.S., Sholomey M.V., Ben' I.i., Yanko N.V., Yatcyna M.D., Gnatyuk O.Y., Kuznetcova H.S., Begal' I.I. Associates natural foci of tick-borne infections in Volyn oblast: proceedings of the Materials of scientific practical conference "Modern problems of epidemiology, microbiologe and hygiene". May 2008, Lviv, Ukraine. Lviv Kolir Pro Servis: (2008).

Chapter 10

Japanese Encephalitis Virus: The Complex Biology of an Emerging Pathogen

Shailendra K. Saxena, Sneham Tiwari, Rakhi Saxena,
Asha Mathur and Madhavan P. N. Nair

Additional information is available at the end of the chapter

http://dx.doi.org/10.5772/54111

1. Introduction

Japanese encephalitis virus (JEV) is a flavivirus, which is an emerging threat globally, majorly being southern and Southeast Asia and Australia. Even though most JEV infections are asymptomatic, it is estimated that only 0.3% leads to disease causing and results in over 35,000 cases including 10,000 deaths annually worldwide, and remaining cases which somehow escape death produce permanent sequelae, proving to be as a persistent threat (Singh et al., 2012). The human infections caused by encephalitic flaviviruses are more often asymptomatic or they cause mild febrile illness but sometimes this low percentage of mild infection turns into a dangerous and life-threatening encephalitis. The conditions which support viral survival are concerned to both viral and host factors that allow virus entry from the blood into the central nervous system (CNS). Host factors play important role in disease susceptibility. Japanese encephalitis, caused by JEV which belongs to arthropod-borne virus family and transmitted through *Culex* mosquito, is centrally a pediatric disease which causes acute infection and inflammation of the brain. Historically, in 1817 JE was first identified in Japan, but the causative agent (JEV) was later isolated from a fetal human case in 1934 (Erlanger *et al.,* 2009). First report of JE in India was in 1955, and since then this deadly virus has engulfed thousands of lives and has shaken several economies. The total numbers of cases reported annually are about 35,000-50,000 (Zheng *et al.,* 2012). Out of these reported cases ~30-50 % patients suffer from neurological sequelae and ~20-40 % cases turn to be fatal (Nett *et al.,* 2009). The actual counts are still higher than reported due to lack of reach of technology and surveillance towards extreme rural areas, which contain more vulnerable and needy population. The natural cycle of JEV consists of pig-mosquito-pig or bird-mosquito-bird (van den Hurk *et al.,* 2009) circulation of virus. When an infected mosquito bites a healthy individual, it may lead to febrile illness or a severe meningoencephalomyelities illness which is life taking. The incidence of the disease intensifies in rainy season as the environment supports the viral growth because of temperature, moistness and dampness which are plus factors letting the virus to bloom and flourish (Saxena *et al.*, 2008) (Fig.1). Today the need is to fight against this reemerging virus by the aid of high level of immunization and therapeutic and preventive measures to slow down the spread of the disease amongst human population.

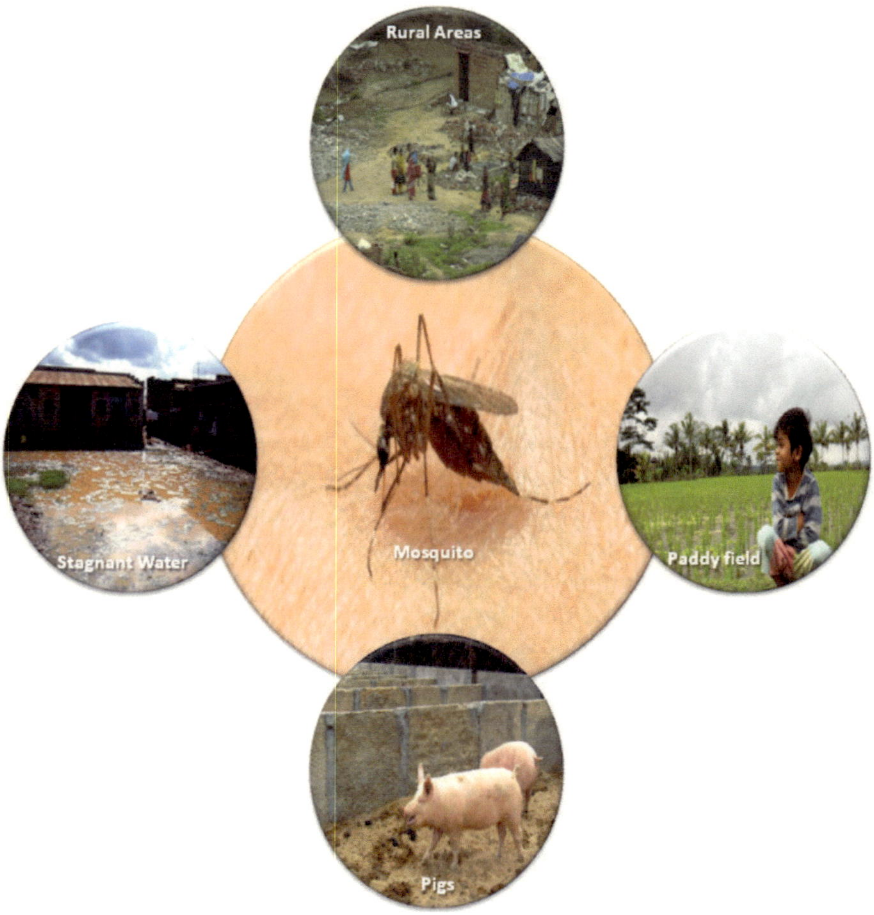

Figure 1. Displaying the contributing factors, which are responsible for the emergence and reemergence of JEV.

2. Genome of the virus

Japanese encephalitis virus belongs to the *Flaviviridae* family, it is an RNA virus measuring ~ 40-50 nm in diameter and structurally it is a spheroid having cubical symmetry. It is an en-

http://dx.doi.org/10.5772/54111

veloped virus having single stranded RNA as a genome which is infectious. The genome is of ~11kb with positive sense and a 5′ cap but it lacks a 3′ poly tail (Vashist et al., 2011). It contains nucleocapsid which is surrounded by a lipid envelope. The genomic RNA contains a single open reading frame (ORF) and codes for a polyprotein of ~3400 amino acids. This polyprotein is cleaved by viral and host proteases into 10 proteins. Structural genes are three in number and are involved in antigenicity since they are expressed on the virus coded by capsid protein and involved in capsid formation: core (C), pre membrane (prM) and envelope (E). Among all three the E gene is the most important and is the most studied one. There are seven non structural genes: NS1, NS2a, NS2b, NS3, NS4a, NS4b, NS5 (Fig.2) and these are involved in virus replication (Saxena et al., 2011). A novel mutation in domain II of the envelop gene of JEV circulating in North India has been reported (Pujhari et al., 2011). The high rate of mutation in JEV is due to RNA dependent RNA polymerase (RdRp) coded by NS5 (Neyts et al., 1999). JEV replicates exclusively in the cytoplasm of infected cells, in a perinuclear location, and matures on intracellular membranes.

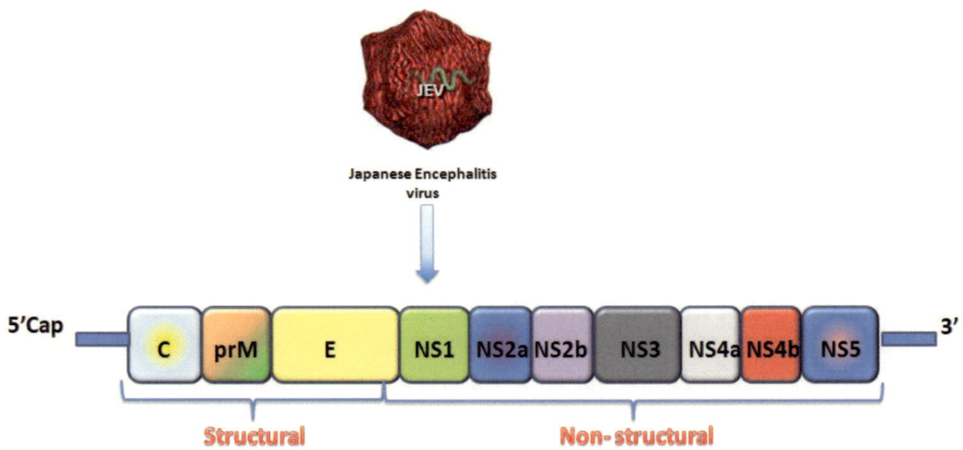

Figure 2. The genome of Japanese Encephalitis Virus, constituting the 3 Structural genes: C, prM, E and 7 Non-structural genes: NS1, NS2a, NS2b, NS3, NS4a, NS4b, NS5.

Japanese encephalitis (JE), caused by Japanese encephalitis virus (JEV), is the most important form of viral encephalitis in Asia. The epidemiology of JE has changed in the past 50 years and the area affected by JEV has expanded to India, China, Southeast Asia and Western Pacific regions. About 50, 000 cases and 10 000 deaths are reported in JEV-endemic areas among a population of 3 billion people. However, the true number is unknown, because most areas where JEV occurs lack diagnostic facilities. Most JEV infections are subclinical. JEV is a member of the JEV serological complex, which causes significant morbidity and mortality. Pigs are the most important biological amplifiers and reservoirs. Generally direct person to person spread of JEV does not or rarely occurs until it is through intrauterine transmission (Guy et al., 2010). Blood and organ transplantation also serve as a mode of transmission. JEV infection transmits from mother to foetus through vertical mode of transmission (Mathur et al., 1982). Symptomatic infections are usually present in the form of non-specific febrile illness, including diarrhoea and rigors followed by headache, vomiting and reduced levels of consciousness and aseptic meningitis or encephalitis. The incubation period after JEV exposure varies from 6 to 16 days (Saxena et al., 2009). One in 200/800 infected people develop clinical signs like high fever and nausea. A quarter of patients with symptoms die; a third of survivors suffer brain damage.

3. Epidemiology

Encephalitis outbreaks have been recorded since early 19th century from countries like Southeast Asia including Japan, Vietnam, Cambodia, Myanmar, India, Nepal, Malaysia, China, Korea, Taiwan, Thailand and reached to the West including Pakistan and the north-east and southwest of India, also the East (New Guinea), the South (Northern Australia Archipelago) and it is estimated theoretically to spread further West (Afghanistan). Between 1978 and 1992, 24 imported cases were reported in above regions due to high transmission. Since the 1990s, the JE is variedly transmitting in humans and is reaching new extended regions encompassing new geographic limits. History tells that a woman in France suffered from JE after she reached Thailand, in 1938. Also JE epidemic was reported in restricted sea-coast of the 'USSR' in 1939. Also in 1946 major outbreaks of JE were recorded in Korea, both in civil in 1949 and in American military personnel in 1950.

Sequencing analysis divides JEV into five genotypes (GI–V) rising from ancestor viruses from Indonesia–Malaysia region. These ancestors have evolved into five genotypes; GI, GII, GIII, GIV and GV, out of them GIV and GV are the most divergent. They always remained confined to their origin region of Indonesia–Malaysia. However GI, GII and GIII are the most recent genotypes which have spread across Asia. All phylogenetic characterization and studies done on a large scale highlights GIII as a predominant genotype of JEV in Japan and Korea since 1935 (Schuh et al., 2009). GI was been isolated in Cambodia and then in China in 1979 and GIII was isolated before the 1970s and then in Vietnam and Japan during 1986 and 1990. Later even GI was reported there in 1995 and 2002 proving that all the strains isolated before 1991 were GIII, and after 1994 were GI. The natural cycle of JEV consists of pig-mosquito-pig or bird-mosquito-bird cycles. GIII was the only widely distributed genotype found in India until till when GI JEV strains were detected and isolated from 66 acute encephalitis syndrome (AES) patients along with GIII strains (Fulmali et al., 2011). This detection indicates their co-circulation and association with humans. In the mid 1990's genetic shift (Nabeshima et al., 2009) had occurred in Japan, Korea and Vietnam that lead to disappearance of GIII and then progressively GI supplanted it (Zhang et al., 2011). In India exact mode of introduction of GI is not clear, but it is possible that it may have been introduced through migratory birds (Huang et al., 2010).

JEV is basically transmitted by *Culex spp* mosquitoes. JEV is distributed in temperate and tropical areas of eastern and southern Asia. Its range has extended from eastern Asia (China, Japan, Korea, maritime Siberia, Taiwan, the Philippines, and Vietnam), to Southeast Asia and northern Australasia (Cambodia, Indonesia, Laos, Malaysia, Papua New Guinea, Thailand, and the Torres Strait islands of northern Australia), and to southern Asia (Bangladesh, Bhutan, India, Myanmar, Nepal, and Sri Lanka) (Fig. 3). Evidences have also been seen for Pakistan. JE is largely a disease of rural areas, especially associated with irrigated rice agriculture. During endemics, no seasonal pattern exists and sporadic cases of encephalitis occur throughout the year, most often in infants and young children. There is a peak in vector density and virus activity during October-December in endemic zones. However, epidemic activity in temperate and subtropical areas occurs most commonly in summer and early autumn (van den et al., 2009).

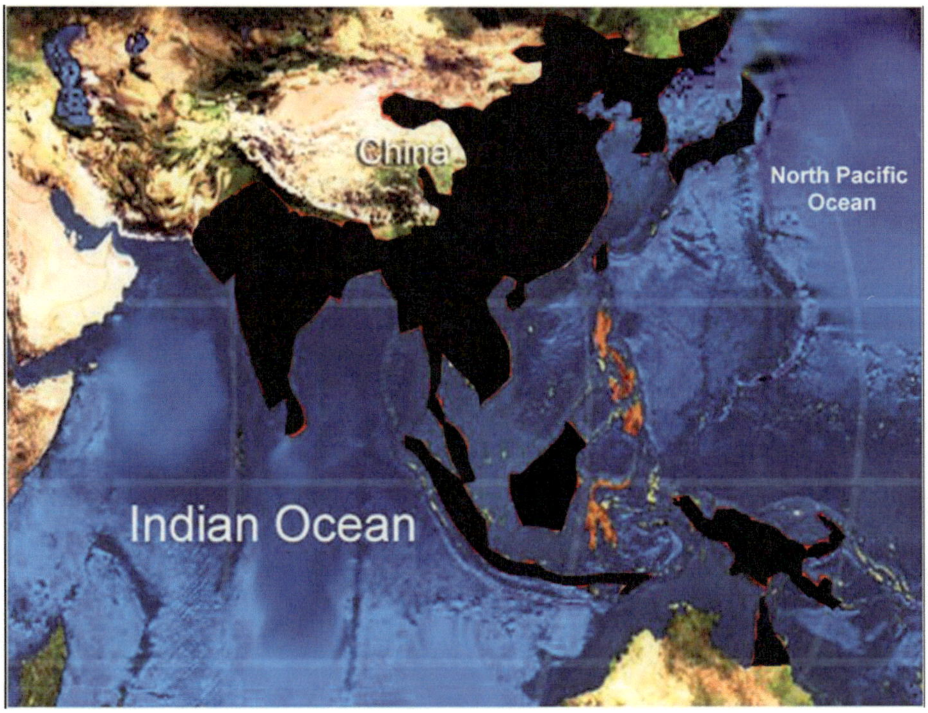

Figure 3. Epidemiology of JE globally. The areas highlighted in black display the regions under the attack of JEV infections and are high infection prone areas.

From past 75 years the major focus of JE coverage was on China and Southeast Asia, but now it has extended its horizons to westward towards India and Pakistan, northern to eastern Russia, eastward towards Philippines and southward to Australia. Occurrence of JE is more closely related to temperature and humidity in the atmosphere (Misra and Kalita, 2010). JEV is also engulfing new geographical regions which are shown by JEV sequencing analysis and results exhibit that JEV is expanding alarmingly to the new regions of Papua New Guinea and Australia. GI strains are often isolated from Northern Thailand, Cambodia, Korea, China, Japan, Vietnam, Taiwan and Australia between 1967 and the present. GII are isolated from Southern Thailand, Malaysia, Indonesia, Papua

New Guinea and Northern Australia. GIII are isolated from temperate regions of Asia. GIV are isolated in Indonesia and GV is isolated in Singapore. Sequence analyses of viral genes are further showing that a "genotype shift" from III to I has occurred in Japan since early 1990s, reasons for which remains unclear (Shimojima et al., 2011). Considering India, rapid spread of Japanese encephalitis (JE) towards the newer areas of northern states of India is also reported (Saxena et al., 2006, 2009).

4. JEV: Infectious agents

The genomic RNA of JEV is ~11 kb in length encoding three structural proteins and seven non-structural proteins. The RNA genome of the virus is infectious which can spread the horizon of disease. The virus genome contains C proteins complexed with the genomic RNA present in a nucleocapsid, and this whole complex is surrounded by enveloped lipid bilayer containing E and prM/M proteins, which is derived from the infected host cells. The prM proteins present in the immature particles, cleave to mature into M proteins. The E protein is the major infectious part which covers the entire surface of the mature virion, and it is the antigen majorly recognized by virus neutralizing antibodies. Further, subviral particles (SVPs), containing prM/M and E proteins enclosed in lipid layers but not surrounded by nucleocapsid, are secreted from flavivirus infected cells, proving these SVPs to be as excellent immunogens. Along with infective E protein, even NS1 protein is also considered as quite infective which may cause lethal effects to hosts when produced and expressed in large quantities. If antiNS1 immunity steps are taken and cytolytic antibodies against NS1 are administered, it would contribute in the reduction of the release of progeny viruses from infected cells. Hence a drug with a mixture of antiE and antiNS1 immunity would definitely pose as a potent fighter against flavivirus infection (Ishikawa et al., 2011).

5. Transmission of disease

JE virus undergoes zoonotic cycles which involve mosquitoes and several vertebrate species as hosts and human beings as dead end hosts. *Culex tritaeniorhyncus* and *Culex gelidus* are reported as principal vectors. These vectors breed in rice fields, irrigation canals and water pools filled with stagnant water and in standing puddles, open sewers, fish ponds etc. These infected mosquitoes (~3%) bite domestic animals and birds, but sometimes they may bite a healthy host (human), which are accidental hosts, facilitating the transmission of the virus to man. Pigs and birds serve as reservoirs and amplifying hosts. Man is an incidental host of the JEV (Fig. 4). In humans, after a bite of infected mosquito, initial viral replication occurs in local and regional lymph nodes. Viral invasion of the central nervous system occurs probably via blood causing infection and subsequent illness.

http://dx.doi.org/10.5772/54111

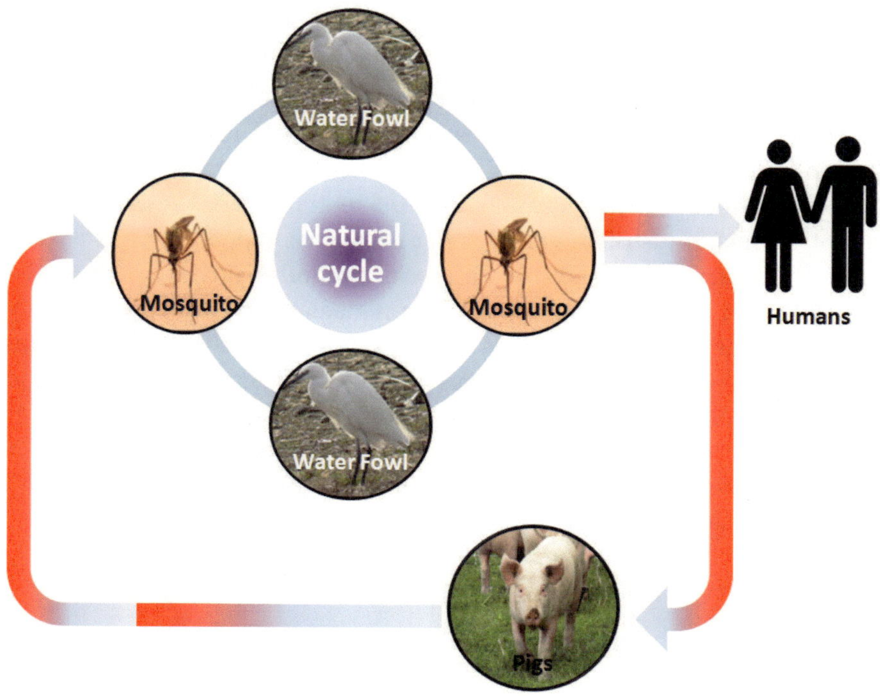

Figure 4. Life cycle of JEV crossing through important vectors and intermediate hosts and finally to dead end reservoirs human hosts.

6. Pathogenesis and pathology

The majority of human infections with encephalitic flaviviruses are asymptomatic or give rise to only a mild febrile illness. However, in a small percentage of infected individuals the mild infection turns into life-threatening encephalitis. Thus, a key question in the pathogenesis of encephalitic flaviviral disease concerns the conditions that allow virus entry from the blood into the central nervous system (CNS). Hypertension, diabetes mellitus, and coinfection with other virus may further deteriorate the infection and can worsen the condition of infected persons by increasing neurological complications which may happen due to facilitation of virus across the blood–brain barrier (Singh et al., 2009). Histological examination shows that virus can affect neurons present in thalamus and brain. Viral antigen is later gets cleared from there due to the induction of adaptive immune. A strong virus-specific antibody response, in CNS may act for recovery from encephalitic infection. Clinical infections with the mosquito-borne encephalitic flaviviruses in humans mostly occur in the absence of detectable viremia consistent with the notion that humans are dead-end hosts in the natural transmission cycle (Müllbacher et al., 2003).

Japanese encephalitis (JE) is now the foremost cause of viral CNS infection. JEV pathogenesis is still unclear (Yang *et al.,* 2011). Since the variation exists in neuro-virulence and peripheral pathogenicity among JE virus strains. After the infected mosquito bite, the virus enters into the reticulo-endothelial system and invades the central nervous system after the transient period of viremia. It distributes itself in hypothalamus, hippocampus, substantia nigra and medulla oblongata regions of brain via vascular endothelial cells by the mechanism of endocytosis which involves cholesterol and clathrin mediated pathways, referred to as lipid rafts acting as portals for virus entry (Das et al., 2010). The virus replicates in neurons and matures in the neuronal secretary system. Nearly 33% of JE infected patients die due to neurocysticercosis (NCC), suggesting that it may somehow predispose to JE (Desai et al., 1997). During acute stages congestion, edema, hemorrhagic symptoms are found in brain. Pathological changes in the neural tissues have also been reported in lymphoid organs and immune cells such as spleen and kupffer cells respectively.

7. Immune response

The pathogenesis of the neurotropic flaviviruses like JEV, involves both virus-mediated damage and the host immune responses. After the mosquito bite, when the virus is inoculated in the host, it replicates in skin dendritic cells, and then is transported to lymph nodes, from where it spreads to peripheral organs, enhancing the viremia. Entry into CNS is an important event which aids viral encephalitis [9]. Roles of both the innate and adaptive immune responses in controlling flaviviral infection are important. IgM and IgG are involved in preventing viral dissemination to the CNS, however CD8+ T cells are important for recovery and immunopathological phases of viral infection.

Infection with flavivirus triggers the host's innate immunity, resulting in signalling pathways and production of interferons (IFN) which are secretory cytokines produced as a response against viral infection. When these IFN bind to the cell-surface receptors, Jak–Stat signaling pathway is activated which in turn induces the transcription of interferon-stimulated genes (ISGs), and the resulting products have potent antiviral, antitumor, and immunomodulatory effects. To win against the IFN defence system, viruses encode viral proteins which are potent enough to block IFN signaling, via various mechanisms (Sen 2001, Weber et al., 2004) like blocking IFN action by preventing Tyk-2 phosphorylation by the production of NS5 protein of JEV (Lin et al., 2004; Lin et al., 2006;Liang et al., 2009).

http://dx.doi.org/10.5772/54111

8. Host immune responses

The virus enters the neuro-parenchyma by crossing capillary walls in the brain and distributes itself in various parts of brain. Initially JE virus is partially destroyed at its site of entry and the remaining virus is disseminated by local and systemic extra neural replication leading to viremia. After primary infection with JEV, presence of IgM antibodies and T-lymphocytes are seen until 2 weeks approximately. But antibodies alone are neither capable of terminating the viremia nor preventing the subsequent infection. Pregnancy is known to cause immunosuppression and persistent maternal infection or pregnancy induced reactivation of the virus which causes foetal infection. Isolation of JEV from human placenta and foetuses has been reported. JEV can establish latency within different organs despite the presence of antiviral antibodies. A significant decrease in serum iron levels, a frequent feature of microbial invasion is observed during JE infection. An early influx of macrophages followed by neutrophils at the site of injury in different organs of humans and mice has been reported, which is correlated with the production of a neutrophil chemotactic macrophage derived factor MDF, with development of hypoglycemia. This chemotactic protein (MDF) has been shown to play a protective role in the host defense against JEV, through production of reactive oxygen intermediates in neutrophils and reactive nitrogen oxide species degrading the virus protein and RNA (Tiwari et al., 2012).

The earliest host response to viral infection is the induction of IFN. Type I IFNs, IFN-α and β are produced by leukocytes and fibroblasts, respectively, in response to infection and activate the transcription of a host of IFN inducible genes that leads to the induction of antiviral pathways. IFN-α has important immunoregulatory functions including the activation of monocytes, enhancement of chemokine expression and MHC class I and II induction. Most of the antiviral activity of IFN-α is mediated by NO radicals synthesized by monocytic phagocytes, mortality in JEV-infected mice increased when the activity of NO synthase was inhibited (Saxena et al., 2000, 2001) as NO blocks mechanism of viral RNA and protein synthesis (Müllbacher et al., 2003). Also natural killer (NK) cells are important part of the innate immune response which is activated at the viral invasion which helps in early defence as NK cells synthesize and regulate cytokines, necessary for adaptive immune response.

9. Adaptive immune response

The importance of humoral response in recovery from encephalitis is demonstrated by several studies showing that administration of antibody during early infection can protect against JE. Studies of the entry process of JEV using electron and confocal microscopy techniques showed that neutralizing mAb strongly inhibits JEV-induced fusion and internalization into cells, but not binding of virus to cells. T cells are of crucial importance for the recovery from most virus infections and individuals deficient in T cells are unable to control virus infections. T cells are necessary for recovery and protection after

JEV infection and also their depletion affects the humoral and cellular, immune defence against flavivirus infections (Müllbacher et al., 2003).

10. RNAi effect on JE

Inhibitory effect of RNAi on JEV replication has been thoroughly studied *in vitro* and *in vivo* (Murakami ET AL., 2005). It is also reported that defective interfering (DI) RNA aids in the persistence of JEV (Yoon et al., 2006). Effectiveness of using siRNA expression based vectors targeting the JEV NS5 gene to inhibit JEV replication, viral protein expression, and RNA levels of JEV E-protein is hot topic of research nowadays. Several studies demonstrate that shRNAs targeting the NS5 gene could specifically and efficiently inhibit JEV replication. Many researchers have shown that siRNA/shRNAs targeting the RdRP coding gene could efficiently inhibit viral replication; the inhibition of viral replication triggered by siRNA/ shRNA targeting of the RdRP gene are reported to be more efficient compared to other genes from the genome (Neyts et al., 1999). Therefore, the NS5 gene which is highly conserved among different strains is often employed as an RNAi target for different studies. shRNAs targeting NS5 gene in the JEV genome are shown to be capable of interfering with JEV replication with very high specificity and efficiency. Hence shRNAs could be used as a potential tool against JEV replication *in vitro*. More research investigating RNAi methodologies to prevent infection or reduce viremia is necessary which may lead to the development of antiviral compounds that are efficacious and inexpensive against Japanese encephalitis infections (Qi et al., 2008).

11. JAK-STAT pathway for JE

IFN-α and IFN-β, play important role in recovery from flaviviral infections. However, they fail sometimes due to ability of JEV to inhibit the JAK-STAT (Janus kinase signal transducer and activator of transcription) pathway (Lin et al., 2006). Studies of DEN-2 antagonism of STAT1 phosphorylation have revealed NS4B as the primary and important antagonist. Still the exact mechanism of IFN antagonism is under study. The specific receptor complex for each IFN-α and IFN-β is composed of two major subunits and several JAK tyrosine kinases constitutively associated with the receptor. Jak1 and Jak2 are required for IFN-α/β signaling. Following binding of the receptor subunits by IFN, the JAKs trans-phosphorylate each other and then phosphorylate critical tyrosine residues within the intracellular domains of the receptor subunits (Lin et al., 2004). These phosphorylated residues serve as recruitment sites for STAT proteins, which bind the activated receptor and are in turn phosphorylated by the JAKs. The phosphorylated STAT proteins then form homodimers, or heterodimers, with other STAT proteins and translocate to the nucleus, where they bind specific DNA sequences within the promoter regions of IFN-stimulated genes (ISGs) (Fig. 5). ISG expression induces an antiviral state within the cell, can modulate cell proliferation and cell death, and modulates immune responses via its roles in activation and maturation of antigen-presenting cells. The ability of the individual non-structural proteins to antagonize JAK-STAT signaling has been studied and results indicated that NS5 blocked STAT1 phosphorylation in response to either IFN-α or IFN-β which highlights the function of NS5 to have a critical role in virus pathogenesis (Best et al., 2005).

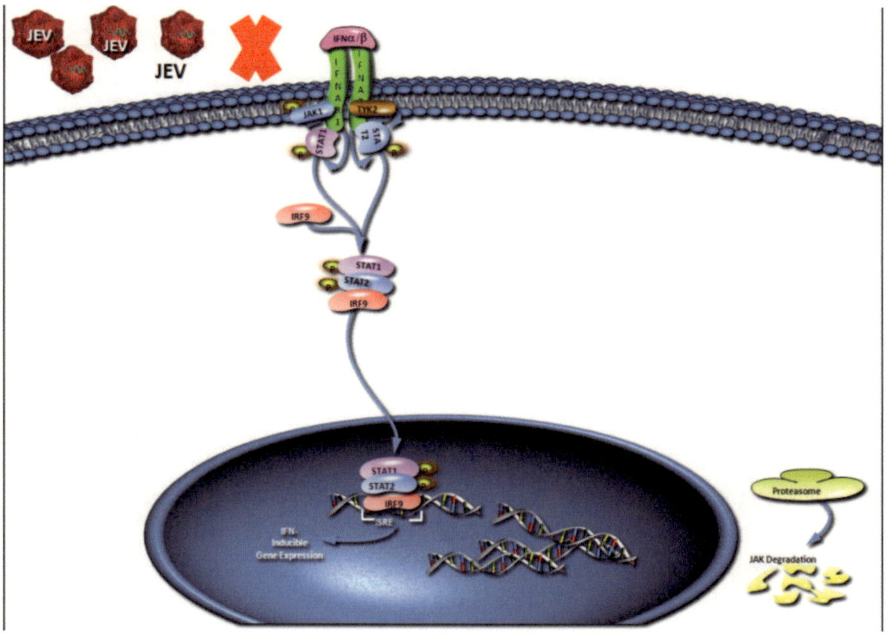

Figure 5. Displaying the JAK STAT Pathway. JAK STAT signaling pathway is important for transduction of information between cells carrying information for cellular differentiation and homeostasis. Cytokines and their receptors are the major activator of JAK/STAT pathway. IFN are antiviral cytokines produced by cells as soon as the onset of viral infection. IFN-α and IFN-β bind to different receptors and, play important role in recovery from flaviviral infections. However, they fail sometimes due to ability of JEV to inhibit the JAK-STAT pathway.

12. Diagnosis

Serology is an important tool for the diagnosis of JE since the virus is difficult to isolate from clinical samples. The hemagglutination inhibition assay also is used but it has practical limitations as it requires paired serum samples from the acute and convalescent phases. The IgM antibody capture ELISA for CSF and serum samples is currently the standard test for diagnosis of JE but still has the drawback of not being able to diagnose about the infection in early stage. Molecular methods using reverse-transcriptase (RT) - PCR techniques have proved to be highly effective for diagnosing infection by RNA viruses. JE viral genome sequences have been detected by RT-PCR in CSF from acute encephalitis cases from several places around the globes. The conventional RT-PCR has shown good specificity in the diagnosis of JEV in both blood and CSF samples but it has poor sensitivity as the virus is often cleared from the peripheral circulation/CSF by the time the test is performed. With the advent of monoclonal antibodies as potential diagnostic tool (Chávez *et al.*, 2010), the rapid detection of JE antigen in cerebrospinal fluid has become possible. The different diagnostic tests have been given in Table 2. However, the most rapid and potential diagnostic tool for JE diagnosis have been shown to be MAC-ELISA (Robinson *et al.*, 2010) and indirect fluorescent antibody. MRI of the brain can also be used in diagnosis. MRI changes can be co-related (Misra *et al.*, 2011) with the type of encephalitis and duration of illness.

13. Vaccines: Immunization against JE

Immunization against JE is cost effective strategy for control and prevention of JE. It has been reported globally that there is a decrease in incidence rates of JE in endemic areas which are administered with high immunization. The 3 most important types of JE vaccines, administered in current era are: the mouse brain derived, purified, inactivated vaccine based on either the Nakayama or Beijing strains of the JE virus; the cell culture derived inactivated JE vaccine based on the viral Beijing P3 strain and the cell culture derived live attenuated JE vaccine based on the SA 14-14-2 strain of the JE virus. In JEV infection, the immunity against prM, E and NS1 proteins is more effective than that of other viral proteins in host defense. (Gao et al., 2010). Currently available vaccines against JE include chemically inactivated vaccines (INV) and a live attenuated vaccine (LAV). Although a mouse brain derived INV produced by BIKEN had been the only internationally approved vaccine and has been used worldwide since the 1960s. But it had a drawback as there were reports of severe adverse events including acute disseminated encephalomyelitis (ADEM) in people vaccinated with it. In early 2009, Vero cell derived INVs produced by Intercell (Austria) and BIKEN (Japan) were licensed. Although these INVs are useful in developed markets, INVs are not ideally suited for nationwide vaccination programs for many endemic countries, since INVs require multiple doses to induce long lasting immunity. LAVs are thus a useful alternative and have been used for decades in China, and other Asian countries, but their substrate and the production methods have still not been approved in other markets, which serve as a drawback to this vaccine. (Ishikawa et al., 2011). Live-attenuated virus vaccines (LAVs) and inactivated virus vaccines (INVs) serve against flaviviral disease, they are potent and economical but do not suit immunocompromised patients. INVs are safer, but are more expensive to produce and less potent. Hence there is an immense need of devicing new and improved products.

Type I IFNs are critical for controlling pathogenic virus infections and can enhance immune responses. Hence their impact on the effectiveness of live-attenuated vaccines involves a balance between limiting viral antigen expression and enhancing the development of adaptive immune responses. The influence of type I IFNs on these parameters has been examined following immunization with RepliVAX WN, a single-cycle flavivirus vaccine (SCFV). Repli-

http://dx.doi.org/10.5772/54111

VAX WN-immunized mice produced IFN-α and displayed increased IFN-stimulated gene transcription (Winkelmann et al., 2012). Multiple vaccines exist to control Japanese encephalitis (JE), but all suffer from problems but this new flavivirus vaccine, a pseudoinfectious virus (RepliVAX WN) that expresses the JE virus (JEV) prM and E proteins prevents flaviviral disease. Engineered second-generation RepliVAX (RepliVAX JE.2) elicited neutralizing antibodies in experimental mice and provided 100% protection from a lethal challenge with JEV (Ishikawa et al., 2008).

Although a licensed vaccine has been available to prevent JE for over 40 years, approximately 20,000 cases are reported annually with 6000 resulting in death. Unfortunately, due to gaps in surveillance, the incidence of JE is also likely to be much higher than reported. A number of different vaccines are available to prevent JE and these have demonstrated an excellent record of efficacy throughout their history. The vaccine that has been in use the longest is the INV prepared from JEV infected mouse brains. This vaccine has been used extensively in East Asia since the 1960s to control JE, and is widely used throughout the world to immunize travellers who visit endemic areas, its protective efficacy is reported to be 80–90% in JEV endemic regions. But still it has a drawback that the product requires a three dose vaccination schedule in order to induce protective immunity and this, along with the recommendation of boosters every 2–3 years which poses as quite expensive for nominal patients from low income group countries and time-consuming too. Furthermore they are also reported for causing allergic reactions and more dangerous side effects like complications including severe neurological disorders such as acute disseminated encephalomyelitis, etc in people being administered by the vaccine (Widman et al., 2008).

Through vaccination in the last five year, JE has been effectively controlled and eliminated in China, Japan, Taiwan, and Korea (Chung et al., 2007; Takahashi et al., 2000; Jelinek et al., 2009). Second generation recombinant vaccines are also being developed, where genes encoding prM and E proteins are packed into vectors. DNA based JEV vaccines which may be very efficient against the virus are under clinical trials. DNAzymes cleave the RNA sequence of the 3′-NCR of JEV genome *in vitro*, on intra-cerebral administration in JE infected mice almost completely (Appaiahgari et al., 2007) and inhibit virus replication in the brain. Use of neutralizing bodies for vaccine designing may also serve the process.

14. Treatment, prevention and control

There is no specific treatment or anti-viral agent for JEV infection, it is proving to be a persistent threat. Monoclonal antibodies (Yamanaka et al., 2010), corticosteroids, interferonα-2a or ribavirin were not that effective in clinical outcome. The effect of rosamarinic acid (RA) has been shown as an effective anti-viral agent that reduces JE viral load along with proinflammatory cytokines in experimental animal. Neutrophils have been also shown to have degradative effect on JEV. Usage of anti-sense molecules (vivo-morpholino) directed against the viral genome, in combating the virus through inhibiting viral replication has been demonstrated (Nazmi et al., 2010). Mycophenolic acid (Sebastian et al., 2011) inhibits JE virus by inhibiting its replication.

Prevention methods are very important for minimizing JE infection (Saxena *et al.,* 2008). Childhood immunization is done by using inactivated mouse brain-derived vaccine which is based on either the Nakayama or Beijing strains of the JE virus, the cell culture derived, inactivated JE vaccine based on the Beijing P-3 strain ; and the cell cultures derived, live – attenuated vaccine based on the SA 14-14-2 strain (Halstead *et al.,* 2011) of the JE virus. Recombinant poxvirus vectors expressing the E and NS1 proteins of the JEV boosting a good immune response in mice models can be used as a vaccine. The prevention of vector –man contact is very good preventive method this can be done by eliminating potential mosquito breeding areas, environmental sanitation, waste water management by treating the water with larvicide either by *Gambusa* (larva-eating fish), drying and wetting of rice fields, frequent vaccination should be implemented, and as well as personal protective measures. Reports have shown that induction of nitric oxide synthase plays a protective role against JEV (Saxena *et al.,* 2001). Diethyldithiocarbamate has been also experimentally shown to inhibit JEV infection. Future predictions of the disease and drug designing can be enhanced by computer aided design databases, which can design *in silico* the most efficient drugs which can be tested experimentally and then can be clinically tried. For the development of appropriate and effective therapy there is an immediate need to understand host factors role in JEV –induced neuropathogenesis (Gupta *et al.,* 2011). Effective anti-viral drugs have yet to be found. Medicines are given mainly to relieve symptoms. Vaccination for people at risk, eliminate mosquito breeding grounds, improve drainage, maintain clean piggeries, use insect repellent and mosquito nets are some of the preventive measures which should be commonly undertaken.

The strategy for prevention and control of JE should include major components such as awareness among general public on the prevention and control of the disease, vector control and immunization. Environmental control is also one important factor as it has been studied that there is a positive impact of urbanization and economic development in the reduction of JE transmission, as clean and sanitized economies will not support environment necessary for mosquito breeding. Land areas under cultivation with impact of agrochemicals may work for reduction of vector density. Along with good environmental strategies vector control is also an important aspect. Maintenance of low vector densities is the need of hour.

Spraying, larviciding and aerial application are the method used for reduction of vector densities. However, alternatives to aerial application like spraying/fogging/Ultra Low Volume (ULV) application are also under consideration. Along with this long term i.e. non-chemical vector control such as water management is also helpful. Use of agrochemicals to control pests may have had indirect effect on vector control. Also, use of larvivorous fish may also be applicable in permanent water bodies. Personal protection is very important as vectors can feed on humans in outdoors, hence over vegetation and shaded humid places should be bit ignored. Minimizing outdoor activity for reducing the exposure time to mosquitoes and wearing long sleeved clothes are some habits needed to be undertaken consideration along with public information and awareness.

http://dx.doi.org/10.5772/54111

15. Conclusion and future implications

Viral encephalitis has proved to be a huge disaster globally, which has engulfed several lives and has shattered various economies. It has been a hot topic amongst the researchers today globally and various ways necessary to combat against the virus are on the way. Intense research for the knowabouts of the virus is carried in several countries, devising strategies to fight with the virus. As a result of severe efforts, JE has been virtually eliminated in most of the countries after the immunization with inactivated mouse brain-derived vaccine, during last four decades. Because of absence of treatment strategies personal protection is the only apt way to reduce disease incidence. Mosquito control is the sole available preventive measure for JEV transmission. Research on JEV needs to be initiated at much wider scale, which should include development of effective anti-viral agents and vaccine strategies. Immunization is needed in JE prone areas. Over use of the vaccines should be avoided otherwise the virus might develop resistance against drugs which are administered frequently. Quarantine checks should be done at international immigration and emigration points, to keep a check on the spread of virus via foreign travelers. Vector control program should be designed in a way that they can control the risk of vectors in an efficient way. General awareness camps should be organized in rural areas to spread alertness in the local population and confronting them with hygiene management and preventive measures. Systematic and combinatorial approach with the joint efforts of scientists, molecular biologists, doctors, drug developers, policy makers and local population is the need of hour. A high sense of urgency is required to address this matter.

Acknowledgements

Authors are grateful to Dr Ch. Mohan Rao, Director, Centre for Cellular and Molecular Biology (Council of Scientific and Industrial Research, India), for the encouragement and support for this work. NIH Awards (R37DA025576; R01MH085259) support S.K.S. and M.P.N.

Author details

Shailendra K. Saxena[1], Sneham Tiwari[1], Rakhi Saxena[1], Asha Mathur[2] and Madhavan P. N. Nair[3]

1 Centre for Cellular and Molecular Biology (CCMB–CSIR), Uppal, India

2 Department of General Pathology & Microbiology, Saraswati Medical & Dental College, Lucknow, India

3 Department of Immunology, Institute of NeuroImmune Pharmacology, Herbert Wertheim College of Medicine, Florida International University, Miami, USA

References

[1] Appaiahgari, M.B. and Vrati, S. (2007). "DNAzyme-mediated inhibition of Japanese encephalitis virus replication in mouse brain." *Mol Ther.* 15(9): 1593-1599.

[2] Best, S.M., Morris, K.L., Shannon, J.G., Robertson, S.J., Mitzel D.N., Park, G.S., Boe,r E., Wolfinbarger, J.B. and Bloom, M.E. (2005). "Inhibition of interferon-stimulated JAK-STAT signaling by a tick-borne flavivirus and identification of NS5 as an interferon antagonist." *J Virol.* 79(20): 12828-12839.

[3] Chávez, J.H., Silva, J.R., Amarilla, A.A. and Moraes Figueiredo, L.T. (2010). "Domain III peptides from flavivirus envelope protein are useful antigens for serologic diagnosis and targets for immunization." *Biologicals.* 38(6): 613-618.

[4] Chung, C.C., Lee, S.S., Chen, Y.S., Tsai, H.C., Wann, S.R., Kao, C.H. and Liu, Y.C. (2007). "Acute flaccid paralysis as an unusual presenting symptom of Japanese encephalitis: a case report and review of the literature." *Infection.* 35(1): 30-32.

[5] Das, S., Chakraborty, S. and Basu, A. (2010). "Critical role of lipid rafts in virus entry and activation of phosphoinositide 3' kinase/Akt signaling during early stages of Japanese encephalitis virus infection in neural stem/progenitor cells." *J. Neurochem.* 115(2): 537-549.

[6] Desai, A., S.K. Shankar, Jayakumar P.N., Chandramuki A., Gourie-Devi, M., Ravikumar, B.V. and Ravi, V. (1997). "Co-existence of cerebral cysticercosis with Japanese encephalitis: a prognostic modulator." *Epidemiol Infect.* 118(2):165-71.

[7] Erlanger, T.E., Weiss, S., Keiser, J., Utzinger, J. and Wiedenmayer, K. (2009). "Past, present, and future of Japanese encephalitis." *Emerg Infect Dis.* 15(1): 1-7.

[8] Weber F., Kochs, G. and Haller, O (2004). "Inverse interference: how viruses fight the interferon system." *Viral Immunol.* 17(4): 498–515.

[9] Fulmali, P.V., Sapkal, G.N., Athawale, S., Gore, M.M., Mishra, A.C. and Bondre, V.P. (2011). "Introduction of Japanese encephalitis virus genotype I, India." *Emerg. Infect. Dis.* 17(2): 319-321.

[10] Sen, G.C. (2001). "Viruses and interferons." *Annu Rev Microbiol.* 55: 255–281

[11] Gao, N., Chen, W., Zheng, Q., Fan, D.Y., Zhang, J.L.., Chen, H, Gao, G.F., Zhou, D.S. and An, J. (2010). "Co-expression of Japanese encephalitis virus prM-E-NS1 antigen with granulocyte-macrophage colony-stimulating factor enhances humoral and anti-virus immunity after DNA vaccination". *Immunol Lett.* 129(1): 23-31.

[12] Gupta, N., Lomash, V. and Rao, P.V. (2010). "Expression profile of Japanese encephalitis virus induced neuroinflammation and its implication in disease severity." *J. Clin. Virol.* 49(1): 4–10.

[13] Guy, B., Guirakhoo, F., Barban, V., Higgs, S., Monath, T.P. and Lang, J. (2010). "Preclinical and clinical development of YFV 17D-based chimeric vaccines against dengue, West Nile and Japanese encephalitis viruses." *Vaccine.* 28(3): 632-649.

[14] Halstead, S.B. and Thomas, S.J. (2011). "New Japanese encephalitis vaccines: alternatives to production in mouse brain. Expert Rev." *Vaccines.* 10(3): 355-364.

[15] Huang, J.H., Lin T.H., Teng, H.J., Su, C.L., Tsai, K.H., Lu, L.C., Lin, C., Yang, C.F., Chang, S.F., Liao, T.L., Yu, S.K., Cheng, C.H., Chang, M.C., Hu, H.C. and Shu, P.Y. (2010). "Molecular epidemiology of Japanese encephalitis virus, Taiwan." *Emerg. Infect. Dis.* 16(5): 876-878.

[16] Ishikawa, T., Wang, G., Widman, D.G., Infante, E., Winkelmann, E.R., Bourne, N. and Mason, PW. (2011). "Enhancing the utility of a prM/E-expressing chimeric vaccine for Japanese encephalitis by addition of the JEV NS1 gene." *Vaccine.* 29(43):7444-7455.

[17] Ishikawa, T., Widman, D.G., Bourne, N., Konishi, E. and Mason, P.W. (2008). "Construction and evaluation of a chimeric pseudoinfectious virus vaccine to prevent Japanese encephalitis." *Vaccine.* 26(22):2772-2781.

[18] Jelinek, T. (2009). "Ixiaro: a new vaccine against Japanese encephalitis." *Expert Rev Vaccines.* 8(11): 1501-1511.

[19] Liang, J.J., Liao, C.L., Liao, J.T., Lee, Y.L. and Lin, Y.L. (2009). "A Japanese encephalitis virus vaccine candidate strain is attenuated by decreasing its interferon antagonistic ability." *Vaccine.* 27(21): 2746-2754.

[20] Lin, R.J., Chang, B.L., Yu, H.P., Liao, C.L. and Lin, Y.L. (2006). "Blocking of interferon-induced Jak-Stat signaling by Japanese encephalitis virus NS5 through a protein tyrosine phosphatase-mediated mechanism." *J Virol.* 80(12): 5908-5918.

[21] Lin, R.J., Liao, C.L., Lin, E. and Lin, Y.L.(2004). "Blocking of the alpha interferon-induced Jak-Stat signaling pathway by Japanese encephalitis virus infection." *J Virol.* 78(17): 9285-9294.

[22] Mathur, A., Chaturvedi, U.C., Tandon, H.O., Agarwal, A.K., Mathur, G.P., Nag, D., Prasad, A. and Mittal, V.P. (1982). "Japanese encephalitis epidemic in Uttar Pradesh, India during 1978." *Indian J Med Res.* 75: 161-169.

[23] Misra, U.K. and Kalita, J. (2010). "Overview: Japanese encephalitis." *Prog Neurobiol.* 91(2): 108-120.

[24] Müllbacher, A., Lobigs, M., Lee, E. (2003). "Immunobiology of mosquito-borne encephalitic flaviviruses." *Adv Virus Res.* 60: 87-120.

[25] Murakami, M., Ota, T., Nukuzuma, S. and Takegami, T. (2005), "Inhibitory effect of RNAi on Japanese encephalitis virus replication *in vitro* and *in vivo*." *Microbiol Immunol.* 49(12): 1047-1056.

[26] Nabeshima, T., Loan, H.T., Inoue, S., Sumiyoshi, M., Haruta, Y., Nga, P.T., Huoung, V.T., del Carmen Parquet, M., Hasebe, F. and Morita, K. (2009). "Evidence of fre-

quent introductions of Japanese encephalitis virus from south-east Asia and continental east Asia to Japan." *J Gen Virol.* 90(Pt 4): 827-832.

[27] Nazmi, A., Dutta, K. and Basu, A. (2010). "Antiviral and neuroprotective role of octaguanidinium dendrimer-conjugated morpholino oligomers in Japanese encephalitis." *PLoS Negl Trop Dis.* 4(11): e892.

[28] Nett, R.J., Campbell, G.L. and Reisen, W.K. (2009). "Potential for the emergence of Japanese encephalitis virus in California." *Vector Borne Zoonotic Dis.* 9(5): 511-517.

[29] Neyts, J., Leyssen, P. and De Clercq, E. (1999). "Infections with flaviviridae." *Verh K Acad Geneeskd Belg.* 61(6): 661-697.

[30] Pujhari, S.K., Prabhakar, S., Ratho, R.K., Modi, M., Sharma, M. and Mishra, B. (2011). "A novel mutation (S227T) in domain II of the envelope gene of Japanese encephalitis virus circulating in North India." *Epidemiol Infect.* 139(6): 849-856.

[31] Qi, W.B., Hua ,R.H., Yan, L.P., Tong, G.Z., Zhang, G.H., Ren, T., Wu, D.L. and Liao, M. (2008). "Effective inhibition of Japanese encephalitis virus replication by small interfering RNAs targeting the NS5 gene." *Virus Res.* 132(1-2): 145-151.

[32] Robinson, J.S., Featherstone, D., Vasanthapuram, R., Biggerstaff, B.J., Desai, A., Ramamurty, N.,. Chowdhury, A.H, Sandhu, H.S., Cavallaro, K.F. and Johnson, B.W. (2010). "Evaluation of three commercially available Japanese encephalitis virus IgM enzyme-linked immunosorbent assays." *Am J Trop Med Hyg.* 83(5): 1146-1155.

[33] Saxena, S.K. (2008). "Japanese encephalitis: perspectives and new developments." *Future Neurol.* 3(5): 515-521.

[34] Saxena, S.K., Tiwari, S., Saxena, R., Mathur, A. and Nair, M.P.N. (2011). 'Japanese Encephalitis: an Emerging and Spreading Arbovirosis: In Flavivirus Encephalitis" (Book), Daniel Ruzek (Ed.), ISBN 979-953-307-775-7, InTech, Croatia (European Union), 295-316.

[35] Saxena, S.K., Mathur, A. and Srivastava, R.C. (2001). "Induction of nitric oxide synthase during Japanese encephalitis virus infection: evidence of protective role." *Arch Biochem Biophys.* 391(1): 1-7.

[36] Saxena, S.K, Mathur, A. and Srivastava, R.C. (2003). "Inhibition of Japanese encephalitis virus infection by diethyldithiocarbamate is independent of its antioxidant potential." *Antivir Chem Chemother.* 14(2): 91-98.

[37] Saxena, S.K., Mishra, N., Saxena, R., Singh, M. and Mathur, A. (2009). "Trend of Japanese encephalitis in North India: evidence from thirty-eight acute encephalitis cases and appraisal of niceties." *J Infect Dev Ctries.* 3(7): 517-530.

[38] Saxena, S.K., Singh, A. and Mathur, A. (2000). "Antiviral effect of nitric oxide during Japanese encephalitis virus infection." *Int J Exp Pathol.* 81(2): 165-172.

[39] Saxena ,S.K., Singh, M., Pathak ,AK. and Mathur, A. (2006). "Reply to 'Encephalitis outbreak finds Indian officials unprepared." *Nat Med.* 12(3): 269-270.

[40] Saxena, V., Mishra, VK, Dhole, TN. (2009). "Evaluation of reverse-transcriptase PCR as a diagnostic tool to confirm Japanese encephalitis virus infection." *Trans R Soc Trop Med Hyg.* 103(4): 403-406.

[41] Schuh, A.J., Li, L., Tesh, R.B., Innis, B.L. and Barrett, A.D. (2010). "Genetic characterization of early isolates of Japanese encephalitis virus: genotype II has been circulating since at least 1951." *J Gen Virol.* 91(Pt 1): 95-102.

[42] Sebastian, L., Madhusudana, S.N., Ravi, V. and Desai, A. (2011). "Mycophenolic acid inhibits replication of Japanese encephalitis virus." *Chemotherapy.* 57(1): 56-61.

[43] Shimojima, M., Nagao, Y., Shimoda, H., Tamaru, S., Yamanaka, T., Matsumura, T., Kondo, T. and Maeda, K. (2011). "Full Genome Sequence and Virulence Analyses of the Recent Equine Isolate of Japanese Encephalitis Virus." *J Vet Med Sci.* 73(6): 813-816.

[44] Singh, A., Saxena, S.K., Mishra, N., and Mathur, A. (2009). "Neuromicrobiology in India." In: Dhawan BN and Seth PK, ed. 'Neurosciences in India' Published by: Indian Academy of Neurosciences (IAN) and Council of Scientific and Industrial Research (CSIR, India), 269-318.

[45] Singh, A., Saxena, S.K., Srivastava, A.K. and Mathur, A. "Japanese Encephalitis: A Persistent Threat."(2012) *Proc Natl Acad Sci.* 82(1): 55-68.

[46] Takahashi, H., Pool V., Tsai, T.F. and Chen, R.T. (2000). "Adverse events after Japanese encephalitis vaccination: review of post-marketing surveillance data from Japan and the United States. The VAERS Working Group. " *Vaccine.* 18(26): 2963-2969.

[47] Tiwari, S., Chitti ,S.V.P., Mathur, A., and Saxena, S.K. (2012). "Japanese encephalitis virus: an emerging pathogen." *American Journal of Virology.* (in press).

[48] van den Hurk, A.F.,. Ritchie, S.A and Mackenzie, J.S. (2009). "Ecology and geographical expansion of Japanese encephalitis virus." *Annu Rev Entomo.* 54: 17-35.

[49] Vashist, S., Bhullar, D. and Vrati, S. (2011). "La protein can simultaneously bind to both 30- and 50-noncoding regions of Japanese encephalitis virus genome." *DNA Cell Bio.* 30(6): 339–346.

[50] Widman, D.G., Frolov, I. and Mason, P.W. (2008). "Third-generation flavivirus vaccines based on single-cycle, encapsidation-defective viruses." *Adv Virus Res.* 72: 77-126.

[51] Winkelmann, E.R., Widman, D.G., Xia J., Ishikawa T., Miller-Kittrell, M., Nelson, M.H., Bourne, N., Scholle, F., Mason, P.W., and Milligan, G.N. (2012). "Intrinsic adjuvanting of a novel single-cycle flavivirus vaccine in the absence of type I interferon receptor signaling." *Vaccine.* 30(8): 1465-1475.

[52] Yamanaka, A., Mulyatno, K.C., Susilowati, H., Hendrianto, E., Utsumi, T. , Amin, M., Lusida, M.I., Soegijanto, S. and Konishi, E. (2010). "Prevalence of antibodies to Japa-

nese encephalitis virus among pigs in Bali and East Java, Indonesia, 2008." *Jpn J Infect Dis*. 63(1): 58-60.

[53] Yang, Y., Ye, J., Yang, X., Jiang, R., Chen, H. and Cao, S. (2011). "Japanese encephalitis virus infection induces changes of mRNA profile of mouse spleen and brain." *Virol J*. 8: 80.

[54] Yoon, S.W., Lee, S.Y., Won, S.Y., Park, S.H., Park, S.Y. and Jeong, Y.S. (2006). "Characterization of homologous defective interfering RNA during persistent infection of Vero cells with Japanese encephalitis virus." *Mol Cells*. 21(1): 112-120.

[55] Zhang, J.S., Zhao, Q.M., Guo, X.F., Zuo, S.Q., Cheng, J.X., Jia, N., Wu, C., Dai,, P.F. and Zhao, J.Y. (2011). "Isolation and genetic characteristics of human genotype 1 Japanese encephalitis virus, China, 2009." *PLoS One*. 6(1): e16418.

[56] Zheng, Y., Li, M., Wang, H. and Liang, G. (2012). "Japanese encephalitis and Japanese encephalitis virus in mainland China." *Rev Med Virol*. doi:10.1002/rmv.1710. [Epub ahead of print].

Chapter 11

Development of Japanese Encephalitis Attenuated Live Vaccine Virus SA14-14-2 and its Charcteristics

Yongxin Yu

Additional information is available at the end of the chapter

http://dx.doi.org/10.5772/ 52980

1. Introduction

Japanese encephalitis (JE) is the most common epidemic viral encephalitis in the world today. It is estimated that the JE virus causes at least 50,000 cases of clinical diseases each year resulting in about 10,000 deaths and 15,000 cases of long-term, neuro-psychiatric sequelae. In recent decades, outbreaks of JE have occurred in several previously non-endemic areas. Nearly 3 billion people live in JE-endemic regions, where more than 70 million children are born each year. For many years, only an inactivated JE vaccine made from infected mouse brain was licensed for use by residents and travelers. However, this vaccine proved to have an unacceptable levels of adverse safety events. Recently a safe and efficacious single-dose, live-attenuated vaccine (SA14-14-2) produced in China has become available to many Asian countries. It was higher immunogenicity, fewer doses of vaccination, less side reaction and cheaper than that of the world wide used mouse brain inactivated vaccine. Since it was licensed in 1989, the vaccine has been used in more than 300 million children with no vaccine-associated encephalitis case ever reported. Currently the vaccine is produced using specific pathogen free (SPF) hamster kidney cell (PHKC) in accordance with WHO technical specifications [47]. This paper reviews the development of the SA14-14-2 vaccine and its characteristics.

1.1. Development of SA14-14-2 attenuated JE live vaccine

1.1.1. History of selecting attenuated vaccine virus SA14-14-2 strain

The vaccine virus strain SA14-14-2 was derived from a wild-type Japanese encephalitis (JE) virus SA14 isolated from pool of *Culex pipiens* mosquito larvae in Xi'an, China. Attenuation was accomplished by serial passages of the SA14 virus in primary hamster kidney (PHK) cell culture at 36 - 37℃. After 100 passages in PHK cells, followed by 3 times of plaque cloning, one clone 12-1-7 was selected from 36 plaque clones, which exhibited lower degree of virulence,LD_{50}>6.0$log_{10}TCID_{50}$ [25]. However its neuroattenuation was unstable and reverted to the virulence of parental SA14 after 1-2 mouse brain or several PHK cell passages [54]. The 12-1-7 clone was further plaque purified for 3 times and another 37 plaque clones were obtained. However those clones still showed unstable after 1-2 mouse brain passages. Then another method was performed for further attenuation. One selected virus clone (SA14-17-4) was peripherally passaged in non-neural tissues (spleen and skin) of mice followed by several times of plaque purification, which resulted in selecting an avirulent and highly stable virus clone, SA14-9-7. However, after human clinical trial, the SA14-9-7 strain showed low immunogenicity in vaccinated children (seroconversion <10%[54]). In order to promote immunogenicity, the SA14-9-7 virus was orally passaged six times in hamster, spleens harvested for two plaque purifications. One selected clone, SA14-5-3, demonstrated higher seroconversion rates in vaccinated children, 86.2% in JE endemic area[54] and 62%in JE non-endemic area[2].The SA14-5-3 strain has been licensed for vaccine production and about five million children were vaccinated. SA14-5-3 vaccine was demonstrated to be safe but low protective efficacy, 64 - 93% in humans in the clinical trial involving 400 thousand children [54].

Methods	**Names**
SA 14 virus isolated from pool of *Culex pipiens* larvae by 11 passages in mouse brain	(SA14)
100 serial passages in PHK cells, followed by three plaque purifications in PCE cells	(SA14 clone 12-1-7)
Two plaque purifications in PCE cells	(SA14 clone 17-4)
One intraperitoneal passage in mice; harvesting of spleen for one plaque purification in PCE cells	(SA14 clone 2)
Three plaque purifications in PCE cells	(SA14 clone 2-1-9)
One passage in mice, harvesting of skin and subcutaneous tissue for one plaque purification in PCE cells	(SA14 clone 9-7)
Six oral passages in hamsters; harvesting of spleens for two plaque purifications in PHK cells	(SA14 clone 5-3)
Five passages in suckling mice; harvesting of skin and subcutaneous tissue for two plaque purifications in PHK cells	(SA14 clone 14-2)*

Table 1. Attenuation history of Japanese encephalitis SA_{14}-14-2 virus strainPCE: primary chick embryo; PHK: primary hamster kidney. * The notation SA14 clone 14-2 is abbreviated to SA14-14-2

To further promote immunogenicity, the SA14-5-3 virus was serially passaged by the subcutaneous route in suckling mice, using injected site skin and local lymph nodes for the subsequent passage materials. After cloning twice in PHK cells, the SA14-14-2 clone was selected [55]. This strain was equally attenuated compared to the SA14-5-3 but more immunogenic in mice, guinea-pigs, and pigs [55]. In human trials SA14-14-2 produced seroconversion rates greater than 90% in JE non-immune subjects living in JE non-endemic region [2]. Besides,

Eckels et al. [7] adapted the SA14-14-2 virus to primary canine kidney cell cultures for 9 passages, SA14-14-2 PDK virus, which showed avirulent in mice and monkeys. However, SA14-14-2 PDK virus resulted in an unacceptably low neutralizing antibody response - 40% seroconversion rate - in childen in China [60]. The passage history is shown in Table1 and the characteristics of the various attenuated virus derivatives are shown in Table2 and 3.

Virus/clones	**Neurovirulence after different mouse brain passages**					
	0	1	2	3	4	5
SA14	6.5[a] (-)[b]	7.7(8.0)	-	-	-	-
SA14-12-1-7	0(5.5)	≥1.5(-)	6.33(-)	-	-	-
SA14-12-1-1	<0.0(7.5)	2.50(6.5)	-	6.00(7.00)	-	-
SA14-9-4-2	<0.0(6.5)	≤1.83(6.0)	-	7.17/6.50	-	-
SA14-17-4	0(-)	≥4.5(≥4.5)	-	-	-	-
SA14-2	0(-)	0(-)	<1.0(5.0)	1.42(6.5)	1.0(6.0)	<1.0(6.5)
SA14-2-1-9	0(4.5)	0(≥6.5)	0(5.0)	<1.0(5.5)	1.30(≥7.5)	≥5.12(7.5)
SA14-9-7	0(6.0)	0(4.0)	0(4.0)	0(5.0)	0(4.0)	0(4.5)
SA14-5-3	0(5.0)	0(5.5)	0.62(4.0)	0(4.75)	0.58(6.5)	2.21(6.5)
SA14-14-2	0(7.0)	1.0(-)	0.58(-)	0.67(-)	0.57(-)	≤2.0(-)

Table 2. Neuroattenuation and its stability (reversibility) of various derivatives of attenuated strains from SA14 virus strainsa., Intracereble (i.c.) inoculation tested in weanling mice, $log_{10}LD_{50}/0.03ml$ b., $log_{10}TCID_{50}/0.2ml$ - not determined

Virus/ clones	**Neurovirulence[a]**		**Reversibility[b]**	**Immunogenicity[c]**
	Dose ($log_{10}pfu/ml$)	**$log_{10}LD_{50}/ml$ or No.dead/ no.tested**		
SA_{14}	8.78	8.50	ND	ND
SA_{14}-12-1-7	7.7[d]	1.65	+	ND
SA_{14}-9-7	6.70[d]	0/10	-	Low
SA_{14}-5-3	6.47	0/10	-	Moderate
SA_{14}-14-2	7.17	0/10	-	High
SA_{14}-14-2 PDK	6.25	0/10	ND	Moderate

Table 3. Summary of the characteristics of various derivatives of attenuated strains from SA_{14} virus strainND not determined a) i.c. inoculation tested in weanling mice b) Reversion to neurovirulence of the parental SA_{14} virus in mice model: +, neuroreversion after one suckling mice or 1-2 weanling mice i.c. passages; -, no neuroreversion after mice i.c. passages. c) Neutralizing antibody seroconversion in humans: low, <10%; moderate, 40%~60%; high, ≥90%. d) $log_{10}TCID_{50}/ml$

1.2. Clinical studies

Vaccine safety has been evaluated in several small-scale studies and in two large-scale studies in China. Studies of 588,512 children aged between 1 and 15 years inoculated with vaccine from one manufacturer [35] and of 60000 children given vaccine from another manufacturer [15] reported no cases of temporally associated encephalitis. The most common adverse effect associated with vaccination was fever, which was reported in less than 0.2% of vaccinated children, with lower rates for rash and other systemic symptoms.

Daily examination of 867 vaccinated children for fever (>38℃) disclosed low rates with onset distributed evenly over the 21-day observation period, without clustering as might have been expected if onset were associated with a specific incubation period. Temperature elevations were limited to a single day in most cases.

A block-randomized coherent study of 13,266 vaccinated and 12,951 nonvaccinated children followed prospectively for 30 days has shown that no cases of encephalitis or meningitis were detected in either groups, and rates of fever, allergic, respiratory symptoms were similar in the two groups [33]. Moreover no case of encephalitis associated with the live vaccine has been reported so far from the large scale vaccination in other areas of China [66] and in countries outside China [38, 4].The vaccine is well tolerated in subjects as young as 8 months.

The immunogenicity and protection efficacy in humans have been studied several times in China and outside China. Neutralizing antibody were produced in 85%~100% of non-immune subjects studied in China [2, 58, 20, 64] and 98%, 92% and 95% studied in Korea [38], Philiphines [12] and Thailand [6], respectively after a single dose of vaccination. Several efficacy trials of SA14-14-2 vaccine in China from 1988 to 1999 in 1 to 10 year-old children have consistently yielded high protection rates, above 95%,[66, 5, 43]. One study in Guizhou province [67] and another in Anhui province [66] have shown the protection efficacy persisted for at least 11 and 5 years respectively following an immunization schedule of one primary dose at one age and one booster dose at two ages. Case-control study for evaluation the efficacy of SA14-14-2 vaccine has been studied. A case control study conducted in 1993 in Sichuan province, China in children <15 years measured vaccine effectiveness of routinely delivered SA14-14-2 vaccine at 80% for a single-dose and 97.5% for a two-dose given at a one year interval [14]. In 1999, the SA14-14-2 vaccine was given as a single dose to over 220000 residents of the Terai region of Nepal in an effort to reduce the impact of an emerging epidemic of JE. A case-control study demonstrated 99.12% efficacy [4] followed by a 5-year efficacy of 96% [41]. In 2000, a case-control study in Chongqing city, China found a 93% efficacy after one dose vaccination [42]. Besides, Kumar [23] reported a case control study in India, where 9.3 million children were immunized with SA14-14-2 vaccine in 2007, demonstrated a 94.5% vaccine efficacy after a single dose.

2. Phenotypic characteristic

2.1. *In vitro* phenotypic characteristics

SA14-14-2 attenuated virus replicates well in primary hamster kidney (PHK) cell, C6/36 mosquito cells, continuous African green monkey kidney (Vero) cells, Rhesus monkey kidney (LLC-MK_2) cells and baby hamster kidney (BHK21) cell lines. SA14-14-2 virus showed homogeneous small plaques (≤1mm) when grown in above - mentioned cells, while SA14 wild strain showed heterogeneous and larger plagues (2-3mm) [57][1].

Many attenuated viruses are temperature-sensitive, often showing restricted growth in vitro at 39-40℃, some strains were even sensitive to 37°C. SA14-14-2 strain was not temperature-sensitive, showing no reduction in infectivity at 37°C or 40°C. SA14-14-2 strain was also thermostable as the parental SA14 virus. In liquid status reduction of virus titer was 3.5log_{10}TCID50 after heated at 50℃ for 50 minutes and virus could be detected 4 hours after further incubation at 50°C, a result similar to that observed with SA14 parent strain. SA14-14-2 was more thermostabe than the SA14-5-3 [57].

2.2. Ability of *in vivo* virus replication

Yu et al. [55] studied the replication ability of SA14-14-2 virus in young mice (2.5 weeks) by subcutaneous (s.c.) inoculation followed by recovering virus from spleens and subcutaneous tissues of the infected mice for 2 weeks post inoculation. In those mice infected with the parent SA14 strain, viruses were recovered from the both tissues from day 4 to day 10 post infections, while those mice inoculated with SA14-14-2 strain, viruses were isolated in both tissues as well but limited within a short period from day 2 to day 4 or day 6 post infections (Table 4). Wu et al. [49] performed a similar study for recovering virus from brains and sera of the infected mice. Mice that infected with as less as 2.7log_{10} pfu/mL of the parent SA14 virus, high titers (≥6.0log_{10} pfu/mL) of virus was detected in the brains and low titers (2.7 – 3.4log_{10} pfu/mL) in the sera, whereas mice inoculated with as high as 6.2log_{10} pfu/mL of the SA14-14-2 , , virus was neither detected in the brains nor in the sera of the mice. Lee et al. [24] examined virus growth of SA14-14-2 live virus and the parent SA14 virus strains in mice after i.p. inoculation. The results showed that SA14 virus was detected in sera and in spleens with peak titers of 3.24log PFU/ml and 4.3 logPFU/g, respectively as well as brains with peak titer of 6.42logPFU/g. On the other hand, SA14-14-2 virus was detected only in the spleens with extremely low titer (1.7logPFU/ml) but not detected in the sera and brains of all ten inoculated mice.

Virus strain	Infected virus titer (log_{10} $TCID_{50}$/mL)	Tissues detected	Virus titers ($log_{10}TCID_{50}$/mL) by days after inoculation					
			2	4	6	7	10	14-15
SA14-14-2	6.7	SC a tissue	3.2	4.2	1.0	ND	ND	ND
		spleen	4.2	4.2	0	ND	ND	ND
SA14	5.7	SC tissue	ND	2.7	ND	≥4.2	0	0
		spleen	ND	2.2	ND	≥4.2	≥3.2	0

Table 4. *In vivo* replication of SA14-14-2 strain in mice. a Subcutaneous tissue

Further investigation for viremia induction of SA14-14-2 virus using guinea pigs animal model has been studied by Liu et al [31]. Guinea pigs intraperitoneally (i.p.) injected with 4.0log_{10} pfu/mL of parent virus SA14 and other 4 JEV virulent strains induced viremia to virus titers of 1.0-3.0log_{10} pfu/mL and lasted for 3 days post infection. However, the animals inoculated with SA14-14-2 strain containing virus titer equal to that of the virulent strains, no viremia was detected from day 1 to day 10 post inoculation (Table 5)

Besides, a viremia clinical study in India has demonstrated the absence of any viremia activity in adult population up to 15 days after administration of a single dose of the live JE SA14-14-2 vaccine.

Virus strain	Animal No.	Viremia titer by day after inoculation (log_{10} pfu/mL)				
		1	3	5	7	10
P3	No.1	2.04	2.18	0	ND	ND
	No.2	2.08	2.59	0	ND	ND
	No.3	2.23	2.56	0	ND	ND
	No.4	1.70	2.21	0	ND	ND
02-41	No.1	1.00	1.78	0	0	0
	No.2	1.78	1.70	0	0	0
	No.3	1.78	1.60	0	0	0
	No.4	1.00	1.90	0	0	0
	No.5	1.30	1.95	0	ND	ND
HLJ02-144	No.1	1.90	1.30	0	0	0
	No.2	2.00	1.00	0	0	0
	No.3	1.95	1.48	0	0	0
	No.4	1.95	1.48	0	0	0
	No.5	2.48	ND	ND	ND	ND
SA14	No.1	2.92	ND	ND	ND	ND
	No.2	2.41	2.85	0	0	0
	No.3	2.94	3.40	0	0	0
	No.4	2.53	3.00	0	0	0
	No.5	3.02	ND	ND	ND	ND
SA14-14-2	No.1	0	0	0	0	0
	No.2	0	0	0	0	0
	No.3	0	0	0	0	0
	No.4	0	0	0	0	0
	No.5	0	0	0	0	0

Table 5. Viremia in guinea pigs after i.p. inoculation with different JEV virus strains. ND, Not determined

These results indicated that growth of the attenuated live virus in vivo was significantly reduced in contrast to the growth of parent SA14 virus, and SA14-14-2 strain showed a lack of viremia and neuroinvasion.

2.3. Neuroattenuation phenotype

Mice and rhesus monkeys are highly susceptible to the wild virulent Japanese encephalitis virus (JEV) inoculated by intracerebral route. Approximately 1~10 plaque forming unit (pfu)

http://dx.doi.org/10.5772/ 52980

of the virus inoculated intracerebrally results in death. Mice are more susceptible than monkey to JE virus following inoculation by the peripheral route. Rhesus monkeys show four grades of response to the different attenuated JE viruses by i.c. inoculation [68]:

1. "death", the inoculation with parental SA14 virus;
2. "survival but showing neurological signs", i.e. the inoculation of SA14 95th PHK cell passage virus (SA14 HKC-95) ;
3. "survival, without showing neurological symptoms, but with fever" i.e. the inoculation with SA14-12-1-7 virus ;
4. "healthy", no fever, no symptom, no death, i.e. when the vaccine virus SA14-14-2 was inoculated.

Neurovirulence of JE SA14-14-2 strain was tested using these animal models with virus titers of 7.0~8.0$\log_{10}$ pfu/ml. Weanling mice inoculated with the virus by i.c. or s.c. inoculation did not cause death. SA14-14-2 was tested by standard intrathalamic and intraspinal combination inoculation method in monkeys. Monkeys showed no mortality or morbidity and only a minimal degree of CNS inflammation around the injection sites [30] (Table 6). Further, neuropathogenicity was tested in immune- deficient or immune-suppressed animals, athymic nude mice or mice treated with cyclophosphamide. No deaths or histopathologic abnormalities were observed after intraperitoneal or subcutaneous inoculation of a viral dose greater than $10^{7.0}$ TCID50/ml. Although cyclophosphamide increases susceptibility of mice to virulent JE strains, immunosuppression with cyclophosphamide did not lead to encephalitis in mice inoculated pheripherally with SA14-14-2 virus [56, 18]. The strain also did not kill weanling hamsters by i.c. inoculations [55].

Virus strain (Virus titer, pfu/ml)	Inoculation route	Mice			Rhesus Monkeys	
		Dilution	Died/tested	Histopathological score (neuronal lesions)[a]	Died/tested	Histopathological score (neuronal lesions)[ab]
SA14 parent (6.15×10^8)	IC	10-1	ND	ND	2/2	2-4
		10-4	8/8	2-4	0/1	2-3
		10-5	ND	ND	2/2	2-4
		10-6	8/8	2-3	2/2	2-4
		10-7	8/8	2-4	2/2	2-4
		10-8	8/8	2-4	ND	ND
	SC	10-1	30/30	2-4(day 5)	ND	ND
SA14-14-2(8×10^6)	IC	1:5	0/30	0-2	0/4	0-1
	SC	1:5	0/30	0(1)[c]	ND	ND

Table 6. Comparative neurovirulence of attenuated SA14-14-2 and parent SA14 Japanese encephalitis viruses in 3-week-old mice and adult rhesus monkeysIC, intracerebral; SC, subcutaneous. ND, Not determineda) 0, No lesion; 1, ≤5%; 2, 6-20%; 3, 21-50%; 4, >50% of neurons died.b) Inoculation in thalami bilaterally (each 0.5ml) and lumbar spinal cord (0.2mL).c) One mouse showed a few dead nerve cells.

2.4. phenotypic stabilities

2.4.1. Stability of plaque morphology

Small homogeneous plaque (≤1mm) morphology was retained through 8 -17 PHK cell passages studied by Jia et al. [17]. As reported by Aihara, plaque-size phenotypes did not change during plaque purification in BHK_{21} cells and propagation in C6/36 cell [1]. Eckels et al. [7] showed that SA14-14-2 strain had a homogeneous small plaque morphology, with no large plaques seen when passed 7 times in LLC-MK_2 cells.

2.4.2. Stability of neuroattenuation

Wang et al. [44] studied neuroattenuation stability by serial passages the SA14-14-2 strain from passage 8 to passage 23 in PHK cells, virulence was tested every 2-3 passages by intracerebral or subcutaneous inoculation in mice (12 ~ 14g). None of the PHK-passaged viruses containing virus doses of 8.0~9.0 log_{10}TCID50 caused death in these mice. Jia et al. [16] passed the SA14-14-2 virus in PHK cells for 17 passages, neurovirulence and neuroinvasion were determined at the 8th, 15th, 17th passage. No animal showed illness at any the passage level.

Eckels et al. [7] performed the neuroattenuation stability by serial passage the SA14-14-2 virus in Beagle canine kidney cells for a total of 15 passages, the passage 15 virus was attenuated for young mice causing no symptoms or death by i.c. inoculation. Wang et al. [45] passaged the SA14-14-2 HKC5 virus in primary dog fetal kidney cell cultures for 11 passages. Each of the passaged virus was tested for its pathogenicity in weanling mice, all the mice survived by either i.c. or s.c. inoculation with a virus dose containing 7.5-8.0 log_{10}TCID50/0.2ml. These results showed that over many passages of the SA14-14-2 virus in PHK cells or primary dog kidney cells, neuroviruence reversed to the virulence of parental SA14 was not observed.

Wu et al [49] studied on the stability of SA14-14-2 vaccine seed virus by i.c. passage in suckling mice, viruses recovered from the mice brain of passage 1 only caused a few weanling mice death following i.c. inoculation with a high dose of 8.7 log_{10}pfu/ml virus (LD50≥7.7 log_{10}pfu), showing no reversion to the virulence of SA14 parent virus (i.c.LD50≥0.28 log_{10}pfu).

Athymic nude mice (nu/nu) inoculated intra-peritoneally with 8.2log_{10}TCID50/ml of SA14-14-2 virus did not fall ill. Attempts to recover virus from brain, liver, spleen, kidney, heart and lymph nodes were made over a period of 3 weeks. In three independent experiments viruses were recovered only in one experiment from brain at the 10th, 14th and 21st day and kidney tissue at 6th day. Virus isolated from the brains on day 21st after intraperitoneal inoculation, was enhanced once in PHK cell to a virus titers of 6.7-7.2 $log_{10}TCID_{50}$/ml and then tested for neurovirulence and neuroinvasiveness in normal mice. Tests were repeated three times and showed that the recovered viruses were avirulent to 10-12g mice by i.c. or intraperitoneal inoculation, maintaining the attenuated phenotype as SA14-14-2 [56].

Neuroattenuation after long-term cold storage has been studied. Fourteen lots of lyophilized live JE vaccines manufactured year by year since 1987 were stored at low temperature (-20℃). After 15 years, neurovirulence of the vaccine viruses were studied in year 2002. The results showed that viruses in the all 14 lots were avirulent for i.c. inoculated mice. [22]

2.5. Growth characteristics and ability of transmission in mosquitoes

Mosquito infection and transmission with SA14-14-2 virus have been done using *Culex tritaeniorhynchus* mosquitoes, the most important JEV vector species, by oral feeding with meals containing the virus or intrathoracial(IT) inoculation with the virus. The mosquitoes did not become infected by oral feeding with meals containing 6.06$\log_{10}$pfu/ml virus and only one of the 34 groups (3.13%) of the infected mosquitoes became infected after feeding with meals containing 6.18 $\log_{10}$pfu/ml virus, reaching a low virus titer of 1.24$\log_{10}$pfu/ml. However, most of the mosquitoes (10 of 14 groups, 71.43%) became infected after feeding meals containing 7.85$\log_{10}$pfu/ml of virulent JE virus strain Nakayama(Nak), reaching higher titers of 3.33-4.79 $\log_{10}$pfu/ml (Table 7) [62]. The result indicated that SA14-14-2 virus is restricted in its ability to infect and replicate in the *Culex tritaeniorhychus* mosquito vector.

Virus strain	Meals containing virus($\log_{10}$pfu/ml)	No. groups tested	Total number of mosquitoes tested	No. group Positive (%)
SA14-14-2	6.06	15(4-31)[1]	345(15-36)[2]	0(0%)
	6.18	34(2-11)	573(10-39)	1(3.13%)(1.24)[3]
Nakayama	7.85	14(3-11)	215(11-26)	10(71.43%)(3.33-4.79)

Table 7. Growth of SA14-14-2 virus and wild virulent JEV Nak strain in *Culex tritaeniorhynchus* mosquitoes by oral infections.

Mosquitoes were exposed to virus-containing meals for oral ingestion. Fully engorged mosquitoes were then collected after a period of extrinsic incubation.

1. Times(days) of extrinsic incubation periods;
2. Numbers of mosquito per group;
3. Virus titers in the mosquito suspensions of the positive groups ($\log_{10}$pfu/ml)

However, virus could replicate at low level by intrathoracical (I.T.) inoculation of the *Cx.tritaeniorhynchus* mosquitoes [62], reaching titers of 2.0~3.72 $\log_{10}$pfu/ml over 2~20 days after inoculation. In contrast, mosquitoes IT infected with its parent SA14 virus exhibited higher ability of replication, reaching titers of 3.0~4.85 $\log_{10}$pfu/ml over the same periods [10].

The ability of transmission by the IT infected mosquitoes was studied later. Two groups of the mosquitoes were infected IT with SA14-14-2 virus, 8 days after infection one group of infected mosquitoes was used to infect suckling mice by direct bite, another group of infected mosquitoes was made in a suspension (M-1), in which the virus content was measured, and used to infect weanling mice by i.c. inoculation. In order to enhance the virus titer of the mosquito suspension (M-1), it was passed once in BHK cells (M-1 C-1) and then infected mice by i.c. and s.c. inoculation. The full E protein gene of the M-1 C-1 virus was sequenced and compared to that of its parent SA14-14-2 virus. As shown in Table 8, none of the mice died after bitten or i.c. inoculation with virus titers of 4.2 and 7.2 log_{10}pfu/ml, and only one nucleotide in the virus E protein gene changed resulting in one amino acid substitution (E447 A→G) which was not reverse mutation. And the eight critical amino acids remained unchanged. The similarity of the virus full E gene sequence compared to that of the parent SA14 was 99.9% [34]. This result demonstrated that the SA14-14-2 virus is phenotypic and genetic stable and could not be transmitted after mosquito passage.

Virus[a]	Virus titer	Virulence tested in				E gene sequence		
		Suckling mice		2.5 weeks mice				
	Pfu/ml	bitten[b]	ic	ic	sc	mutation		similarity
SA_{14}-14-2 M-1	$10^{4.2}$	0/16[c]	0/16					
M-1C-1	$10^{7.2}$			0/10	0/10	0/8[d]	E-447 (A→G)	99.9%

Table 8. Virulence and E gene sequence of the SA_{14}-14-2 virus after *Culex tritaeniorhynchus* mosquitoes IT passage. a One intrathoracical passage (SA_{14}-14-2 M-1) and one BHK-21 cell passage (M-1 C-1).b By the infected mosquitoes c No. dead /no. testedd No. reversion/no. attenuating amino acidSC Subcutaneously

3. Genotypic characteristics

3.1. Gene sequence of SA14-14-2 compared to its parent SA14 and other attenuated derivatives.

When the full-length gene sequence of SA_{14}-14-2 was compared to parental $SA_{14,}$ 57-66 nucleotide substitutions were found to be scattered all over the genome except prM. These coded for 24-31 amino acid substitutions, of which 8 were in E protein[1, 61] and were studied to be the critical amino acid mutations involved in virus attenuation [3, 13] (Table 9). Among the 8 substituted amino acids observed in SA14-14-2 virus, only 3 substitutions appeared in the unstable virus SA14-12-1-7; while those highly and stable strains, SA_{14}-9-7, SA_{14}-5-3 and SA_{14}-14-2 PDK viruses had 6 changes of the 8 amino acids [Ni H et al.,1994, 8]. Two of the 8 amino acid substitutions at position E-177 (T,Threonine→A,Alanine) and E-264 (Q, Glutamine→H, Histudine) were unique to SA_{14}-14-2 virus [8] (Table 10). The contribution of these two amino acid changes to the biological properties of SA_{14}-14-2 virus requires further study.

http://dx.doi.org/10.5772/ 52980

Position		**SA14-14-2**		SA14
aa	nt	Zeng	Aihara	
C-65	292	S	S	L
E-107	1296	F	F	L
E-138	1389	K	K	E
E-176	1503	V	V	I
E-177	1506	A	A	T
E-264	1769	H	H	Q
E-279	1813	M	M	K
E-315	1921	V	V	A
E-334	1977	P	S	S
E-439	2293	R	R	K
NS1-292	3351	S	S	G
NS1-339	3493	M	M	R
NS1-351	3528	H	H	D
NS1-354	3539	K	K	N
NS1-392	3652	V	V	A
NS2B-63	4403	D	D	E
NS2B-65	4408	G	G	D
NS2B-87	4475	F	L	L
NS3-59	4782	V	V	M
NS3-73	4825	K	K	R
NS3-105	4921	G	G	A
NS3-343	5634	R	W	R
NS4A-27	6634	I	T	I
NS4B-106	7227	V	V	I
NS5-31	7768	G	A	A
NS5-45	7809	S	R	R
NS5-195	8261	I	M	M
NS5-386	8832	Y	Y	H
NS5-636	9593	H	Q	Q
NS5-671	9688	A	A	V
NS5-731	9898	G	D	D
NS5-759	9954	P	A	A
NS5-767	9978	V	L	L

Table 9. Comparison of amino acid differences between JE attenuated vaccine SA14-14-2 and its parent SA14 strain reported by Aihare and Zeng

Sequences were reported by [1] and [61]

3.2. Stability of gene sequence of SA14-14-2 virus strain

SA14-14-2 virus at PHK cells passage 8 (PHK_8) was serially passed to PHK17 or given one i.c. passage in suckling mouse (HKC_8SM_1). The E protein gene of the viruses was sequenced and compared to that of SA14-14-2 PHK_8 and parental SA_{14}. At passage 17, all the 8 attenuating amino acid residues in SA14-14-2 PHK_8 were retained no change, while two new nucleotide mutations were found at NT-1970 (T ▪ G), and NT-2169 (A ▪ G), which resulted in two amino acid changes at positions E-331 (S ▪ R) and E-398 (K ▪ E)(Table 11). The two substituted amino acids, Arg(R) and Glu(E), were not the residues of parental SA14, Ser(S) and Lys(K), this suggests that the two changes were not reverse mutation [9]. After one passage of the PHK_8 virus in suckling mouse brain (SA14-14-2 HK_8SM_1), 7 of the 8 amino acids remained unchanged, one at E107 (F→L) was reverse mutation, while 3 other amino acid mutations appeared at E-83, E-318 and E-327, which were not reverse mutations (Table 11).

Virus	Mutation sites							
	107	138	176	177	264	279	315	439
SA_{14}-14-2 PHK	F	K	V	A	H	M	V	R
SA_{14}-12-1-7	F	E	V	T	Q	K	A	R
SA_{14}-9-7	F	K	V	T	Q	M	V	R
SA_{14}-5-3	F	K	V	T	Q	M	V	R
SA_{14}-14-2 PDK	F	K	V	T	Q	M	V	R
Parental SA_{14}	L	E	I	T	Q	K	A	K

Table 10. Comparison of the amino acid differences in the E protein gene of JE SA_{14}-14-2 PHK vaccine virus with the other attenuated derivatives and the parental SA14

Site	SA_{14} V_2	SA14-14-2		
		HKC_8V_2	$HKC_{17}V_2$	HKC_8SM_1
E-83	E	E	E	Q
E-107	L	F	F	L
E-138	E	K	K	K
E-176	I	V	V	V
E-177	T	A	A	A
E-264	Q	H	H	H
E-279	K	M	M	M
E-315	A	V	V	V
E-318	G	G	G	D
E-327	S	S	S	F
E-331	S	S	R	S
E-398	K	K	E	K
E-439	K	R	R	R

Table 11. Substitutions of amino acid of SA14-14-2 strain after passage in PHK cell or suckling mice. HKC_8V_2, HKC 8 passages, vero cells 2 passages ;$HKC_{17}V_2$, HKC 17 passages, vero cells 2 passages ;HKC_8SM_1, HKC 8 passages, suckling mice one i.c. passage

Li et al. [27] and Gao et al.[11] performed similar studies by additional passage of the SA14-14-2 vaccine seed virus (early passage) in PHK cell culture to passage 20 and passage 18, respectively. The E protein gene sequences of the various passaged viruses were sequenced and compared to the original seed virus.The results demonstrated no reverse mutation of the 8 attenuating amino acids.

Xu et al [52] studied full-length sequence stability of the SA14-14-2 virus by passing the early passages seed virus(PHK_8) on PHK cells to passage 22 ($PHKC_{22}$) and its full-length genome was sequenced. By comparing the full sequences of the $PHKC_{22}$ with the original primary seed virus of SA14-14-2 in Genbank (D90195), the result showed that there were only 8 nucleotide differences (one in E, 5 in non-structure-region and 2 in 3'-NTR) leading to 4 amino acids changed, which were not reverse mutations. The homology of the nucleotides and amino acids between the viruses of passage 22 viruses and the primary seed virus in Genbank was 99.93% and 99.88%, respectively (Table 12). These results demonstrated that the genotype of SA14-14-2 vaccine virus was very stable during multiple cell culture passages.

Position		Nucleotide change	Amino acid change
Nt	Aa		
2142	E-389	a→c	D→N
3929	NS2a-69	t→c	none
5634	NS3-343	t→a	W→R
6634	NS4a-57	c→t	T→I
7655	NS4b-130	g→t	none
9593	NS5-639	g→t	Q→H
10701(3'-NCR)		-→g	
10784(3'-NCR)		t→c	

Table 12. Nucleotide and amino acid changes in the PHK cells passage 22 compared to the sequence of SA14-14-2 in Genbank (D90195)

4. Immunogenicity

4.1. Humoral immune response

Wills et al. [48] investigated the ability of SA14-14-2 (PHK) and other 4 attenuated vaccine clones SA14-2-8, SA14-5-3, SA14-14-2 (PDK) to induce a humoral immune response in Balb/c mice. The mice, 6-8 weeks old, were inoculated by intraperitoneal route with 10^3 and 10^6 pfu of the live viruses. Mice were bled 14 and 28 days postinoculation. Anti-JE serum antibody levels were measured using hemagglutination inhibition (HAI) and neutralization (N) tests. The results demonstrated that the live SA14-14-2 (PHK) elicited good HAI and N responses at dose of 10^3 and 10^6 pfu at 14 days postinoculation, with the 28-days sera showing no reduction in N titer. In comparison, 10^6 pfu of the SA14-14-2 (PDK) virus evoked only a poor N response by 14 days postinoculation and neutralizing antibody was not detectable with a dose of 10^3 pfu either 14 or 28 days postinoculation (titre ≤20). The two early vaccine clones SA14-2-8 and SA14-5-3 both produced results very similar to SA14-14-2 (PDK) in terms of HAI and N responses at the given dose (Table 13).

Lee et al. [24] reported that mice vaccinated with one dose of SA14-14-2 virus (4.0$\log_{10}$pfu/ml) produced N antibody (titer 1:60), HAI antibody(22.2), complement fixation (CF) antibody (11.2) and were protected against a lethal JEV i.c. challenge (90% protection). Meanwhile, the anti-NS1(non-structural NS1) antibody was detected in sera of the vaccinated mice, which may also be responsible for the protection.

Virus strains	Titre at day 14 for dose (Log_{10} pfu)				Titre at day 28 for dose (Log_{10} pfu)			
	3		6		3		6	
	N	HAI	N	HAI	N	HAI	N	HAI
SA14-14-2(PHK)	320	320	640	80	320	NT	640	320
SA14-14-2(PDK)	<20	40	80	320	<20	160	80	NT
SA14-2-8	80	NT	160	NT	160	NT	160	NT
SA14-5-3	40	NT	80	NT	160	NT	160	NT

Table 13. Humoral immune responses (N and HAI) derived from Babl/c mice inoculated with attenuated vaccine strains. Note: N, neutralization titre, taken as the highest dilution of serum to neutralize 50% of plaque numbers of homologous virus;HAI, Haemagglutination inhibition titre, taken as the highest dilution of serum to inhibit 4 HA units of homologous virus;NT, not tested.

4.2. Protection efficacy

Several studies have demonstrated that SA14-14-2 live vaccine induced high and broad protection against challenge by various JEV virulent strains in mice. Wang et al. [46] performed a study comparing the protective efficacy of 3 kinds of JE vaccine, the SA14-14-2 attenuated vaccine, the PHK derived P3 inactivated Vaccine (iPHKV) and the mouse brain purified inactivated Nak vaccine (MBV) in mice by i.p. inoculation with one dose of live vaccine, or 2 doses of the 2 kinds of inactivated vaccines respectively followed by i.p. challenge with 2 virulent JEV P3 and Nak strains. The results indicated that despite levels of neutralizing antibodies (N) developed by the vaccination with live vaccine and MBV were equal at the day of pre-challenge, mice receiving the live vaccine were protected against the 2 challenging strains at higher rates than mice receiving the 2 inactivated vaccines (Table 14). Yu et al.[59] compared the immunogenicity of the SA14-14-2 live vaccine and iPHKV in mice by i.p. vaccination followed by i.p. challenge with 14 wild strains isolated from different areas and years in China. The results indicated that live vaccine induced higher and broader protection levels than that induced by the iPHKV. In another study, Jia et al. [21] demonstrated that mice s.c. inoculated with a single dose of 34 or 340 pfu/mL SA14-14-2 virus, mice were protected (80-100%) against i.p. challenge of the 22 JEV strains (11 isolated in China and the other 11 from Thailand, Vietnam, Indonesia, India, Philippines and Japan).

Vaccine	N titers at pre-challenge against		Protection against			
			P3		Nak	
	P3	Nak	i.p.	i.c.	i.p.	i.c.
SA14-14-2	20[a]	40	10/10[b]	8/10	10/10	4/10
iPHKV P3	10	5	7/10	ND	5/10	ND
MBV(Nak)	20	40	8/10	3/10	4/10	1/10
Control	ND	ND	2/10	1/10	2/10	3/14

Table 14. Protection of three kinds of JE vaccine in mice. Note: ND, Not determineda) Reciprocal of the highest dilution of serum that resulted in 50% reduction of plaque numbers.b) Number surviving challenge/number challenged i.p. intraperitoneally

No.	Challenge Virus strain	Genotype	Dose (pfu)				
			2340	234	23	Control	Challenge virus dose ($log_{10}LD_{50}$)
1	SH-53	I	10/10[a]	10/10	9/10	2/10	3.58
2	SH-101	I	10/10	10/10	10/10	2/10	3.17
3	LN02-102	I	10/10	8/10	4/10	1/10	3.84
4	SH03-127	I	10/10	8/10	7/10	1/10	3.71
5	HN04-11	I	10/10	10/10	5/10	2/10	2.75
6	SC04-17	I	10/10	9/10	10/10	2/10	4.00
7	SH05-24	I	10/10	9/10	4/10	1/10	3.77
8	02-29	III	10/10	10/10	7/10	2/10	3.50
9	02-41	III	10/10	10/10	6/10	2/10	4.50
10	HLJ02-134	III	9/9	10/10	6/10	2/10	2.88
11	HLJ02-144	III	10/10	8/10	4/10	0/10	3.00
12	DL04-06	III	10/10	9/10	9/10	2/10	3.24
13	P3	III	9/10	9/10	9/10	1/10	3.78
14	SA14	III	9/10	9/10	9/10	1/10	3.65
15	SA4	III	10/10	10/10	4/10	2/10	3.42
16	KT	III	10/10	9/10	5/10	1/10	3.31

Table 15. Protection efficacy of SA14-14-2 against intraperitoneal challenge with different heterologous JE virus strains. Mice were immunized with either 2340 pfu, 234 pfu or 23 pfu of SA14-14-2 virus;a) Number surviving challenge/number challenged.

However, since 1970's, a new genotype I of JEV has circulated in China while the genotype III JEV are still circulating in nature. In order to further categorize the degree of immunogenicity conferred by the SA14-14-2 vaccine against the both wild-type JEV genotypes (I and III) currently circulating in China. Liu et al [32] examined the protective efficacies of the SA14-14-2 live vaccine in mice by a single s.c.vaccination followed by i.p. challenge with 16 JEV isolates of the both genotype. As shown in Table 15,mice immunized with 2340 pfu of the live vaccine virus conferred an 80-100% protection rate against challenge with the 16 heterologous JE virus strains. Protection efficacy was 70-80% with vaccination dose as low as 234 pfu.

This result was consistent with previous data indicating SA14-14-2 vaccine conferred strong and broad protections against JEV challenge[59][21].

4.3. Suppression of viremia induction

As shown in Table 16, guinea-pigs immunized with a single SA14-14-2 dose of 5.87 pfu/mL virus induced low neutralizing antibody levels(<10 by PRNT) 14 days after vaccination, but viremia was significantly suppressed in all vaccinated animals after i.p. challenge with P3 virulent JE strain compared to control animals in which all developed high levels of viremia (2.0-3.54$\log_{10}$ pfu/mL) that last 4 days. Interestingly, despite the neutralizing antibody levels of the vaccinated animals at the day of challenge (day0) were low, higher levels antibody developed rapidly beginning at day 4 post challenge compared to the control animals that developed slowly with low level antibodies beginning at day 7 post challenge [19].

Vaccine	No. testing	Viremia by day after challenge					Titer of N antibody by day after challenge						
		2	3	4	5	7	0	2	3	4	5	7	14
SA14-14-2	1	0/2[a]	ND	ND	0/2	0/2	<4-4[c]	<4-4	ND	ND	256	1024	2048
	2	0/3	0/3	0/3	ND	0/3	<4-16	<4-16	<4-16	16-64	ND	128-1024	1024-2048
None (control)	1	3/3 (2.1-2.8)[b]	ND	ND	0/3	0/3	< 4	< 4	ND	ND	<4	<4-8	32-64
	2	4/4 (2.0-2.7)	4/4 (1.7-2.8)	2/2 (1.0-1.7)	ND	0/4	< 4	< 4	< 4	< 4	ND	8	128

Table 16. Viremia suppression in guinea-pigs after vaccination with SA14-14-2 vaccine followed by challenge with virulent JEV. a, No. viremia positive/ no. tested; b,Viremia titre,$\log_{10}$ pfu/mL; c, Reciprocal of the highest dilution of serum that resulted in 50% reduction of plaque numbers

4.4. Evidence of cellular immune responses

Several studies have shown evidence of cellular immunity induced by vaccination of SA14-14-2 vaccine in mice. Li et al.[28] studied the specific cytotoxic T lymphocyte (CTL) mediated immune responses in mice by vaccination with SA14-14-2 live vaccine and PHK inactivated vaccine. In the three testings, the average percentage of the specific CTL activity induced by mice vaccinated with one dose of live vaccine was higher (79.2%) than the mice immunized with twice doses of the inactivated vaccine (29.0%). Jia et al. [17] studied adoptive immunity in mice and demonstrated that mice received transfer of immune spleen cells from mice immunized with SA14-14-2 live vaccine was protected better (50% protection) than that from mice immunized with 2 doses of inactivated vaccine (10% protection).Another study was performed for examining the elicitation of cellular immunity by SA14-14-2 vaccine using an enzyme-linked immunospot (ELISPOT) assay. BALB/C mice were s.c. vaccinated with one dose of the live vaccine or 2 doses of a commercial SA14-14-2 inactivated PHK vaccine. Fourteen days after the initial immunization, mice were sacrificed and the the spleenocytes were isolated for detection of INF-◉ and IL-2 spot forming cells (SFC) by

ELISPOT assay. Serum samples were collected from the mice and pooled for detecting neutralizing antibody. Another group of immunized mice were i.p. challenged by virulent JEV P3 strains 14 days postvaccination. The results demonstrated that mice immunized with SA14-14-2 live vaccine produced more IFN-γ SFC (89/10^6 cells) and IL-2 SFC (70-100/10^6 cells) than mice immunized with the inactivated vaccine (<10/10^6 cells), respectively, the positive conversion rates of mice producing IFN-γ and IL-2 SFC following the vaccination with live vaccine compared to the vaccination with inactivated were significant i.e, 100% and 100% vs 20% and 40% respectively. However, neutralizing antibody levels in mice following vaccination with the both vaccines were similar, but higher protection effects were observed for the live vaccine immunized mice (100% vs 80%) (Table 17) [26]. These data suggested the protection correlated better with cellular immunity than neutralizing antibody responses following live vaccine vaccination. Moreover, Li et al. [29] investigated the interaction of SA14-14-2 virus with mouse bone marrow-derived dendritic cells (bmDCs). The results showed that the infection of bmDCs with SA14-14-2 resulted in viral replication and upregulation of bmDCs maturation marker molecules(CD40,CD80,CD83 and MHC1). The infection also stimulated the production of interferon-α(IFN-α),monocyte chemoattractant protein-1 (MCP-1/CCL2), tumor necrosis factor-α(TNF-α) and interleukin-6 (IL-6) of bmDCs. Furthermore, the SA14-14-2 infected bmDCs impaired the expansion of Foxp3+ regulatory T (Treg) cells with immunosuppressive potential, suggesting that SA14-14-2 infection induced antiviral immunity rather than immunosuppression. Taken together, the results indicated that SA14-14-2 infection caused bmDCs maturation, changed the expression profiles of several cytokines, and triggered T cell activation. This offered an insight in the immunologic mechanisms associated with the high efficacy of the SA14-14-2 vaccine.

Vaccine	Vaccinated dose (log_{10}pfu/ml)	ELISPOT assay		Protection	NAb
		IFN-r	IL-2		
SA14-14-2 PHK live	6.31	10/10a	10/10b	10/10c	40d
	3.31	10/10	10/10	9/10	40
	2.31	9/10	10/10	5/10	10
SA14-14-2 inactivated	Undiluted	2/10	4/10	8/10	40
Control	-	0/10	0/10	0/10	10

Table 17. Results of ELISPOT assay, protections and neutralizing antibody (NAb) responses in mice vaccinated with SA14-14-2 live and inactivated JE vaccines. a No. IFN-γ positive/no. tested mice; b No. IL-2 positive/no. tested mice; c No. survival/no. mice tested;d Reciprocal of the highest dilution of serum that resulted in 50% reduction of plaque numbers

Recently, Zhang et al.[65] investigated cytokine and chemokine responses in humans recipients (34 subjects) of SA14-14-2 live attenuated vaccine, the results indicated that levels of interleukin (IL-8), monocyte chemoattractant protein (MCP)-1, macrophage inflammatory protein (MIP)-α and MIP-1β were significantly higher in the vaccinees than in a control group. IL-6 was detectable in 64.7% of vaccinees, but was not detectable in any of the controls. Therefore, IL-6, IL-8, MCP-1,MCP-1α and MIP-1β may play important roles in the immune response to JE live attenuated vaccine in the humans.

Besides Xu et al.[51] reported that mice immunized with SA14-14-2 virus non-structural NS1 protein, which expressed and purified from SA14-14-2 virus NS1 recombinant *E.coli* BL21 (DE3), were protected against a lethal JEV challenge (50-70% protection). Guinea-pigs vaccinated with the NS1 protein presented with reduced viremia following challenge with virulent JE virus (Table 18)

Tested groups	No. animals	Viremia (pfu/ml) by days postchallenge						
		0	1	3	5	7	10	14
SA14-14-2 NS1	1	0a	0	0	0	0	0	0
	2	0	0	0	0	0	0	0
	3	0	0	2. 5	0	0	0	0
	4	0	7. 5	20	0	0	0	0
	5	0	17. 5	145	15	0	0	0
Unimmunized controls	1	0	7. 5	> 579	208	0	0	0
	2	0	47. 5	260	0	0	0	0
	3	0	22. 5	318	230	2. 5	0	0
	4	0	7. 5	225	0	0	0	0
	5	0	0	> 750	ND	ND	ND	ND

Table 18. Viremia suppression in guinea pigs vaccinated with SA14-14-2 NS1 protein followed by challenge with virulent JEV. ND, Not determinedGuinea pigs were intraperitoneally (i.p.) vaccinated with NS1 protein, each 60 ug, at day 0 and 7 respectively. Fourteen days after the first vaccination, each vaccinated and unvaccinated animal was i.p. challenged with virulent JEV P3 strain (each 2.5ml).a No virus detected in the undiluted serum

5. Discussion

Japanese encephalitis is a neuroinvasive virus, which is destructive of neural tissue. Loss of neurovirulence is an important consideration in live JE vaccine development. It is well known that the mice and Rhesus monkeys are highly sensitive animals for testing neurovirulence of JE virus. Both were used during development of live JE vaccine. The process of derivation of the SA14-14-2 strain has demonstrated fine balances between stable neuroattenuation and immunogenicity.

The principal issue surrounding the clinical application of the SA14-14-2 live virus vaccine candidate is safety, especially absence of neurovirulence and stable even passage in brain tissue. During development of the SA14-14-2 strain, it was demonstrated that unstable attenuated virus clones i.e. SA14-12-1-7 and SA14-12-1-1 could be detected by several passages in PHK cells or one i.c. mouse passage. Using this method, SA14-14-2 vaccine virus was selected for its neuroattenuation stability. To ensure vaccine safety, absence of neuroreversion after one ic passage in suckling mice is required in the quality control for vaccine production.

Compared with other live attenuated viral strains, SA14-14-2 has the following characteristics:

1. Not temperature sensitive. During the course of attenuation the SA14 parental virus was cultured at 37°C, while other live vaccine strains were cultured and passaged at lower temperature (24℃ or 32-35°C);

2. Homogeneity. SA14-14-2 strain exhibits as homogeneous small plaques and is stable after several tissue culture passages. The virus strain has been purified by 14 times by a plaque picking technique. Many licensed live vaccines were developed without clonal purification, i.e. the yellow fever 17D vaccine or insufficient purification, i.e. polio vaccine strains. It was reported that the yellow fever 17D vaccine and polio Sabin vaccine virus particles may be heterogeneous [36, 40], as they were not or insufficient cloned. The mixtures may contain neurovirulent virus particles;

3. Highly attenuated for experimental animals: SA14-14-2 strain is avirulent following inoculation by intracerebral or subcutaneous routes in 2.5-week old mice. Monkeys inoculated by the combination of intrathalamic and intraspinal routes developed no signs or death, and on histopathological examination, exhibited minor inflammatory reaction only along the needle track. While the yellow fever vaccine strain 17D, in world-wide use for 70 years, may cause up to 10% death in monkeys while lethal dose in an i.c. mouse test is as high as $3.0\log_{10}$LD50. Also, polio vaccine viruses cause more histopathological lesions in monkeys than did SA14-14-2 virus;

4. Numerous substitutions of nucleotide and amino acid in the virus genome: mutation of virus genome is the molecular basis of attenuation. Molecular studies indicate that the SA14-14-2 vaccine strain differs from that of the virulent parental SA14 strain at 57-66 nucleotide locations resulting in 24-31 amino acid changes. The number of mutations observed is similar to the most stable Polio vaccine virus type I, with 56 nucleotide mutations resulting in 21 amino acid changes. Polio vaccine virus type III, which is unstable, has only 10 nucleotide mutations involving 2-3 amino acids. Polio virus type II, has 23 nucleotide mutations, also fewer than SA14-14-2. More than 70% Vaccine Associated Paralytic Poliomyelitis has been caused by Type III polio vaccine virus, which has the fewest amino acid changes from parental virus [40].

As for the immunogenicity of the SA14-14-2 vaccine, studies have demonstrated that protection efficacy of the live attenuated vaccine was mediated by the presence of neutralizing antibodies and by potent cell-mediated immunity as well as the NS1 protein induced immunity, which associated with the high efficacy of the SA14-14-2 vaccine. Besides anamnestic immune response will give quick rise of neutralizing antibody and provide long-term protection against JE infection among subjects who become seronegative after immunization with SA14-14-2 live vaccine [39]

Live JE vaccine (SA14-14-2) has been used in more than 300 million children since large scale production began in 1989. To date no vaccine associated JE cases has been reported in China and outside.The safety of live JE vaccine is due to a high degree of neuroattenuation and a number of stable phenotypic and genotypic characteristics. The combination of lack of viremia in the vaccinees and the absence of virus replication and dissemination in the mosquito vector make the likelihood of transmission of JE vaccine virus and the risk of environment highly unlikely. Therefore the exceptional safety, stability, immunogenicity and long-term protective efficacy present a strong case for the expended use of this live attenuated JE vaccine in the world.

Author details

Yongxin Yu*

Address all correspondence to: yuyongxin@nicpbp.org.cn

Department of Arbovirus Vaccines, National Institutes for Food and Drug Control, P.R. China

References

[1] Aihara, S., Rao, C. M., Yu, Y. X., Lee, T., Watanabe, K., Komiya, T., et al. (1991). Identification of mutations that occurred on the genome of Japanese encephalitis virus during the attenuation process. *Virus Genes*, 5, 95-109.

[2] Ao, J., Yu, Y. X., Wu, H. Y., Wu, P. F., Wang, Z. W., & Zhang, G. M. (1983). Selection of a better immunogenic and highly attenuated live vaccine virus strain of Japanese encephalitis II. Safety and immunogenicity of live JE vaccine SA14-14-2 observed in inoculated children. *Chin J Microbiol Immunol*, 3, 245-248.

[3] Arroyo, J., Guirakhoo, F., Fenner, S., Zhang, Z. X., Monath, T. P., & Chambers, T. J. (2001). Molecular basis for attenuation of neurovirulence of a yellow fever virus/Japanese encephalitis virus chimera vaccine (ChimeriVax-JE). *J Virol*, 934-942.

[4] Bista, M. B., Banerjee, M. K., Shin, S. H., Tandan, J. B., Kim, M. H., & Sohn, Y. M. (2001). Efficacy of single-dose SA14-14-2 vaccine against Japanese encephalitis: a case control study. *Lancet*, 358(9284), 791-5.

[5] Chen, P. Q., Zhou, B. L., Ma, W. X., et al. (1992). study on the epidemiological efficacy of live Japanese encephalitis vaccine (SA14-14-2). *Chin J Biologicals*, 5, 135-7.

[6] Chotpitayasunondh, T., Sohn, Y. M., Yoksan, S., et al. (2011). Immunizing children aged 9 to 15 months with live attenuated SA14-14-2 Japanese encephalitis vaccine in Thailand. *J Med Assoc Thai*, 94(3), s195-s197.

[7] Eckels, K. H., Yu, Y. X., Dubois, D. R., Marchett, N. J., Trent, D. W., & Johnson, A. J. (1988). Japanese encephalitis virus live-attenuated vaccine, Chinese strain SA14-14-2; adaptation to primary canine kidney cell cultures and preparation of a vaccine for human use. *Vaccine*, 6, 513-8.

[8] Fan, X. L., Yu, Y. X., Li, D. F., & Yao, Z. H. (2002a). Comparison of nucleotide and deduced amino acid sequences of E protein gene of the wild-type Japanese encephalitis virus strain SA14 and its different attenuated derivatives. *Virologica Sinica*, 17, 216-220.

[9] Fan, X. L., Yu, Y. X., Li, D. F., & Yao, Z. H. (2002b). The stability of E protein gene of the Japanese encephalitis live-attenuated vaccine virus SA14-14-2. *Chin J Virology*, 18, 39-47.

[10] Feng, Y., Zhang, H. L., Yu, Y. X., Zhang, Z. Y., Yang, W. H., Dong, G. M., et al. (2007). Observations on the replication of virus and stability of virulence in Culex tritaeniorhynchus after intrathoracically inoculation with attenuated Japanese encephalitis virus SA14-14-2 vaccine strain. *Chin J Zoonoses*, 23, 278-281.

[11] Gao, X. J., Zhao, Y. J., Liu, C. M., Zou, Y., Wei, Y., Zheng, X. G., et al. (2006). The stability of E gene of the Japanese encephalitis attenuated virus strain SA14-14-2. *Prog in Microbiol Immunol*, 34, 1-11.

[12] Gatchalian, S., Yao, Y., Zhou, B., et al. Comparison of the immunogenicity and safety of measles vaccine administered alone or with live, attenuated Japanese encephalitis SA14-14-2 vaccine in Philippine infants [J]. *Vaccine*, 26(18), 2234-2241.

[13] Guirakhoo, F., Zhang, Z. X., Chambers, T. J., Delagrave, S., Arroyo, J., Barrett, A. D. T., et al. (1999). Immunogenicity, genetic stability, and protective efficacy of a recombinant, chimeric yellow fever-Japanese encephalitis virus (ChimeriVax-JE) as a live, attenuated vaccine candidate against Japanese encephalitis. *Virology*, 257, 363-372.

[14] Hennessy, S., Liu, Z. L., Tsai, T. F., et al. (1996). Effectiveness of live-attenuated Japanese encephalitis vaccine (SA14-14-2): a case control study. *Lancet*, 347, 1583-87.

[15] Huang, Z. L., Li, X. G., & Wu, J. N. (1998). Observation on the side reaction after vaccination with Japanese encephalitis live vaccine. *Chin J Zoonoses*, 14, 60-61.

[16] Jia, L. L., Zheng, Z., & Yu, Y. X. (1992). Study on the immune mechanism of JE attenuated live vaccine(SA14-14-2 strain). *Chin J Microbio Immuno*, 12, 364-366.

[17] Jia, L. L., Zheng, Z., Guo, Y. P., & Yu, Y. X. (1992). Stability of live-attenuated Japanese encephalitis vaccine strain SA14-14-2. *Chin J Biologicals*, 5, 174-6.

[18] Jia, L. L., Zheng, Z., & Yu, Y. X. (1993). Pathogenicity and Immunogenicity of attenuated Japanese encephalitis vaccine (SA14-14-2) in immune-inhibited mice. *Virologica Sinica*, 8, 20-4.

[19] Jia, L. L., Zheng, Z., Wang, Z. W., et al. (1995a). Protective effect and antibody response in guinea-pigs immunized with Japanese encephalitis attenuated live vaccine after challenge with virulent virus. *Prog Microbiol Immunol*, 23, 73-76.

[20] Jia, L. L., Zheng, Z., Yu, Y. X., et al. (1995b). Neutralizing antibody response of Japanese encephalitis live vaccine in children residing in JE endemic area. *Chin J*, 11, 343-4.

[21] Jia, L. L., Yu, Y. X., Tsai, T. F., et al. (2000). Immunity of live attenuated Japanese encephalitis (JE) vaccine to different wild JE virus strains. *Chin J Biologicals*, 13, 208-210.

[22] Jia, L. L., Yu, Y. X., Huang, Ying., Wang, Z. W., Yue, G. Z., Zheng, Z., et al. (2004). Stability of phenotype and E Protein gene of primary virus seed and final product of live attenuated Japanese encephalitis vaccine. *Chin J Biologicals*, 17, 12-5.

[23] Kumar, R., & Rizvi, A. (2009). Effectiveness of one dose of SA14-14-2 vaccine against Japanese encephalitis. *N Engl J Med*, 360, 4465-66.

[24] Komiya, Lee T., Watanabe, K., et al. (1995). Immune response in mice infected with the attenuated Japanese encephalitis vaccine strain SA14-14-2. *Acta Virologica*, 39, 161-164.

[25] Li, H. M., Yu, Y. X., Ao, J., & Fong, T. (1966). Studies on the variation of Japanese encephalitis virus : the pathogenicity and immunogenicity of SA14-A clone viruses. *Acta Microbiologica Sinica*, 12, 41-49.

[26] Li, M. G., Yu, Y. X., Liu, X. Y., Xu, H. S., Jia, L. L., Wang, Z. W., et al. (2010). Comparative study on the cellular immune response induced by live attenuated SA14-14-2 Japanese encephalitis vaccine and inactivated Japanese encephalitis vaccine in mice. *Chin J Vaccines Immunization*, 16(4), 339-44.

[27] Li, Y. H., Liu, J., Wang, W., Niu, J. C., Wu, Y. L., Liu, R., et al. (2003). Study of the genetic stability of Japanese encephalitis attenuated virus strain SA14-14-2 after passaging on primary hamster kidney cells. *Chin J Biologicals*, 16, 333-335.

[28] Li, Y. L., Li, S. Y., Wang, H. B., et al. (1999). Comparison of antibody and cell-mediated immune responses induced by live attenuated and inactivated Japanese encephalitis vaccine in mice. *Chin J Biologicals*, 12, 229-230.

[29] Li, Y. M., Ye, J., Yang, X. H., et al. (2011). Infection of mouse bone marrow-derived dendritic cells by live attenuated Japanese encephalitis virus induces cells maturation and triggers T cells activation. *Vaccine*, 29, 855-862.

[30] Ling, J. P., Zhu, Y. G., Du, G. Z., Lang, S. H., Jia, L. L., & Yu, Y. X. (2000). Comparison of pathogenicity and pathology between wild Japanese encephalitis virus SA14 and attenuated strain SA14-14-2 in Rhesus monkey and mouse models. *Progress in Microbiology and Immunology*, 28, 1-4.

[31] Liu, X. Y., Yu, Y. X., Xu, H. S., et al. (2010). Comparison of viremia formation between guinea-pigs infected with wild and attenuated (SA14-14-2) Japanese encephalitis viruses. *Chin J Exp Clin Virol*, 24, 343-5.

[32] Liu, X. Y., Yu, Y. X., Li, M. G., et al. (2011). Study on the protective efficacy of SA14-14-2 attenuated Japanese encephalitis against different JE virus isolates circulating in China. *Vaccine*, 29, 2127-2130.

[33] Liu, Z. L., Hennessy, S., Strom, B. L., Tsai, T. F., Wan, C. M., & Tang, S. C. (1997). Short-term safety of live attenuated Japanese encephalitis vaccine (SA14-14-2): results of a randomized trial with 26,239 subjects. *J Infect Dis*, 176, 1366-9.

[34] Liu, Z. W., Yu, Y. X., Zhang, H. L., Wang, Z. W., Jia, L. L., Zhang, Z. Y., et al. (2007). Biological and molecular characteristics of live attenuated Japanese encephalitis vaccine virus strain SA14-14-2 inoculated intrathoracically to Culex tritaeniorhynchus. *Chin J Biologicals*, 20, 419-421.

[35] Yu, W. X., Wang, Y. X., Zhou, S. G., Ma, B. L. Y. H., Feng, S. Y., et al. (1993). Observation of safety and serological efficacy from large-scale field trial on Japanese encephalitis live vaccine. *Chin J Biologicals*, 6, 188-191.

[36] Monath, T. P. (2004). Yellow fever vaccine. *In: Plotkin SA, Orenstein WA, editors. Vaccines.4th ed. USA: Saunders*, 667-670.

[37] Burns, N. I. H., Chang, N. J., -J, G., Zhang, J., Wills, M. R., Trent, D. W., et al. (1994). Comparison of nucleotide and deduced amino and sequence of non-coding regions and structural protein genes of the wild-type Japanese encephalitis virus strain SA14 and its attenuated vaccine derivatives. *J gen virol*, 75, 1505-1510.

[38] Sohn, Y. M., Park, M. S., Rho, H. O., Chandler, L. J., Shope, R. E., & Tsai, T. F. (1999). Primary and booster immune responses to SA14-14-2 Japanese encephalitis vaccine in Korean infants. *Vaccine*, 17, 2259-64.

[39] Sohn, Y. M., & Tandan, J. B. (2008). A 5-year follow- up of antibody response in children vaccinated with single dose of live attenuated SA-14-14-2 Japanese encephalitis vaccine: Immunogenicity and anamnestic responses [J]. *Vaccine*, 26, 1638-43.

[40] Sutter, R. W., & Cochi, S. L. (2004). Live attenuated poliovirus vaccine. *In: Plotkin SA, Orenstein WA, editors. Vaccines. 4th ed. USA: Saunders*, 667-670.

[41] Tandan, J. B., Ohrr, H., Sohn, Y. M., Yoksan, S. Jim, Nam, C. M., et al. (2007). Single dose of SA14-14-2 vaccine provides long-term protection against Japanese encephalitis: A case-control study in Nepalese children 5 years after immunization. *Vaccine*, 25, 5041-5045.

[42] Tang, W. G., Zhao, D. H., Zhou, S., et al. (2003). A case control study on the effectiveness of live attenuated Japanese encephalitis vaccine. *Chin J Vaccines Immunization*, 9, 213-4.

[43] Wang, J. R., Na, J. Q., Zhao, S. S., et al. (1993). Study on the epidemiological efficacy of live Japanese encephalitis vaccine. *Chin J Biological*, 6, 36-37.

[44] Wang, S. G., Yang, H. J., Deng, Y. Y., Wang, F. B., Zheng, Q. W., & Yu, Y. X. (1990). Studies on the production of live-attenuated Japanese encephalitis vaccine SA14-14-2. *Chin J Virology*, 6, 38-43.

[45] Wang, S. G., Yu, Y. X., Zheng, Q. W., Zhang, D. Q., Jia, L. L., & Li, Y. H. (1992). Study on adaption of attenuated Japanese encephalitis virus strain (SA14-14-2 PHK) to primary fetal dog kidney cell cultures. *Chin J Biologicals*, 5, 49-51.

[46] Wang, Z. W., Jia, L. L., Yue, G. Z., et al. (1999). Study on the comparison of protective effect in mice with three kinds of JE vaccine made in China and Japan. *Chin J Public Health*, 18, 69-71.

[47] WHO Technical Report Series No.910. (2002). Guidelines for the the production and control of Japanese encephalitis vaccine (live) for human use. *In: WHO Expert Committee On Biological Standardization, Fifth-first report. Geneva.World Health Organization. Annex 3.*

[48] Wills, M. R., Singh, B. K., Debnath, N. C., et al. (1993). Immunogenicity of wild-type and vaccine strains of Japanese encephalitis virus and the effect of haplotype restriction on murine immune responses. *Vaccine*, 11, 761-6.

[49] Wu, Y. L., Liu, J., Yang, H. Q., Zhao, N., Mou, J. C., Huang, Y. X., et al. (2007). Genetic property of attenuated Japanese encephalitis virus strain SA14-14-2 after subculture in suckling mouse brain. *Chin J Biologicals*, 20, 19-21.

[50] Wu, Y. L., Zhou, Y., Huang, Y. X., et al. (2007). Dynamic distribution of attenuated Japanese encephalitis virus strain SA14-14-2 in mice. *Chin J Biologicals*, 20, 204-5.

[51] Xu, H. S., Yu, Y. X., Jia, L. L., Huang, Y., Dong, G. M., & Yu, W. Y. (2010). Prokaryotic expression and immunogenicity of NS1 and E proteins of Japanese encephalitis virus SA14-14-2 strain. *Chin J Biol*, 23(2), 118-23.

[52] Xu, L. Y., Xu, W. Q., Xu, F. H., Wang, B., & Zhang, X. J. (2008). Biological and genetic stability of attenuated Japanese encephalitis vaccine virus strain SA14-14-2. *Chin J Biologicals*, 21, 833-837.

[53] Yu, Y. X., Ao, J., Lei, W. X., & LI, H. M. (1962). Studies on the variation of Japanese encephalitis virus: Pathogenicity and immunogenicity in mice and monkeys after serial passages in primary hamster kidney cells. *Acta microbiologica Sincica*, 8, 260-269.

[54] Yu, Y. X., Ao, J., Zhu, Y. G., Fong, T., Huang, N. J., & Liu, L. H. (1973). Studies on the variation of Japanese encephalitis virus. V. The biological characteristics of an attenuated live vaccine virus strain. *Acta Microbiologica Sinica*, 13, 16-24.

[55] Yu, Y. X., Wu, P. F., Ao, J., & Liu, L. H. (1981). Selection of a better immunogenic and highly attenuated live vaccine virus strain of Japanese B encephalitis I. Some biological characteristics of SA14-14-2 mutant. *Chin J Microbiol Immunol*, 1, 77-83.

[56] Yu, Y. X., Wang, J. F., Zhuang, G. M., & Li, H. M. (1985). Response of normal and athymic mice to infection by virulent and attenuated Japanese encephalitis viruses. *Chin J Virology*, 1, 20-39.

[57] Yu, Y. X., & Wang, J. F. (1986). In vitro Characteristics of attenuated Japanese encephalitis viruses. *Chin J Virology*, 2, 197-201.

[58] Yu, Y. X., Zhang, G. M., Guo, Y. P., Ao, J., & Li, H. M. (1988). Safety of a live-attenuated Japanese encephalitis virus vaccine (SA14-14-2) for children. *Am J Trop Med Hyg*, 39, 214-217.

[59] Yu, Y. X., Zhang, G. M., & Zheng, Z. (1989). Immunogenicity of live and killed Japanese Encephalitis (JE) vaccine to challenge with different Japanese Encephalitis virus strains. *Chin J Virology*, 6, 106-10.

[60] Yu, Y. X., Ma, W. X., Jia, L. L., Jiang, X. K., Wang, H. Q., & Yue, G. Z. (1994). Clinical and serological studies of Japanese encephalitis live vaccine, SA14-14-2 PDK strain, in humans. *Chin J Biologicals*, 7, 52.

[61] Zeng, M. Y. U. Y. X., Dong, G. M., Jia, L. L., Yao, Y. F., & Li, D. F. (2001). Sequence analysis of the full-length genome of Japanese encephalitis virus vaccine SA14-14-2. *Chin J Microbiol Immunol*, 21, 535-9.

[62] Zhang, Y. Z., Zhang, H. L., Yu, Y. X., Feng, Y., Dong, G. M., Yang, W. H., et al. (2005a). Studies on Culex tritaeniorhynchus and Culex pipiens quinquefascitatus infected orally by Japanese encephalitis SA14-14-2 vaccine virus. *Chin J Zoonoses*, 21, 584-591.

[63] Zhang, Y. Z., Zhang, H. L., Yu, Y. X., Feng, Y., Dong, G. M., Yang, W. H., et al. (2005b). Research on Culex tritaeniorhynchus and Culex pipiens quinquefascitatus intrathoracically infected with attenuated Japanese encephalitis virus SA14-14-2 vaccine strain. *Chin J Exp Clin Virol*, 19, 344-346.

[64] Zhang, H. R., Wang, L. Y., Chen, L. J., et al. (2002). Analysis on the immune effects and safety of the live attenuated and inactivated Japanese encephalitis vaccines. *Chin J Vaccines Immunization*, 8, 248-50.

[65] Zhang, J. S., Zhao, Q. M., Zuo, S. Q., et al. (2012). Cytokine and chemokine responses to Japanese encephalitis live attenuated vaccine in a human population. *International J Infectious Disease*, 16, 285-288.

[66] Zhou, B. L., Jia, L. L., Xu, X. L., Wang, H. M., Cai, Z. Y., Zhang, Z. J., et al. (1999). A large-scale study on the safety and epidemiological efficacy of Japanese encephalitis (JE) live vaccine (SA14-14-2) in the JE endemic areas. *Chin J Epidemiol*, 20, 38-41.

[67] Zhou, B. L., Zhang, M., Chen, P. Q., Jiang, X. K., Zhang, L. B., Quan, B. H., et al. (2001). An 11 years follow-up of epidemiological effect of live attenuated Japanese encephalitis vaccine (SA14-14-2). *Chin J Biologicals*, 14, 183-185.

[68] Zhu, Y. G., Li, H. M., & Zang, X. (1966). Pathology of attenuated Japanese encephalitis virus. *Chin J Pathology*, 10, 113-6.

Chapter 12

Yellow Fever Encephalitis: An Emerging and Resurging Global Public Health Threat in a Changing Environment

Kaliyaperumal Karunamoorthi

Additional information is available at the end of the chapter

http://dx.doi.org/10.5772/46041

1. Introduction

Emergence and re-surgence of vector-borne diseases still constitute an important threat to human health in the 21st century, causing over a million death and considerable mortality and morbidity worldwide. Vector-borne diseases are linked to the environment by the ecology of the vectors and of their hosts, including humans. In the recent decades, climate change is a global phenomenon which has greatly influenced the emergence and resurgence of several infectious diseases such as malaria, dengue fever, plague, filariasis, trypanosomiasis, leishmaniasis and arbo-viral diseases, particularly yellow fever. Indeed, arbo-viruses will represent a threat for the coming century too. The resource constrained developing countries are the foremost sufferer and the major victims of several vector-borne diseases [1], including yellow fever.

Yellow fever (YF) is one of the great infectious scourges of humankind. It is a zoonosis indigenous to some tropical regions of South America and Africa which has caused numerous epidemics with high mortality rates throughout history [2]. Approximately 200,000 cases of YF occur annually, resulting in about 30 000 deaths; 90% of cases occur in Africa. Large epidemics, with over 100,000 cases, have been recorded repeatedly in Sub-Saharan Africa, and multiple outbreaks have occurred in the Americas. The virus has never appeared in Asia or in the Indian subcontinent [3].

YFV is endemically transmitted in forests and savannas of South America and Africa, periodically emerging from enzootic cycles to cause epidemics of hemorrhagic fever [2],with reported fatality rates ranging from 20% to 80% due to two principal syndromes: YEL-AND (yellow-fever associated neurologic disease, which includes encephalitis, myelitis or myeloencephalitis [ADEM]), and YEL-AVD (yellow-fever associated viscerotropic disease, which usually involves multi-organ failure including liver, renal and circulatory failure) [4].

Although YF has undoubtedly been endemic in tropical Africa for thousands of years, it was only after the arrival of the European migrants in the New World at the end of the fifteenth century that this scourge emerged in the form of devastating epidemics. The term 'vomito-negro' was used in those days to describe clinical aspects of this pathological condition, because death was frequently preceded by black vomit or by partially digested blood. Other terms used to designate yellow fever included 'Yellow Jack' and 'Safran scourge,' with reference to the jaundice observed in many patients [5].

Griffin Hughes was the first to use the term "yellow fever" to describe the disease in his book in 1750 [6]. At different stages of human development, YF has caused untold hardship and indescribable misery among different populations in the Americas, Europe, and Africa. Hundreds of thousands of people have been affected by the disease throughout ages among which tens of thousands have died. YF brought economic disaster in its wake, constituting a stumbling block to development too [7].

YF is known for bringing on a characteristic yellow tinge to the eyes and skin, and for the terrible "black vomit" caused by bleeding into the stomach [8,9]. It was one of the most feared lethal diseases before the development of effective vaccine. Today the disease still affects as many as 200,000 persons annually in the tropical regions of Africa and South America, and poses a significant hazard to unvaccinated travellers to these areas [10]. Recent increases in the density and distribution of the urban mosquito vector, *Ae. aegypti*, as well as the rise in air travel has increased the risk of introduction and spread of yellow fever to North and Central America, the Caribbean and Asia [10].

In East Africa, yellow fever remains as a disease of increasing epidemic risk. The most recent yellow fever outbreak in the region was reported by the WHO in the late 2010 and included the first human cases reported in Uganda in almost 50 years [11]. Prior to this, outbreaks occurred in Sudan (2003 and 2005) and were the first reports of yellow fever from that country in approximately 50 years. These events were preceded by the first outbreak ever reported in Kenya (1992–1993), which were the first reported human cases in East Africa for close to 25 years [11].

Over the last 20 years the number of yellow fever epidemics has risen and more countries are reporting cases. Mosquito numbers and habitats are increasing. Nevertheless, in both Africa and the Americas, there is a large susceptible, unvaccinated population. Changes in the world's environment, such as deforestation and urbanization, have increased contact with the mosquito/virus. Widespread international travel plays an important role in spreading the disease. The priorities are vaccination of exposed populations, improved surveillance and epidemic preparedness [12]. During the 20th century yellow fever has reemerged as a cause of human suffering. The recent epidemics are clearly indicating the vulnerability and potentiality of the YF as a global public health threat in the changing environment. In this context, the present chapter becomes more significant and pertains.

http://dx.doi.org/10.5772/46041

2. Global public health impact

The virus is endemic in tropical areas of Africa and Latin America, with a combined population of over 900 million people [13]. During the past decade, official reports of YF incidence (50-120 cases a year from South America and 200–1200 cases a year from Africa) probably underestimate the true number of cases. Many cases of jaundice and fever (a surveillance definition of yellow fever) are not assessed, unexplained deaths go unreported, symptoms suggest alternative diagnoses, and, in some countries, surveillance systems for yellow fever are not in place [14]. The case-fatality rate ranges from 20% to 50% and is partly dependent on case recognition and testing practices [15,16]. The continued presence and epidemic potential of yellow fever virus make it a global health threat. The growth of international travel to endemic areas annually has increased the number of travelers potentially exposed to the virus and consequently it has increased the risk of introduction into other new areas where competent vectors are present [10].

3. A brief history of YF

The cause of YF was unknown, but it was thought to be contracted either by coming into contact with "effluvia" from those stricken by the disease or with fomites such as clothing, sheets, and other articles that patients had used. Fear of contracting the contagion led people to shun their neighbours and friends and even to abandon loved ones. "It just tore society apart" [17]. Known today to be spread by infected mosquitoes, yellow fever was long believed to be a miasmatic disease originating from rotten vegetable matter and other putrefying filth, and most believed the fever to be contagious. There were many debates regarding the agent that caused YF and Carlos Findlay was the first to suggest that mosquitoes transmitted the disease [8,9]. Text box 1 indicates some of the key milestones in the history of YF [18].

The earliest description of yellow fever is found in a Mayan manuscript in 1648, but by genome sequence analysis it appears that yellow fever virus evolved from other mosquito-borne viruses about 3000 years ago [19]. Yellow fever originated in Africa and in the 1500s yellow fever virus was probably introduced into the New World via ships carrying slaves from West Africa. Epidemics soon became common in the coastal communities of South and Central America and along the southern and eastern seaboard of North America as far north as Boston. Between 1668 and 1893, there were more than 135 epidemics in the USA [17]. Large epidemics occurred throughout the 18th and 19th centuries in the Caribbean islands, the United States, Africa, Europe, West Indies, and South America.

4. Geographical distribution

YF is present in both the rural and urban tropical areas of 45 endemic countries in Africa and Latin America, with a potential combined population of over 900 million individuals

[20]. The vast majority of cases and deaths take place in sub-Saharan Africa, where yellow fever is a major public health problem occurring in epidemic patterns. Africa also experiences periodic yet unpredictable outbreaks of urban yellow fever. Thirty-two African countries are now considered at risk of yellow fever, with a total population of 610 million people, among which more than 219 million live in urban settings [21]. The countries in Africa and the Americas to be at the risk of yellow fever is given in text box 2 [22].

Year	Description of events
1648	An epidemic of probable yellow fever erupts in the Yucatan Peninsula (Mexico)
1750	Griffin Hughes was the first to use the term " yellow fever " to describe the disease in his book
1793	An epidemic in Philadelphia kills about 10% of the population and sparks debate between ''contagionists'' and ''anti-contagionists.''
1802	StubbinsFfirth, a Philadelphia medical student, begins self-experiments to disprove the theory of contagion.
1854	Luis Daniel Beauperthuy of Venezuela suggests that a mosquito might transmit yellow fever.
1881	Carlos J. Finlay of Havana publishes his hypothesis that a specific mosquito (*Cubex cubensis* now *Aedes aegypti*) might transmit yellow fever.
1880s	Yellow fever in Panama kills tens of thousands of French workers, causing Ferdinand DeLesseps to abandon his attempt to build a canal across the isthmus.
1901	The Reed Commission publishes its definitive proof of the mosquito hypothesis based on the data obtained at Camp Lazear.
1902	William Crawford Gorgas supervises on the eradication of yellow fever from Havana by controlling *Ae. aegypti*.
1916	The Rockefeller Foundation begins its commitment to eradicate yellow fever.
1925	The Rockefeller Foundation opens a laboratory in Yaba, Nigeria, to investigate the etiology of yellow fever.
1927	The causative agent of YF disease, YFV, was first isolated from a Ghanaian patient named Asibi
1930	Max Theiler demonstrates that white mice are susceptible to yellow fever by intracerebral inoculation, which leads to a ''mouse protection test'' for seroepidemiologic studies and to an effective vaccine.
1933	Fred L. Soper and colleagues report an outbreak of yellow fever in a rural area of Brazil in which *Ae. aegypti* was not present, suggesting other vectors.
1937	Large-scale immunizations with the 17-D yellow fever vaccine are begun.
1940s	Due to mass vaccination campaigns and efforts to remove *Ae. aegypti* breeding sites, urban YF was dramatically controlled in Africa, particularly in French speaking West African countries
1951	Theiler receives the Nobel Prize for his work that led to the discovery of the 17D vaccine.
2002	The World Health Organization estimates that yellow fever affects each year up to 200,000 persons with up to 30,000 deaths.

Text Box 1. Key Milestones in the History of Yellow Fever (Bryan et al., 2004) [18]

http://dx.doi.org/10.5772/46041

Africa	
West Africa	Benin, Burkina Faso, Cape Verde, Coˆ te d'Ivoire, Equatorial Guinea, Gambia, Ghana, Guinea, Guinea-Bissau, Liberia, Mali, Mauritania, Niger, Nigeria, Sao Tome and Principe, Senegal, Sierra Leone, Togo
Central Africa	Angola, Burundi, Cameroon, Central African Republic, Chad, Democratic Republic of the Congo, Gabon, Rwanda
East Africa	Ethiopia, Kenya, Somalia, Sudan, Tanzania, Uganda
America	
Central America	Panama
South America	Argentina, Bolivia, Brazil, Colombia, Ecuador, Guyana, French Guyana, Paraguay, Peru, Suriname, Trinidad and Tobago, Venezuela

Text Box 2. Countries in Africa and the Americas at the risk of yellow fever

The yellow fever endemic countries in the tropical region of Africa and America are shown in the map (Figure 1) [23]. YF is endemic in ten South and Central American countries and in several Caribbean islands. Bolivia, Brazil, Colombia, Ecuador, and Peru and Venezuela are considered to be at greatest risk. Although the disease usually causes only sporadic cases and small outbreaks, nearly all the major urban centers in the American tropics have been reinfested with *Ae. aegypti* and most urban dwellers are vulnerable because of the low immunization coverage. Latin America is now at greater risk of urban epidemics than at any time in the past 50 years [21].

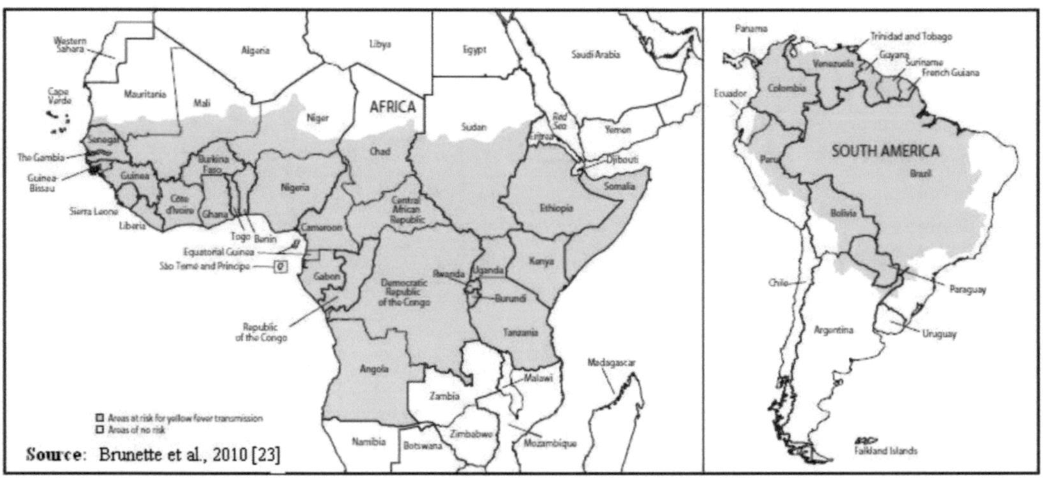

Figure 1. Yellow fever endemic countries in the tropical regions of Africa and America

5. The paradoxical absence of yellow fever from Asian countries

YF has never been reported from Asia, but, should it be accidentally imported, the potential for outbreaks, as the appropriate mosquito vector is present over there [21]. The lack of YFV in Asia is not clearly understood, although a number of hypotheses have been put forward [24]. The mosquito vector *Ae. aegypti* is prevalent in Asia and Pacific countries and has been important in the rapid emergence of dengue as a major public health problem in the twentieth century [25]. Laboratory studies indicate that Asian strains of *Ae. aegypti* can transmit YFV but are less competent than strains from the Americas. Demographic factors, including the remote location of sylvatic YF transmission and the cross-protective immunity provided by prior exposure to dengue and other flaviviruses, likely play a role in the lack of YF in Asia [26].

6. History of human YF outbreaks

At the beginning of the 20th century, a large number of yellow fever epidemics were recorded in both African and American cities, and these occurred against a background of annual cases. Table 1 and 2 lists an overview on the historical outbreaks in both tropical Africa and America by year and countries. Yellow fever epidemics are re-emerging in Africa and America, and the occurrence of repeated rural outbreaks increases the risk for major urban epidemics. The first disease outbreak that can reliably be regarded as YF was documented in 1648 and occurred in the Yucatan, Mexico and Guadeloupe [27].

Year	Countries	Name of City	Cases	Deaths
1668	United States America	New York and Philadelphia	NA	NA
1793	United States America	NA	NA	NA
Between 1668 and 1870 nearly 15 epidemics	United States America	New York	NA	In 1798, 1 500 people died
between 1668 and 1867 30 epidemic in 1793	United States America	Philadelphia	NA	3500
1793 outbreak	United States America	Philadelphia	NA	4000
1853	United States America	New Orleans	NA	7849
1854	United States America	Charleston	NA	682 persons
1878	United States America	Mississippi Valley	NA	13,000 people
1795 outbreak	West Indies	European troops stationed there	NA	3 1,000 people died
1905	United States America	New Orleans	4000	423
1647		Barbados	NA	6000
1802	Haiti	NA	NA	29000

http://dx.doi.org/10.5772/46041

Year	Countries	Name of City	Cases	Deaths
1878	United States America	Over 100 American towns	NA	20000
1942	Brazil	NA	NA	NA
1981-1982	Bolivia	NA	NA	NA
2003	Colombia	States of Cesar, Magdalena and La Guajira	28	11

Table 1. The history of Yellow fever outbreaks in subtropical regions of America

7. Recent emergence and resurgence of YF

In the 18th and 19th centuries, YF was a huge public health problem until mosquito control measures and production of an effective vaccine brought the epidemics under control in the 20th century. Yet as we enter the 21st century this virus is once again a significant public health problem [15,26,28] and is classified as a reemerging disease. Urban YF has not been reported from the Americas since 1954, but jungle yellow fever transmitted by Haemagogus vectors increasingly affects forest dwellers in Bolivia, Brazil, Columbia, Ecuador, and Peru, and periodically causes small outbreaks [15, 29,30]. The reinvasion of South America by *Ae. aegypti* after relaxation of the eradication programme in the 1970s, and presence of *Ae. aegypti* in cities near areas in which sylvatic yellow fever is endemic, poses a threat of urbanisation of yellow-fever transmission [25,29]. Following several decades of relative calmness, YF reappeared in Africa in the 1980s, endangering populations not only in the so-called endemic countries but in the rest of the world too [31]. The resurgence of YF is also closely connected with changes in the modern world and with the interaction of various economic, climatic, social and political factors [32].

8. Compounding factors for emergence and resurgence of YF

YF has been subjected to partial control for decades, but there are signs that case numbers are now increasing globally, with the risk of local epidemic outbreaks [33]. The agent of YF, yellow fever virus, can cause devastating epidemics of potentially fatal, hemorrhagic disease. We rely on mass vaccination campaigns to prevent and control these outbreaks. However, the risk of major YF epidemics, especially in densely populated, poor urban settings, both in Africa and South America, has greatly increased due to: (1) reinvasion of urban settings by the mosquito vector of YF, *Ae. aegypti*; (2) rapid urbanization, particularly in parts of Africa, with populations shifting from rural to predominantly urban; and (3) waning immunization coverage. Consequently, YF is considered an emerging, or reemerging disease of considerable importance [22].

Year	Countries	Number of cases	Year	Countries	Number of cases
1912	Zaire	NA	**1994**	Gabon	28
1917	Zaire	NA	**1994**	Ghana	79
1927-1928	Zaire	NA	**1994**	Kenya	7
1936	Sudan, Uganda, Kenya	NA	**1994**	Nigeria	1227
1940	Sudan, Uganda, Kenya	NA	**1995**	Gabon	16
1958	Zaire	NA	**1995**	Liberia	360
1959	Sudan	NA	**1995**	Senegal	79
1960-1962	Ethiopia	100,000	**1995**	Kenya	3
1965	Senegal	20,000	**1995**	Sierra Leone	1
1966	Ethiopia, Sudan	10,000	**1996**	Benin	120
1969	Nigeria	NA	**1996**	Ghana	27
1971	Angola	NA	**1996**	Senegal	128
1972	Zaire	NA	**1997**	Benin	18
1978	Gambia	8400	**1997**	Ivory Coast	11
1983	Upper Volta	NA	**1997**	Ghana	6
1988	Angola	NA	**1997**	Nigeria	7
1992-1993	Kenya	NA	**1997**	Liberia	1
Epidemics between 1986 and 1994	Nigeria	Approximately 120,000	**1998**	Burkina Faso	2
1990	Cameroon	20,000	**2000**	Nigeria	2
1992	Kenya	NA	**2000**	Liberia	102
1993	Ghana	39	**2000**	Guinea	512
1993	Kenya	27	**2001**	Ivory Coast	203
1993	Nigeria	152	**2001**	Guinea	18
1994	Cameroon	10	**2005**	Sudan	491

Table 2. The history of Yellow fever outbreaks in the subtropical regions of Africa

8.1. Unchecked and unplanned urbanization

It is one of the key determinant in terms emergence and resurgence of many vector-borne diseases particularly YF. With an annual growth rate of nearly 4%, Africa's cities are the fastest expanding in the world. Not only are more and more people living in the cities but the number of cities is also increasing. Whereas today 62.1% of Africa's population lives in rural areas, it is predicted that by 2020 this proportion will be reversed, i.e. that 63% of the continent's population will be urban dwellers. Between now and 2015, it is estimated that the number of cities with more than 1 million inhabitants will increase from 43 to 70 in Africa [34]. On the edge of modern cities, shanty towns with no access to basic sanitation (running water and waste disposal) are also developing rapidly. Domestic water containers and all manner of refuse littering the streets (aluminium and tin cans, old tyres, etc.) favor the multiplication of breeding sites for mosquito larvae [35].

8.2. Climate change

Climate change affects the spread of vector borne diseases both directly and indirectly. Global warming and increased rainfall contribute to the abundance and distribution of vectors like mosquitoes. Current evidence suggests that inter-annual and inter-decadal climate variability have a direct influence on the epidemiology of vector-borne diseases [36]. It is estimated that average global temperatures will have risen by 1.0-3.5°C by 2100 [37], increasing the likelihood of many vector-borne diseases [36]. If the water temperature rises, the larvae take a shorter time to mature [38] and consequently there is a greater capacity to produce more offspring during the transmission period.

The extrinsic incubation period of dengue and yellow fever viruses is also dependent on temperature. Within a wide range of temperature, the warmer the ambient temperature, the shorter the incubation period from the time the mosquito imbibes the infective blood until the mosquito is able to transmit by bite. The implication is that with warmer temperatures not only would there be a wider distribution of *Ae. aegypti* and faster mosquito metamorphosis, but also the viruses of dengue and yellow fever would have a shorter extrinsic incubation period and thus would cycle more rapidly within the mosquito. A more rapid cycle would increase the speed of epidemic spread [39].

8.3. Globalization

Kelley Lee (2000) [40] has defined globalization as 'the process of closer interaction of human activity across a range of spheres, including the economic, social, political and cultural, experienced along three dimensions: spatial, temporal and cognitive'. The recent emergence and resurgence of vector-borne diseases are the result of human activities-transportation of goods and people-and will continue with increasing globalization of trade [41]. The increasing phenomenon of globalization has been observed to alter the YF disease pattern.

8.4. International travel and trade

Every year, about 9 million people from Asia, Europe, and North America travel to countries where yellow fever is endemic; the number of travellers who actually visit areas within these countries where transmission of the virus occurs might exceed 3 million in the coming years [42]. In Africa yellow fever was mainly a problem of the sub-Saharan countries of West Africa, but reached as far east as central Sudan and Kenya [43-46]. A large number of outbreaks were reported in eastern Mexico and other Central American countries. At this time, YF was an epidemic disease mainly of port cities [35].

8.5. Rural-urban migration

West Africa is witnessing significant migratory flows owing to rural exodus, movements of religious groups such as the Mourides in Senegal, cross-border movements of seasonal workers and nomadic pastoral communities, trade routes stretching from the Sahel to the coast of the Gulf of Guinea, the phenomenon of new urban dwellers returning regularly to their rural communities of origin, and migration by populations fleeing armed conflicts.

These human movements increase the risk of contamination of non-immune persons travelling in areas where contaminated vectors persist and, conversely, favour the introduction of the disease into previously YF free zones [47].

8.6. Genetic and behavioral variation

YF outbreaks are common in Africa despite the current knowledge of the disease transmission and the availability of a vaccine. In Africa, YF cases are not uniformly distributed throughout the endemic area; rather, more cases are reported in West Africa compared to East and Central Africa. Genetic differences between genotypes of YF in Africa probably contribute to the observed distribution of YF outbreaks. Genetic and behavioral variation in mosquito vectors may also play a major role in the distribution of YF outbreaks. The other factors also contribute to the epidemiology of YF, including host genetic background, climate, vaccination coverage, vertebrate hosts and movement of vertebrate hosts [48].

9. Yellow fever vectors

Yellow fever virus is transmitted principally by insects (mosquitoes), but ticks (*Amblyomma variegatum*) may play a secondary and minor role in Africa. It was not until 1901 that yellow fever transmission to humans was associated with the blood-feeding by the *Ae. aegypti* mosquito (Figure 2), which was a major breakthrough in understanding this dreadful disease. Dispatched to Cuba by the United States government to investigate the cause of YF, Walter Reed and colleagues confirmed that the primary mode of YF transmission to humans was the *Ae. aegypti* mosquito (Figure 2) and the in ground-breaking virologic studies demonstrated that the disease was caused by an agent that could be filtered from the blood of infected individuals [49]. The reservoirof yellow fever virus is the susceptible vector mosquito species that remains infected throughout its life and can transmit the virus transovarially. Yellow fever can persist as a zoonosis in the tropical areas of Africa and America, with nonhuman primates responsible for maintaining the infection. Man and monkey play the role of amplifiers of the amount of virus available for the infection of mosquitos [50].

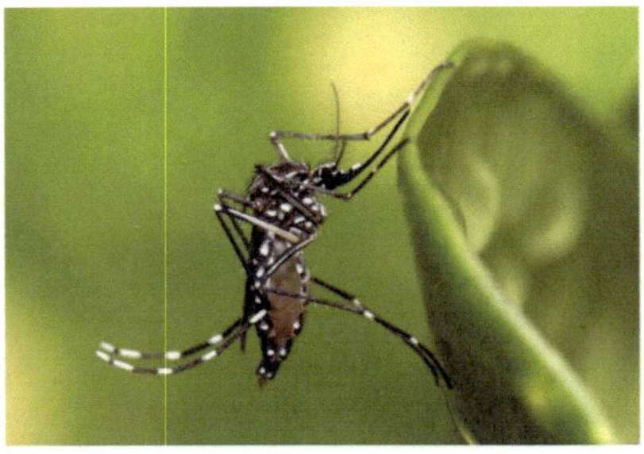

Figure 2. *Aedes aegypti*, the primary disease vector for yellow fever (Photo by Muhammad Mahdi Kharim, published under the GNU free documentation licences)

10. Yellow fever virus

Ever since the causative agent of YF disease YFV, was first isolated in 1927 from a Ghanaian patient named Asibi [50], the Asibi YFV strain is still widely used by the scientists of today. YFV is the prototype member of the family Flaviviridae(from the Latin flavus, meaning yellow), and genus Flavivirus, which get their name from the Latin word for yellow (flavus). The genome is a single-stranded, positive-sense RNA, 10,500 - 11,000 nucleotides in length. The genus Flavivirus contains approximately 70 viruses, and the major flavivirus diseases are yellow fever (YF), dengue, West Nile, Japanese encephalitis, and tick-borne encephalitis [51]. Unlike other mosquito-borne flaviviruses, YFV has a tropism for the liver and causes a viscerotropic disease whereas many other mosquito-borne flaviviruses have a tropism for the brain, or in the case of the DEN viruses they target cells of reticuloendothelial origin [52].

It was one of the earliest viruses to be identified and linked to human disease. Although substantial variation exists among strains, they can be grouped into monophyletic geographical variants, called topotypes. African isolates are usually grouped into two topotypes, associated with East and West Africa [53,54], although some studies have argued for up to five [55]. Two more have been identified from South America, although one has not been recovered since 1974, suggesting that it may be extinct in the wild. There is no evidence for a difference in virulence between the topotypes [56]. YF activity often occurs in areas after increases in temperature and rainfall that will favor increased biodiversity, including increased numbers of animals and arthropods while reduced rainfall limits mosquito vector density [49]. It has been known for over 50 years that increased temperatures are associated with enhanced transmission of YF virus [56] due to shortened extrinsic incubation period and increased biting by mosquitoes of vertebrate hosts [49].

11. Epidemiology

The virus is maintained in endemic areas of Africa and South America by enzootic transmission between mosquitoes and monkeys, and obviously the epidemiology of the disease reflects the geographical distribution of the mosquito vectors [57].

11.1. Transmission

The enzootic transmission cycle involves tree-hole-breeding mosquitoes such as *Aemagogus janthinomys*(South America) and *Ae. africanus*(Africa), and nonhuman primates. Infection of mosquitoes begins after ingestion of blood containing a threshold concentration of virus (~3.5 log 10 $ml^{-}1$), resulting in infection of the midgut epithelium. The virus is released from the midgut into the hemolymph and spreads to other tissues, notably the reproductive tract and salivary glands. A period of 7-10 days is required between ingestion of virus and virus secretion in saliva (the extrinsic incubation period), after which the female mosquito is capable of transmitting virus to a susceptible host.

Vertical transmission of virus occurs from the female mosquito to her progeny and from congenitally infected males to females during copulation. Virus in the egg stage provides a mechanism for virus survival over the dry season when adult mosquito activity and horizontal transmission abate. The virus is maintained over the dry season by vertical transmission in mosquitoes. Ova containing virus survive in dry tree-holes and hatch infectious progeny mosquitoes when the rains resume [58].

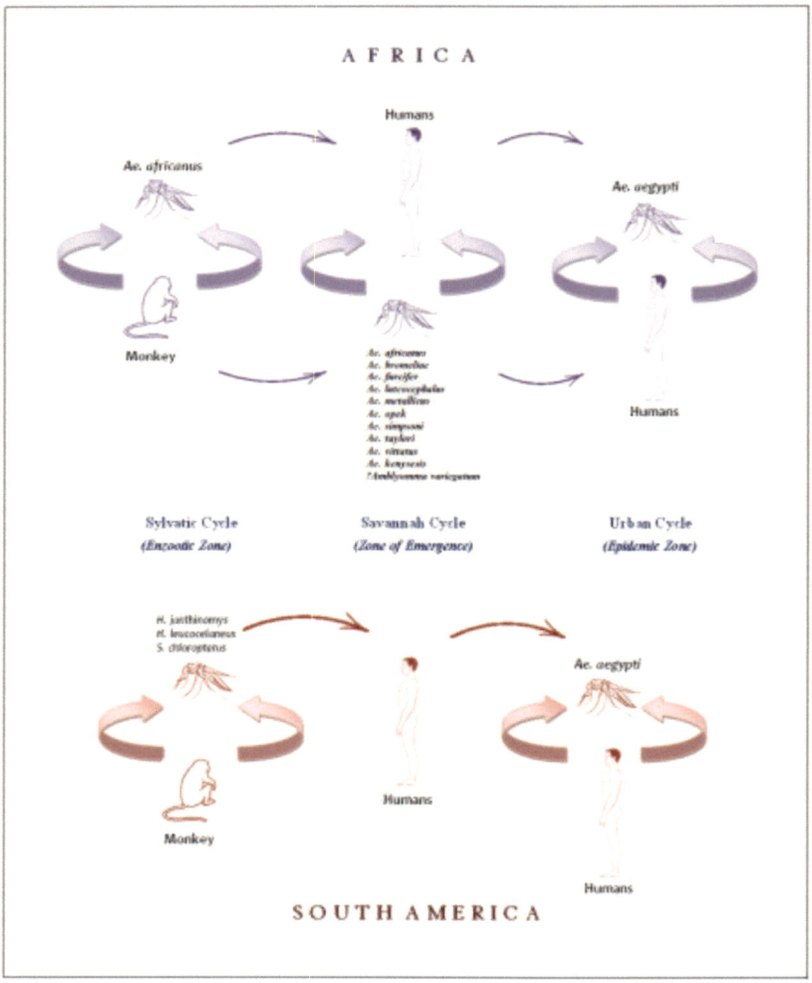

Figure 3. Yellow Fever Transmision cycles in Africa and South America

http://dx.doi.org/10.5772/46041

11.2. Transmission cycle patterns and ecology

In Africa, three transmission cycles can be distinguished: the sylvatic, urban, and savannah cycles. In South America, only sylvatic and urban cycles have been identified (Figure 3). In all the three cycles, yellow fever virus is transmitted between primates by diurnally active tree hole-breeding mosquitoes. Neither the virus nor the clinical disease differs in these three cycles, but identifying the type of transmission cycle is important for disease control. In all of these cycles, endemic and epidemic disease patterns can occur [59]. Sylvatic yellow fever (YF) in South America is maintained in an epizootic cycle between non-human primates and Haemagogus and Sabethes mosquitoes, tree-hole breeding species that reside in the forest canopy. Humans are infected incidentally in the sylvatic cycle when they inhabit or work in the forest where infected mosquitoes are present [60].

In the "Jungle" or "Sylvatic" cycle, the virus is transmitted among monkeys by tree-hole breeding mosquitoes. Humans are infected incidentally when entering the area (e.g., to work as foresters) and have what is termed "jungle yellow fever". The main vector in Africa is *Aedes africanus*, while in South America it is Haemagogus species. Other mosquito species involved in transmission include *Ae. africanus, Ae. furcifer, Ae. vittatus, Ae. luteocephalus, Ae. opok, Ae. metallicus,* and *Ae. simpsoni* in Africa, and Sabetheschloropterus in South America. The primate species acting as vertebrate hosts of the virus also differ by geographic area.

The "Urban" cycle involves transmission of YF virus between humans by *Ae. aegypti*, a domestic vector that breeds close to human habitation in water, and scrap containers including used tires in urban areas or dry savannah areas. In this situation, the disease is known as "urban yellow fever" [49]. YF is transmitted in urban cycles between humans and the container-breeding, anthropophilic mosquito *Aedes aegypti* [15]. In Africa, a third cycle is recognized, the intermediate or savannah cycle, where humans in the moist savannah regions come into contact with the jungle cycle. This has been referred to as the "Zone of Emergence." Although YF is considered to be a mosquito-borne disease, Amblyommavariegatum ticks have been shown to be naturally infected with the virus in central Africa [61]. The significance of this observation in the ecology of YF virus has yet to be determined.

Urban cycle epidemics develop from anthroponotic, also known as human-to-human, transmission in which humans serve as the sole host reservoir of the peridomestic *Ae. aegypti* mosquito vector. Urban epidemics occur when anicteric but viremic persons who are not yet severely ill, travel from jungles and savannas to cities where they infect local *Ae. aegypti* mosquitoes, a species that is abundant in urban areas and in areas where humans store water. When YF is identified in any setting, the likelihood that it resulted from human-to-human transmission or its possible introduction into an urban setting must be rapidly assessed to determine the need for emergency vaccination [62]. The intrinsic incubation period in human beings is between two and six days. The extrinsic incubation period in a mosquito varies from four to 18 days (average 12 days), with the temperature and humidity. Once the mosquito becomes infective, it remains so for the rest of its life [63].

12. Clinical signs and symptoms

YF is the original viral haemorrhagic fever (VHF), a pansystemic viral sepsis with viraemia, fever, prostration, hepatic, renal, and myocardial injury, haemorrhage, shock, and high lethality. Patients with yellow fever suffer with a terrifying and untreatable a clinical disease as yellow fever is responsible for 1000-fold more illness and death than Ebola. Yellow fever stands apart from Ebola and other VHFs in its severity of hepatic injury and the universal appearance of jaundice [10]. It is difficult to distinguish YF' clinically from many other tropical diseases and often impossible when the condition is mild or atypical. The clinical symptoms associated with the early stages of YF infection are indistinguishable from those of malaria, and where the two diseases coexist, YF should not be ruled out even in the absence of jaundice or the finding of malaria parasites in a blood smear [64,65]. The clinical disease varies from non-specific abortive illness to fatal haemorrhagic fever [66]. Disease onset is typically abrupt, with fever, chills, malaise, headache, lower back pain, generalised myalgia, nausea, and dizziness. On physical examination the patient is febrile and appears acutely ill, with congestion of the conjunctivae and face and a relative bradycardia with respect to the height of fever (Faget's sign). The average fever is 39° C and lasts for 3.3 days.

13. Diagnosis of YF

Clinical diagnosis of yellow fever is possible when the pathognomonic features of biphasic/triphasic acute illness and typical clinical features occur in unvaccinated individuals with a compatible exposure history. Unfortunately, these features are present only in a minority of patients [67]. Laboratory confirmation of YF is pivotal to diagnosis, but unfortunately requires highly trained laboratory staff with access to specialized equipment and materials.

Laboratory diagnosis of YF is made by detection of either virus or virus antigen or genome (by enzymelinkedimmunosorbent assay (ELISA), polymerase chain reaction (PCR), or inoculation virus into suckling mice, mosquitoes, or cell cultures), or by serology (immunoglobulin M capture ELISA), though cross-reactions with other flaviviruses complicate serologic methods of diagnosis. Postmortem examination of the liver reveals pathognomonic features of YF, including mid-zonal necrosis, and definitive diagnosis can be made by immunohistochemical staining of tissues (liver, heart, kidneys) for yellow fever antigen. It is important to note that liver biopsy should never be used for diagnosis during YF illness because of the risk for fatal hemorrhage at the biopsy site [67].

14. Treatment

In the absence of specific therapy, treatment of YF is chiefly supportive. Because most YF cases occur in areas lacking basic hospital facilities and where patients do not have access to modern intensive care. In the early stages of the disease, therapy should focus on controlling the fever and vomiting, relieving the headache and abdominal pains, and correcting the dehydration. During the hepatorenal phase, suitable therapy based on careful patient monitoring should be administered to control the bleeding and manifestations associated with hepatorenal damage. Appropriate treatment to control malaria and secondary bacterial infections should be administered when necessary [64,65].

15. Prevention and control

Because no antiviral treatment exists for the disease, prevention through use of personal protection measures and vaccination is crucial to lower disease risk and mortality [14]. A number of approaches have been taken to control YF. Historically, the development of live vaccines was used to control the disease in Africa, whereas mosquito vector control was used in the Americas. Following the demonstration that YFV is transmitted by *Ae. aegypti* came the realization that it should be possible to control the disease by controlling mosquito populations [26]. The re-emergence of yellow fever in Africa and South America during the past decade tempers previous optimism that this disease as a public health problem could be eliminated during the twentieth century [15]. Vaccination and eradication of *Ae. aegypti* are the only effective strategies to reduce YF morbidity and mortality in the affected areas.

15.1. Yellow fever vaccine

Yellow fever vaccine is given for two reasons: to protect travellers visiting areas with the risk of yellow fever virus transmission and to prevent the international spread by minimizing the risk of importation and translocation of the virus by viraemictravellers [14]. Following the successful isolation of YFV in 1927 by American (strain Asibi) and French (strain French viscerotropic virus) workers, researchers placed great effort on the development of vaccines. The development of two live vaccines in the 1930s represents a milestone in the control of the disease. Strain Asibi was passaged through chicken tissue to develop the 17D vaccine strain, whereas strain French viscerotropic virus was passaged through mouse brain to develop the French neurotropic vaccine (FNV). Both vaccines are highly efficacious and they dramatically reduced the number of YF cases in Africa. Unfortunately, the FNV caused cases of postvaccinal neurotropic disease in vaccinees and was discontinued in 1971, whereas 17D is still used today throughout the world [26].

Although immunity from vaccination probably lasts for a lifetime [68,69], a 10 year interval between vaccinations is stipulated in the International Health Regulations (2005) for individuals travelling to countries with a yellow fever vaccination entry requirement. The International Certificate of Vaccination or Prophylaxis is a traveler's official documentation and it becomes valid 10 days after vaccination and remains so for 10 years [36]. Re-immunization is required every 10 years to maintain a valid international vaccination certificate. The World Health Organization recommends vaccination of children at 9 months old, concomitant with measles vaccination, because of better cost/benefit analysis than campaign vaccinations to control outbreaks [70]. It is recommended that the yellow fever vaccine be administered at 12 months of age. In the case of outbreaks, it can be administered as early as 6 months of age [71]. Yellow fever vaccine is a live vaccine, so theoretically it should not be given to pregnant women or to immunosuppressed individuals. A single fatal adverse reaction (encephalitis) has been reported in an immunosuppressed individual with HIV/AIDS.

15.2. Vector control

Vector control is defined as measures of any kind directed against a vector of disease and intended to limit its ability to transmit the disease [72]. In yellow fever control specifically in certain circumstances, mosquito control is vital until vaccination takes effect.

15.2.1. Source reduction

The risk of yellow fever transmission in urban areas can be reduced by eliminating potential mosquito breeding sites and applying insecticides to water where they develop in their immature stages [13]. Indeed, source reduction is one of the key components in the vector control programme since the target is exceptionally specific unlike adult control [73]. Vector-control strategies that were once successful for elimination of yellow fever from many regions have faltered, leading to reemergence of the disease[3]. Application of spray insecticides to kill adult mosquitoes during urban epidemics, combined with emergency vaccination campaigns, can reduce or halt yellow fever transmission and the "buying time" for vaccinated populations to build immunity [13].

Historically, mosquito control campaigns successfully eliminated *Ae. aegypti*, the urban yellow fever vector, from most mainland countries of central and South America. However, this mosquito species has re-colonized urban areas in the region and poses a renewed risk of urban yellow fever. Mosquito control programmes targeting wild mosquitoes in forested areas are not practical for preventing jungle (or sylvatic) yellow fever transmission [13]. The period between about 1950 and the 1970s was one of the complacency about the control of YF, probably arising from the feeling that YF vaccination had solved the problem. *Ae. aegypti* control was reduced and overall disease record keeping appears to have diminished. For the period 1960–2005, only 110 yellow fever points were recorded in Africa and 171 in South America. In both regions, these records more or less fall within the same areas of risk shown for the first half of the last century, although there is a noticeable lack of new records in Central America and proportionately more cases within the Amazon basin [33].

15.2.2. Insect repellents

Ae. aegypti, has adapted their peak biting activities in the early evening and early morning, when their potential hosts are less protected. Mosquito repellents have a unique role under these conditions. Easily accessible, safe and effective mosquito repellents provide a valuable supplement to IRS and ITN use, and in areas with day-biting, exophagic vectors, this may be the only option for reducing the level of disease transmission [74]. The core principle of repellents usage is that they are extremely useful and helpful whenever and wherever other personal protection measures are impossible or impracticable [75]. Insect repellents are ex-

http://dx.doi.org/10.5772/46041

ceptionally helpful to the travelers, who visit for a short-span of time in the disease endemic areas. The main advantage is that the repellents are relatively cheap, highly effective and can be applied as a short-term measure [76].

A laboratory study was carried out to evaluate the relative efficacy of N-N-diethylm-toluamide (DEET) and N,N-diethyl-phenylacetamide (DEPA)-treated wristbands against three major vector mosquitoes. Overall, both DEET and DEPA have shown various degrees of repellency impact against all three vector mosquitoes. DEPA treated wristbands did not show any significant differences in terms of reduction in human landing rate and the mean complete protection time against *An. stephensi* and *Ae. aegypti* were between 1.5 and 2.0 mg/cm^2 [77]. A study revealed the repellent efficacy of dimethyl-phthalate (DMP) treated wristband against *Ae. aegypti* under the laboratory conditions. It is estimated that 74.4 and 86.5% of reduction of man landing rates were obtained against *Ae. aegypti* at concentrations of 1.5 and 2.0 mg/cm2 respectively [1]. These studies results suggest that repellent-treated fabric strips could serve as a means of potential personal protection expedient to avoid insect's annoyance and to reduce vector-borne disease transmission.

However, generally synthetic repellents have several limitations, including reduced efficacy owing to sweating, unpleasant odor, relatively expensive and can cause allergic reactions [72]. Plants have been used since ancient times to repel/kill blood-sucking insects in the human history and even now, in many parts of the world, people use plant substances to drive-away the mosquitoes and other blood-sucking insects [78]. Currently repellents of plant origin have been receiving massive attention due to their environmental and user friendly nature [79].

It is unlikely that vector control strategies alone will result in the elimination of yellow fever; such strategies must be combined with effective vaccination programs. Besides, in YF endemic countries, people particularly travelers should take precautions to avoid mosquito bites to reduce the risk of yellow fever. Besides, using insect repellents, people must use permethrin-impregnated clothing, and bed nets and staying in the screened room could be advisable.

16. Conclusion

YF has played a central role in the history of infectious diseases. It was the first disease to be demonstrated to be transmitted by an arthropod, one of the first diseases to be shown to be caused by a virus, and one of the first infectious agents to be controlled by the development of a live vaccine [80]. Indeed, the challenges and dangers posed by yellow fever remain formidable. It is mainly contributed by the global warming, land use changes, uncontrolled population growth, unchecked urbanization, rural - urban migration, international trade, conflict and civil disruption. Although the tools for diagnosis, vector control, vaccine and surveillance are available, their implementation is extremely poor or inadequate in many of the resource-constrained YF endemic countries. In addition, the global-warming concomitant effect immensely contributed to the high reproduction rate and the capacity of insect vectors to establish and to adapt to new environmental conditions.

Certainly, the present scrutiny clearly suggests that the yellow fever encephalitis is emerging and resurging as a global public health threat in a changing environment. It contributes to remain as a disease of increasing epidemic risk. Therefore, the following issues such as high population density, development of peri-urban areas with rural interfaces, urban construction in forest areas, inconsistent vector control programme, spread of new pathogens, inadequate coverage and short-supply of yellow fever vaccine, must be addressed effectively for the betterment of humankind, eventually to build a yellow fever free world in the near future.

Acknowledgement

I would like to thank Mrs. Melita Prakash for her sincere assistance in editing the manuscript. My last but not the least heartfelt thanks go to my colleagues of our Department of Environmental Health Science, College Public Health and Medicine, Jimma University, Jimma, Ethiopia, for their kind support and cooperation.

Author details

Kaliyaperumal Karunamoorthi[1,2]

Address all correspondence to: k_karunamoorthi@yahoo.com

1 Unit of Medical Entomology & Vector Control, Department of Environmental Health Sciences & Technology, College of Public Health & Medical Sciences, Jimma University, Jimma, Ethiopia

2 Research and Development Centre, Bharathiar University, Coimbatore, Tamil Nadu, India

References

[1] Karunamoorthi K, Sabesan S. Laboratory evaluation of Dimethyl phthalate treated wristbands against three predominant mosquito (Diptera: Culicidae) vectors of disease. European Review of Medical and Pharmacological Science 2010;14(5): 443-448.

[2] Monath T, Cetron M, Teuwen D. Yellow fever vaccine. In: Plotkin S, Orenstein W, Offit P, editors. Vaccines. 5th ed. Saunders Elsevier; 2008. Pp. 959-1055.

[3] Barnett ED. Yellow Fever: Epidemiology and Prevention. Clinical Infectious Diseases 2007;44: 850-6.

[4] Barrett AD, Monath TP, Barban V, Niedrig M, Teuwen DE. 17D yellow fever vaccines: new insights. A report of a workshop held during the World Congress on medicine and health in the tropics, Marseille, France, Monday 12 September 2005. Vaccine 2007;25(15):2758-65.

[5] Chastel C. Yellow Fever, Historical. In: Plotkin S, Orenstein W, Offit P, editors. Vaccines. 5th ed. Saunders Elsevier; 2008. Pp. 959-1055.

[6] Garrison FH. An Introduction to the History of Medicine with Medical Chronology, Suggestions for Study and Bibliographical Data. Philadelphia: W.B. Saunders Company, 1929.

[7] Tomori O. Impact of yellow fever on the developing world. Advances in Virus Research 1999; 53: 5-34.

[8] Findlay C. El mosquito hipot é ticamenteconsideradocomoagente de transmissi ó n de la fiebreamailla.Anuals of Royal Academy. De cien.m é d. de la Habana 1881;18: 147-169.

[9] Chastel C. Centenary of the discovery of yellow fever virus and its transmission by a mosquito (Cuba 1900 – 1901). Bulletin de la Soci é t é de PathologieExotique (1990) 2003;96: 250-256.

[10] Monath TP. Yellow fever: an update. Lancet Infectious Diseases 2001;1: 11-20

[11] Ellis BR, Barrett ADT. The enigma of yellow fever in East Africa. Reviews in Medical Virology 2008;18: 331-46.

[12] US Dep. Health and WHO. Yellow fever. 2008. Available at: http://www.allcountries.org/health/yellow_fever.html (accessed on 16th June 2012).

[13] WHO. Yellow fever Fact sheet N°100, January 2011. Available at: http://www.who.int/mediacentre/factsheets/fs100/en/ (accessed on 16th June 2012).

[14] Jentes ES, Poumerol G, Gershman MD, Hill DR, Lemarchand J, Lewis RF, Staples JE, Tomori O, Wilder-Smith A, Monath TP. The revised global yellow fever risk map and recommendations for vaccination, 2010: consensus of the Informal WHO Working Group on Geographic Risk for Yellow Fever. Lancet Infectious Diseases 2011;11: 622-32.

[15] Robertson SE, Hull BP, Tomori O, Bele O, LeDuc JW, Esteves K. Yellow fever: a decade of reemergence. Journal of the American Medical Association 1996;276: 1157-1162.

[16] WHO. Yellow fever vaccine: WHO position paper. WHO Weekly Epidemiological Record 2003;78: 349-59.

[17] McCarthy M. A century of the US Army yellow fever research. The Lancet 2001;357: 1772

[18] Bryant JE, Holmes EC, Barrett, AD. Out of Africa: a molecular perspective on the introduction of yellow fever virus into the Americas. PLoS Pathogen 2007;3: 668-673.

[19] Zanotto PM de A, Gould EA, Gao GF, et al. Population dynamics of flaviviruses revealed by molecular phylogenies. Proceedings of the National Academy of Sciences of the United States of America 1996;93: 548-53.

[20] Thomas RE, Lorenzetti DL, Spragins W, Jackson D, Williamson T. Active and passive surveillance of yellow fever vaccine 17D or 17DD-associated serious adverse events: Systematic review. Vaccine 2011;29: 4544-4555

[21] WHO. Global Alert and Response (GAR). Yellow fever: a current threat. 2012. Available at: http://www.who.int/csr/disease/yellowfev/impact1/en/index.html (accessed on 3rd June 2012).

[22] Gardner CL, Ryman KD. Yellow Fever: A Reemerging Threat. Clinics in Laboratory Medicine 2010;30: 237-260.

[23] Brunette GW, Kozarsky PE, Magill AJ, Shlim DR, Whatley AD, eds. CDC health information for international travel 2010. Atlanta. GA: US Department of Health and Human Services, Public Health Service, CDC; 2009.

[24] Monath TP. The absence of yellow fever in Asia-cause for concern? Virus information exchange newsletter for South-East Asia and the Western Pacific 1989;6:106-7

[25] Gubler DJ. The changing epidemiology of yellow fever and dengue, 1900 to 2003: full circle? Comparative Immunology, Microbiology and Infectious Diseases 2004;27: 319-30.

[26] Barrett ADT, Higgs S. Yellow fever: a disease that has yet to be conquered. Annual Review of Entomology 2007;5: 209-229.

[27] Carter HR. Yellow Fever: An Epidemiological and Historical Study of Its Place of Origin. Baltimore: The Williams and Wilkins Company, 1931.

[28] WHO. Yellow fever, 1996-1997. WHO Weekly Epidemiological Record 1998a;73: 354-359.

[29] Brès PLJ. A century of progress in combating yellow fever. Bulletin of World Health Organization 1986;64: 775-86.

[30] Anon. Yellow fever, 1996-1997 Part 1. WHO Weekly Epidemiological Record 1998;13;73(46): 354-5.

[31] WHO. Assessment of yellow fever epidemic risk - a decision making tool for preventive immunization campaigns. WHO Weekly Epidemiological Record 2007;18(82): 153-160. Available at: http://www.who.int/wer (accessed on 18th June 2012).

[32] Cardona OD. The need for rethinking the concepts of vulnerability and risk from a holistic perspective: a necessary review and criticism of effective risk assessment,

2003. In: Bankoff G. et al. Mapping vulnerability: disasters, development and people. London, Earthscan Publishers, 2003.

[33] Rogers DJ, Wilson AJ, Hay SI, Graham AJ. The Global Distribution of Yellow Fever and Dengue. Advances in Parasitology 2006;62: 182-220.

[34] World Urbanization Prospects: the 1999 revision. New York, United Nations Population Division, 2001 (ST/ESA/SER.A/194).

[35] Hinrichsen D, Salem RM, Blackburn R. Meeting the Urban Challenge. Baltimore, Johns Hopkins Bloomberg School of Public Health, Population Reports, Series M, No. 16. 2002.

[36] GithekoAK, Lindsay SW, Confalonieri UE, Patz JA. Climate change and vector-borne diseases: a regional analysis. Bulletin of the World Health Organization 2000;78(9): 1136-1147.

[37] Watson RT et al., eds. Climate change 1995; impacts, adaptations and mitigation of climate change: scientific-technical analysis. Contribution of Working Group II to the Second Assessment Report of the Intergovernmental Panel on Climate Change. Cambridge, Cambridge University Press, 1996.

[38] Rueda LM et al. Temperature-dependent development and survival rates of Culex-quinquefasciatus and Aedes aegypti (Diptera: Culicidae). Journal of Medical Entomology 1990;27: 892-898.

[39] Shope RE. Global climate change and infectious diseases. Environmental Health Perspectives 1991;96: 171-74.

[40] Lee K. Globalization and health policy: a review of the literature and proposed research and policy agenda In: Health Development in the New Global Economy PAHO: Washington. 2000.

[41] Reiter IP. Yellow fever to Chikungunya – the globalization of vectors and vector borne diseases. Vector-Borne Diseases: Impact of Climate Change on Vectors and Rodent Reservoirs. Berlin, 27 & 28 September 2007

[42] Monath TP, Cetron MS. Prevention of yellow fever in persons traveling to the tropics. Clinical Infectious Diseases 2002;34: 1369-78.

[43] Soper FL. The unfinished business of Yellow Fever. A speech given at a Symposium in Commemoration of Carlos Juan Finlay. Jefferson Medical College of Philadelphia. 1955.

[44] Haddow AJ. Yellow fever in central Uganda, 1964. Part I. Historical introduction. Transactions of the Royal Society of Tropical Medicine and Hygiene 1965;59: 436-441.

[45] Reiter P, Cordellier R, Ouma JO, Cropp CB, Savage HM, Sanders EJ, Marfin AA, Tukei PM, Agata NN, Gitau LG, Rapuoda BA, Gubler DJ. First recorded outbreak of yellow fever in Kenya, 1992-1993. II. Entomologic investigations. American Journal of Tropical Medicine and Hygiene 1998;59: 650-656.

[46] Bell H. Frontiers of Medicine in the Anglo-Egyptian Sudan, 1899-1940. Oxford Historical Monographs. Oxford: Oxford University Press. 1999.

[47] WHO. World Health Organization Weekly Epidemiological Record 2006;33(81): 317-324. Available at: http://www.who.int/wer/2006/wer8133.pdf (accessed on 2nd June 2012).

[48] Mutebi J, Barrett ADT. The epidemiology of yellow fever in Africa. Microbes and Infection 2002;4: 1459-1468.

[49] Staples JE, Monath TP. Yellow fever: 100 years of discovery. Journal of the American Medical Association 2008;300(8): 960-2.

[50] WHO. Prevention and Control of Yellow Fever in Africa. Geneva, Switzerland, WHO, 1986.

[51] Barrett ADT, Weaver SC. Arboviruses: alphavirusesflaviviruses and bunyaviruses. In Medical Microbiology, ed. D Greenwood, RCB Slacks, JF Peutherer, pp. 482–94. Edinburgh: Churchill Livingstone. 16th ed. 2002.

[52] Volk DE, May FJ, Gandham, SHA, Anderson A, Von Lindern JJ, Beasley DWC, Barrett ADT, Gorenstein DG. Structure of yellow fever virus envelope protein domain III. Virology 2009;394: 12-18.

[53] Deubel V, Digoutte JP, Monath TP, Girard M. Genetic heterogeneity of yellow fever virus strains from Africa and the Americas. Journal of General Virology 1986;67: 209-213.

[54] WHO Yellow Fever. Vol. 2005. WHO; Geneva: 2001. pp. WHO fact sheet 100.

[55] Mutebi JP, Wang H, Li L, Bryant JE, Barrett AD. Phylogenetic and evolutionary relationships among yellow fever virus isolates in Africa. Journal of Virology 2001;75(15): 6999-7008.

[56] Strode GK. Yellow Fever. McGraw-Hill, New York. 1951.

[57] Galbraith SE, Barrett ADT. Vaccines for Biodefense and Emerging and Neglected Diseases. Yellow Fever. Academic Press, 1 Edition, ISBN-13: 978-0123694089. 2009. pp753-785.

[58] Monath TP. Yellow fever. Insect Ecology: an Ecosystem Approach,Schowalter, T.D. (Ed.), 2nd Ed. Elsevier/Academic, San Diego, CA. 2006.

[59] Marfin AA, BarwickEidex R, Monath TP. Yellow Fever. In :Guerrant RL, Walker DH, Weller PF, eds. Tropical Infectious Diseases : Principles, Pathogens, & Practice. 2nd ed. Philadelphia: Elsevier; 2005a.

[60] Monath T. Yellow fever and dengue-the interactions of virus, vector and host in the re-emergence of epidemic disease. Seminars in Virology 1994;5: 133-145.

[61] Germain M, Saluzzo JF, Cornet JP, Hervé JP, Sureau P, Camicas JL, Robin Y, Salaün JJ, Hème G. Isolement du virus de la fièvrejaune à partir de la ponte et de lar-

vesd'unetiqueAmblyommavariegatum. ComptesRendus des Seances de l Academie des Sciences. Serie D, Sciences Naturelles1979;289(8): 635-637.

[62] Huhn GD, Brown J, Perea W, Berthe A, Otero H, LiBeau G, Maksha N, Sankoh M, Montgomery S, Marfin A, Admassu M. Vaccination coverage survey versus administrative data in the assessment of mass yellow fever immunization in internally displaced persons-Liberia, 2004. Vaccine 2006;24: 730-737

[63] Marfin AA, Eidex RSB, Kozarsky PE, Cetron MS. Yellow Fever and Japanese Encephalitis Vaccines: Indications and Complications. Infectious Disease Clinics of North America 2005b;19: 151-168

[64] WHO. Prevention and Control of Yellow Fever in Africa. World Health Organization, Geneva. 1986.

[65] Monath TP, Heinz FX. Flaviviruses. In "Fields Virology" (B.N. Fields, D.M. Knipes, P.M. Howley, R.M. Chanock, J.L. Melnick, T.P. Monath, B. Roizman, and S.E. Straus, eds.), 3rd ed., pp. 961-1034. Lippincott-Raven, Philadelphia. 1995.

[66] Kerr JA. The clinical aspects and diagnosis of yellow fever. In, Strode GK, ed. Yellow fever. New York: McGraw-Hill, pp629-40. 1951.

[67] Monath TP. Yellow fever vaccine. In: Plotkin SA and Orenstein WA (eds.) Vaccines, 4th ed., pp. 1095–1176. Philadelphia, PA: WB Saunders. 2004.

[68] Poland JD, Calisher CH, Monath TP, Downs WG, Murphy K. Persistence of neutralizing antibody 30-35 years after immunization with 17D yellow fever vaccine. Bulletin of World Health Organization 1981;59: 895-900.

[69] Rosenzweig EC, Babione RW, Wisseman CL. Immunological studies with group B arthropod-borne viruses, IV: persistence of yellow fever antibodies following vaccination with 17D strain yellow fever vaccine. American Journal of Tropical Medicine and Hygiene 1963;12: 230-35.

[70] WHO. Global programme for vaccines. Yellow fever. Fact Sheet No. 100. World Health Organization, Geneva: Mimeo; August 1998b, pp. 5.

[71] PAHO. Control of Yellow Fever Field Guide. Scientific and Technical Publication No. 603. PAN American Health Organization, Regional Office of the World Health Organization, Washington, D.C. 20037. 2005.

[72] Karunamoorthi K. Vector Control: A Cornerstone in the Malaria Elimination Campaign. Clinical Microbiology and Infection, 2011a;17(11): 1608-1616.

[73] Karunamoorthi K, Ilango K. Larvicidal activity of Cymbopogoncitratus(DC) Stapf. and Croton macrostachyusDel. against Anopheles arabiensisPatton (Diptera: Culicidae),the principal malaria vector. European Review of Medical and Pharmacological Science 2010;14(1): 57-62.

[74] Moore SJ. Guidelines for Studies on plant-based insect repellents. In Traditional Medicinal Plants and Malaria. Edited by Wilcox M, Bodeker G, Rasoanaivo P. London: CRC Press, Taylor and Francis; pp365-372. 2004.

[75] Karunamoorthi K, Sabesan S. Field trials on the efficacy of DEET impregnated anklets, wristbands, shoulder, and pocket strips against mosquito vectors of disease. Parasitology Research 2009a;105(3): 641-45.

[76] Karunamoorthi K. Systems Thinking: Prevention and Control of Japanese Encephalitis - "The Plague of the Orient", Flavivirus Encephalitis, Daniel Ruzek (Ed.), ISBN: 978-953-307-669-0. 2011b. InTech Open Access Publisher. Available at: http://www.intechopen.com/articles/show/title/systems-thinking-prevention-and-control-of-japanese-encephalitis-the-plague-of-the-orient (accessed on 5th June 2012).

[77] Karunamoorthi K, Sabesan S. Relative efficacy of repellents treated wristbands against three major mosquitoes (Insecta; Diptera: Culicidae) vectors of disease, under laboratory conditions. International Health 2009b;1(2):173-177.

[78] Karunamoorthi K, Ramanujam S, Rathinasamy R. Evaluation of leaf extracts of Vitex-negundo L. (Family: Verbenaceae) against larvae of Culextritaeniorhynchus and repellent activity on adult vector mosquitoes. Parasitology Research 2008;103(3): 545-550.

[79] Karunamoorthi K, Ilango K, Endale A. Ethnobotanical survey of knowledge and usage custom of traditional insect/mosquito repellent plants among the Ethiopian Oromo ethnic group. Journal of Ethnopharmacology 2009;125: 224-229.

[80] Barrett ADT. Yellow fever A deadly disease poised to kill again. The Journal of Clinical Investigation 2006;116(10):2566.

Chapter 13

The Fatal Case of Lyssavirus Encephalitis in the Russian Far East

Galina N. Leonova, Larisa M. Somova,
Sergei I. Belikov, Il'ya G. Kondratov,
Natalya G. Plekhova, Natalya V. Krylova,
Elena V. Pavlenko, Mikhail P. Tiunov and
Sergey E. Tkachev

Additional information is available at the end of the chapter

http://dx.doi.org/10.5772/52869

1. Introduction

Lyssaviruses represent the Lissavirus genus belonging to the family Rhabdoviridae [Warrell, Warrell, 2004]. This genus includes 7 genotypes. Genotype 1 is Rabies virus, which is widespread all over the world [Hughes, 2008; Iseni et al., 1998]. Genotypes 2 (Lagos bat virus) [Boulger, Porterfield, 1958; Sureau et al., 1980], 3 (Mokola virus) [Shope et al., 1970; Familusi et al., 1972; Kemp et al., 1972] and 4 (Duvenhage virus) [Meredith et al., 1971; Van der Merwe, 1982] are widespread in Central and South Africa. In European countries as well as in European part of Russia there are European bat lyssaviruses of subtypes 1 and 2 (EBLV-1 и EBLV-2) belonging to genotypes 5 and 6, which were isolated from bats and humans bitten by them (for EBLV-1: [Boulger, Porterfield, 1958; Schneider, Cox, 1994; Selimov et al., 1989; Selimov et al., 1991], for EBLV-2: [Lumio et al., 1986; King et al., 1994]). Australian bat lyssavirus (ABLV) belongs to genotype 7, which is also known to be isolated from humans [McCall et al., 2000; Fraser et al., 1996]. Four genotypes have been recently discovered which are Aravan Virus (Kyrgyzstan) [Botvinkin et al., 1996; Kuzmin et al., 1992], Khujand virus (Tajikistan) [Kuzmin et al., 2001], Irkut virus (Eastern Siberia) and West Caucasian Bat virus (Caucasus) [Botvinkin et al., 2003].

The risk of bat virus infection in humans is low. Every three months the single cases of chiropteran and human virus infection are reported in Europe (France, Spain, Slovenia, Germany, Romania, Ukraine, Russia, etc.) [Rab. Bull. Europe, 2008]. The confirmed cases of rabies following the bat bite were reported in Ukraine and Russia [Botvinkin et al., 2005]. These cases were associated with European bat virus type 1 (EBLV-1). Human cases of Lyssavirus infection in Siberia and Russian Far East were undiscovered so far.

This paper reviews the epidemiological and clinico-morphological characteristics of the fatal human case of not previously described lyssavirus infection identified in Asian Russia as well as results of virological and molecular genetic analysis of its infection agent.

2. Methods of diagnosis

2.1. Virological tests

The brain samples taken postmortem from the patient were used to prepare 10% suspension. To isolate the virus two-day-old noninbred white mice were used. These animals were challenged with 0.01 ml of 10% brain suspension both intracerebrally and subcutaneously. The isolated strain was called Ozernoe after the place where the dead patient was infected.

The titer of virus with 10-fold dilution was determined using intracerebral inoculation of the two-day-old and three-week-old white mice as well as pig embryo kidney (PEK) cell cultures.

2.2. Immunological methods

The IgG antibodies were determined by ELISA using a Vector-TBE-IgG kit ("Vector-Best", Novosibirsk, Russia). We used the conventional methods for determine hemagglutinating properties of the isolated strain and haemagglutination-inhibition (HI) antibodies in the patient's blood.

For the indirect immunofluorescent (IF) antibody method Ozernoe strain was used to infect continuous PEK cell culture; the slides were prepared on the second day after infection. The luminescent sera against human globulins (manufactured by Gamaleya Institute of Epidemiology and Microbiology RAMS, Moscow, Russia) were used to detect the specific luminescence of the antigen–antibody complexes. The titer of specific antibodies was determined by the bright green intraplasma granular fluorescence of the specific complex using the end-point dilutions of the blood serum.

2.3. Morphological methods

Conventional methods were used for pathohistological examination of the cadaveric material fixed in 8% neutral buffered formalin. The samples were fixed in paraffin wax according to the standard technique [Pearse, 1968], and sections with five micron thickness were cut using a hand-driven microtome and transferred to egg albumin coated slides. Then the sections were dewaxed in xylene, stained in hematoxylin and eosin, mounted in DPX, and viewed under light microscope and photographed (Axioscope A1, Zeiss, Germany).

2.4. Electron Microscopy (EM)

The passaged PEK cell culture was infected with Ozernoe strain. After one day the monolayer was separated from the glass using 0.2 ml of 0.25% tripsin solution after each removal of supernatant fluid for 5 minutes. The PEK cells (2 X10^6), after infection for 1, 2 and 3 days with Ozernoe virus strain, were placed into the combined fixator for 1 h at room temperature [Ito, Karnovsky, 1968]. The fixator was prepared on the basis of 0.2 M cacodylate buffer (pH 7.4) with 3% paraformaldehyde and 0.02% picric acid. After centrifugation the cells were postfixed in 1% buffered OsO4 (Serva, USA) at room temperature for 2 hours. Later on, the dehydration of samples was performed in ethanol solution of increasing density and embedded in epon-araldite resin (Serva, USA). The ultra thin microscopic sections were prepared with ultramicrotome LKB-V (LKB, Sweden) in a plane parallel to the cells monolayer. Samples were contrasted with lead citrate by standard method and examined with Libra 200 FE (Carl Zeiss, Germany) transmission electron microscope.

2.5. Molecular genetic methods

2.5.1. Extraction of RNA, PCR and sequencing

Total RNA was extracted from the brain of infected suckling mice using a RIBO-zol-A kit (AmpliSens, Russia) according to the manufacturer's protocol. Reverse transcription reaction was carried out using random hexanucleotide primers and Reverta-L-10 kit (InterLabService, Russia) according to the manufacturer's recommendations. For initial detection of virus we used primers previously described by Heaton et al. (1997) for nucleoprotein-encoding genes with minor modifications (JW12 – ATGTAACACCCCTACAATGG, JW6(DPL) – CAATTTGCACACATTTTGTG, JW6(M) – CAGTTAGCGCACATCTTATG, JW6(E) – CAGTTGGCACACATCTTGTG). Amplification was performed with common forward primer JW12 and one of the backward primers (JW6(DPL), JW6(M), JW6(E)) alternately. The length of amplification product of the lyssavirus nucleoprotein gene fragment was equally 605 bp. The set of primers for complete genome sequencing has been constructed on the basis of full genome sequence of strain Irkut (GeneBank Accession EF614260), so the amplified fragments were 600-700 nucleotides in length, and overlapping areas of the adjacent fragments were 70-100 nucleotides in length. PCR was carried out in the final volume of 20 µl. PCR buffer contained 4.0 – 6.0 mM magnesium chloride, 65 mM Tris-HCl (pH 8.8), 20 mM $(NH_4)_2SO_4$, 0.01% Tween-20, 200 mM of each dNTP, 0.5 units of Taq-polymerase (AmpliSens, Russia), 10 pmol of each primer and 0.5 – 2 µl of cDNA mixture (template). The amplification was performed with DNA Engine Dyad (MJ Research, USA) using initial denaturation at 96°C for 30 sec followed by 35 cycles of amplification (5 sec – 96°C, 5 sec – 53°C, 1 min – 72°C). All PCR products were analyzed in 0.8 % agarose gel in TAE buffer contained ethidium bromide and DNA amplicons were extracted from gel slices with QIAquick gel extraction kit (Qiagen). In purified PCR products the both strands were directly sequenced using the same set of primers. Sequencing was performed with Genome Lab DTCS-Quick Start Kit (Beckman Coulter, USA) and automated sequencer CEQ-8800 (Beckman Coulter, USA).

2.5.2. Phylogenetic analysis

Phylogenetic trees were constructed by: (i) maximum-parsimony (MP) using algorithms from the DNAPARS and PROTPARS programs of the PHYLIP package; (ii) neighbour-joining (NJ) using the evolutionary distance correction statistics of Kimura (1980) and Tajima & Nei (1984); and (iii) maximum-likelihood (ML) using the PAUP* phylogenetic program [Swofford, 2001].

Bootstrap resampling analysis [Felsenstein, 1985] was carried out using 1000 data replications to evaluate the robustness of the phylogenetic groupings observed. Bootstrap values gave a strong evidence for a particular phylogenetic grouping [Hillis, Bull, 1993]. All ABL nucleotide sequences obtained in this study have been submitted to GeneBank and their accession numbers are listed in Table 1. All other lyssavirus nucleotide sequences used for phylogenetic analysis and sequence comparison were obtained from GenBank; their accession numbers and appropriate references are listed in Table 1.

3. The results of a comprehensive study of virus infection case

3.1. Clinical and epidemiological diagnosis

The patient was a twenty-year-old girl named Zh. who was the resident of Ozernoye village (Yaroslavsky Region, Primorye Territory, Far East of Russia). She's got an acute disease on the 10th of September, 2007 (medical record No11063). The epidemiological anamnesis contained two facts to be paid attention to. Firstly, on July 12 – 13, 2007 the patient was bitten by a tick into lumbar region while being in forest zone of Yaroslavsky Region. Prior to this, she had been vaccinated against tick-borne encephalitis (TBE) and had routine revaccinations. Secondly, on August 10, 2007 in Ozernoe the girl ran into the bat which entered into the house. Being frightened by a loud music the bat has bumped into the girl and wounded her underlip left two thin parallel slightly bleeding stripes. The bat species was unknown. The wounds healed in a short period of time. During one month the girl's mother who was a health-care worker, did not notice any inflammatory infiltration in the wound or increase of regional lymph nodes. The girl felt well and did not have any complaints. She was not vaccinated against rabies.

One month later (on September 10, 2007) the girl got an acute disease caused by hypothermia (she sopped in the rain). Her body temperature rose up to 38°C and intensive headache, repeated vomiting, diplopia, head and hand tremor occurred. On September 11, 2007 she was hospitalized to infectious disease ward of Ussuriysk hospital. The patient has got worse: the general brain symptomatology (constricting diffuse headache and multiple vomiting without any relief) and toxic syndrome increased (the body temperature reached 38.6°); the photophobia occurred. The bulbar disturbances (chocking when swallowing, baryphonia) added and increased; profuse discharge of phlegm from the upper respiratory tract was noticed; meningeal symptoms and depression of consciousness (soporific state) occurred. On September 13, 2007, the patient with a diagnosis of meningoencephalitis was tak-

http://dx.doi.org/10.5772/52869

en into the Primorye Clinical Hospital No.1 of Vladivostok. On her arrival at hospital department of resuscitation and intensive care the patient was in deep sopor. She was found to have three-finger stiff neck. Kernig's sign was not observed. Pupils with the diameter of 3 mm were sluggish in respond to the light, D<S. The diagnosis set was infectious (virus) meningoencephalitis of unknown origin, an acute stage with a severe course attended by deep flaccid paresis and bulbar syndrome. On September 14, 2007, the patient was examined by a neurologist who indicated poor general state and depressed consciousness up to the level of superficial coma. The skin of arms, legs and upper shoulder girdle was covered with punctulated hemorrhagic rash (D=1–1,5 mm). There was Kernig's sign of 160° – 170° on both sides. Pupils were mydriatic, D=S; pupillary reactions were lively. Amyotonia of limbs was observed. Deep reflexes were very weak, D=S; pathological reflexes were not recorded. An assumption of rhabdovirus infection was made upon epidemiological anamnesis, presence of hemorrhagic rash on the skin, ecchymoses at sites of injection, bloody vagina discharges, hypersalivation, and neurologic symptomatology, as well as lack of vaccination against rabies. Development of infection was probably caused by abrupt hypothermia.

As seen in Tabl. 1, blood test revealed the decrease in hemoglobin level (from 149.7 g/L to 116.7 g/L), erythrocyte content (from 4.9 $\times 10^9$ cells per liter to 3.5 $\times 10^9$ cells per liter), the hematocrit (from 48 to 32) and increase in erythrocyte sedimentation rate (ESR) (from 20 mm/hr to 65 mm/hr). At all times a stable leukocytosis (10 – 13 $\times 10^9$ cells per liter) was observed. To estimate a degree of neutrophil shift in blood which reflects the severity of pathologic process, an index of neutrophil shift, which normally is 0.06, was counted. On arrival of the patient at hospital department the index of neutrophil shift was 0.2 that is 3.3 times higher than normal. At the day when patient died the index of neutrophil shift was 0.4, that is 6.7 times higher than normal. The value of leukocyte intoxication index (LII) by Calf-Caliph is representative for the estimation of an intoxication degree. Normally, the LII is 0.3 – 1.5 units and the values ≥1.5 indicate the intoxication. After the hospitalization of the patient the LII was 3.8 units, and by the time of death it was 8.3 units indicating the high stage of intoxication.

Parameters	**13.09.2007**	**21.09.2007**
Hemoglobin	149,7 g/l	116,7 g/l
Erythrocytes	4,9.10^9cells/l	3,5.10^9cells/l
Hematocrit	48	32
ESR	20 mm/h	65 mm/h
Leukocytes	10-13.10^9 cells/l	10-13.10^9 cells/l
(DNI) delta neutrophil index (normal - 0.06)	0,2	0,4
(LI) Leukocyte index of intoxication (normal - 0,3-1,5 u.)	3,8 u.	8,3 u. (high toxicity)

Table 1. Dynamics of the hematological parameters.

Moreover, the determination of total serum immunoglobulin levels (IgM, IgG, IgA) in the patient's blood (on the arrival at hospital) showed the dis-immunoglobulinemia with IgM level 2.4 times higher than normal (3.15 g/L and 1.30 g/L, respectively), and IgG and IgA levels 1.5 and 1.8 times, respectively, lower than normal. The number of circulating immune complexes (CIC) of small sizes was 1.7 times higher than normal (123 and 72 arbitrary units, respectively). The results of hematomancy indicated increasing intensity of intoxication, overall inflammatory reaction, and multiple organ failure.

Despite the intensive therapy (antibacterial, antiviral, neurometabolic, symptomatic, and artificial lung ventilation (ALV) via bronchostomy) the patient was getting worse every day due to the increase of general brain symptoms coupled with multiple organ failure, bilateral hypostatic pneumonia, arterial blood pressure (ABP) fall up to 60/40 mm Hg, and apparent tachycardia of 140 – 160 beats per minute. On the eleventh day, September 21, 2007, the disease resulted in fatal outcome.

3.2. Pathologic diagnosis

The pathologic diagnosis was an acute stage of meningoencephalitis as an underlying disease with complications of edema, swelling and dislocation of brain as well as bilateral hypostatic pneumonia and parenchymatous degeneration of myocardium, liver and kidney. The post-mortem analysis indicated an acute spongy endema in brain and hemocirculatory disorders in all parts of the central nervous system (CNS) (Fig. 1). A significant vascular disruption of the microvasculature was due to plethora, fibrinoid necrosis of vascular wall and the presence of fibrin in the vascular lumen (1 a, b, c), as well as erythrostasis (1 d), hyaline thrombi (1 f) and a small amount of mononuclear cells in many vascular lumen. Around some lumen a sparse perivascular lymphohistiocytic infiltrate was observed (1 a). The spongy edema was found in all parts of the brain. It was the mostly evident in the cerebellum with fiber dissociation of the medullary substance; also the small diapedetic hemorrhages were found. In the cerebellar cortex a total loss of Purkinje cells was observed without any evident proliferation of Bergmann glia. Besides, a dramatic depletion and atrophy of granular layer was found. The mild proliferating and infiltrating components of inflammation stood out particularly due to severe destructive changes of the inflammatory process structure in the CNS. Along with the vascular disruption a total chromatolysis and necrobiosis of nerve cells were found, as well as the formation of many neuronophagic nodules like "rabies nodules" mainly in the subcortical brain (Fig. 1g). In the lung a vascular plethora, erythrostasis, red thrombi in vascular lumen, destructive changes of many vascular walls and an evident serohemorrhagic edema of pulmonary tissue were presented. A polymorphic cellular exudate was observed in the lumen of some large bronchi. In the lung parenchyma a damage of alveolar septa followed by formation of emphysematous areas filled with serofibrinous contents were found. A focal inflammatory polymorphic cellular infiltration was observed. In the spleen the pathohistological changes characterizing a severe immunodeficiency state as delymphatization of white pulp follicles which were not almost visualized were found. At the same time, lymphocyte aggregations were identified only in periarteriolar follicular area (T-dependent zone). A cellular depletion with nonuniform tissue atrophy and denudation of stroma were observed in red pulp. Also the vascular plethora, erythrostasis, fibrinoid swelling, fibrinoid necrosis and hyalinosis of vascular walls, as well as thickening and hyalinosis of septa were found. In the liver the extended distrophic and necrobiotic changes of parenchyma coupled with diffuse sparse proliferation of Kupffer cells and friable polymorphic cellular infiltration along the portal tracts followed by destruction of blood vessel walls were presented. In the kidney a severe necrotic glomerulonephrosis was found. In the cortical substance a necrosis and destruction of the vessels in malpighian tufts, as well as hemorrhages were observed. In the medullary substance a vascular plethora and hemorrhages were found. Also a total necrobiosis and tubular epithelium necrosis were observed along the nephrons. The results obtained by histological study indicated the severe multipleorgan pathology coupled with systemic destructive-dystrophic changes of blood vessels with predominance of edematous and destructive changes in CNS and parenchymatous organs. The pathological process was accompanied by the development of a severe immunodeficiency and a suppression of cell-mediated inflammatory response.

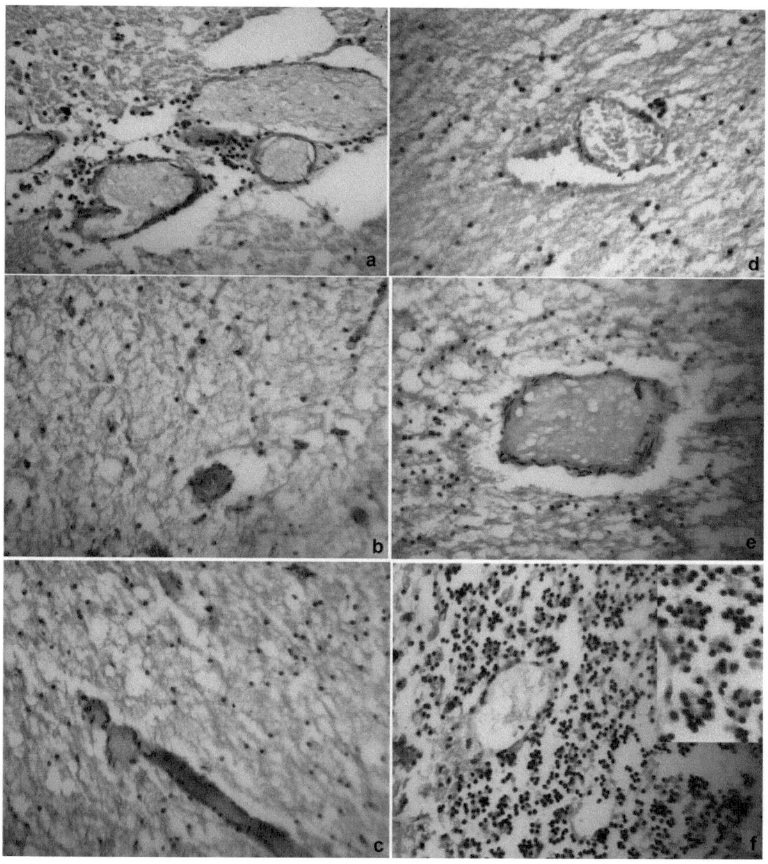

Figure 1. The pathomorphological changes in brain of patient Zh. deceased because of Lyssavirus infection. A – a sparse perivascular found round some lumen; B, C – lymphohistiocytic infiltrate significant vascular disruption of the microvasculature with the fibrinoid necrosis of vascular wall and the presence of fibrin in the vascular lumen; D – erythrostasis; E – hyaline thrombi and a small amount of mononuclear cells in many vascular lumen; F – neuronophagic nodules like "rabies nodules" in the subcortical brain. Gemotoxiline-eozine; X 200.

3.3. The laboratory diagnostics

The brain samples taken postmortem were used to prepare 10% suspension for the infection of two-day-old noninbred white mice. All mice have fall ill on the seventh day; and during the reisolation the symptoms appeared on the sixth day (physical inactivity and respiratory impairment followed by death) (Fig. 2). With the first passage the incubation period shortened to 5 – 6 days.

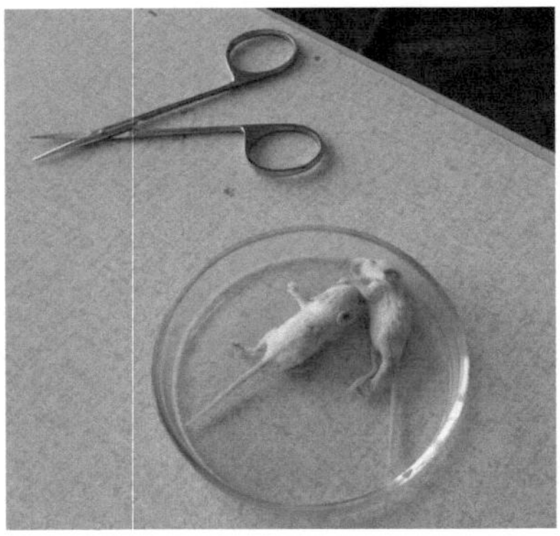

Figure 2. The clinical picture of infection for 6-7 days in mice infected with a 10% suspension of the brain of dead patient Zh.

The two-day-old white mice challenged intracelebrally showed high susceptibility to the isolated virus. Its titer content in the brain of the dead patient was 3.7 lg LD_{50}, and on the first passage it has reached 6.0 lg LD_{50}. At the same time, the susceptibility of the three-four-week-old white mice was much lower; in the first passage the virus titre has hardly reached 2.5 $lgLD_{50}$. The virus antigen showed an evident hemagglutinating activity; in the brain of the dead patient it was 32 a.u., and in the brain on the suckling mice it was 64-128 a.u. The isolated virus strain was named Ozernoe, and the conclusion about the virus etiology of disease was made.

On the fourth day after the onset of disease the patient blood was tested by ELISA for antibodies against tick-borne encephalitis virus (TBEV) and borrelia because the anamnesis had the fact of tick bite in the endemic part of Primorskiy region. The IgM class antibodies against both pathogens were not found, but IgG antibodies against TBEV were revealed with titer 1:800 that was estimated as antibodies after earlier anti-TBEV vaccination. The hemagglutinating antigen was obtained from the brains of infected mice and used in hemagglutination-inhibition reaction test (HIRT); in this test the homologous antibodies were revealed in patient blood sera with titer 1:20. But belonging of this antigen to the particular virus wasn't known, so PEK cells cultures were infected with Ozernoe strain and then the slides with antigen were prepared for virus identification by indirect immunnofluorescence test (IIFT). To get the evidence of homologous antigen specifity in IIFT the blood sera of patient Zh. was used. Both in HIRT and in IIFT the titer were low (the titer 1:40 by specific fluorescence in IIFT). Moreover, the blood serum of person triple-immunized against rabies virus was used for antigen detection in IIFT. Using the slides with Ozernoe strain antigen the antibodies with titer 1:160 were found in this blood serum that could indicate the close antigen relationship between studied strain and vaccine strain of rabies virus. Based on the obtained data we considered that this fatal case could be prevented with timely course of vaccine prophylaxis against rabies virus.

3.4. Electron Microscopy (EM)

The electron microscopy study revealed that the cytoplasm of infected PEK cells contained multivesicular and lamellar bodies. The granular electron-dense structures with fibrillar inclusions were observed around of the cellular nucleus or very close to the plasma membrane during all periods of infection. The number of these structures increased with time and a larger number of them were found at 72 h post-infection (Figs 3b). The granular electron-dense structures were localized very close to the plasma membrane or fused to it (Figs 3c). Each infected cell contained from 2 to 8 cytoplasmic inclusions which seemed to be Negri body-like (viral ribonucleoprotein (RNP)) structures as a strongly electron-dense matrix. The assembled viral particles with 100 nm in diameter and variable lengths (approximately 670 nm) were observed around such structures (Figs 3d). The viral particles were also associated with vesicles close to the endoplasmic reticulum or Golgi apparatus.

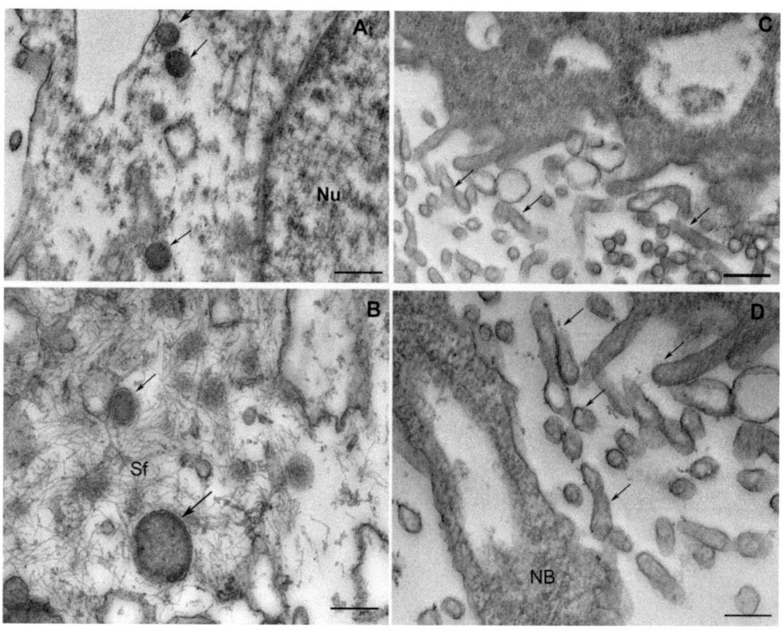

Figure 3. Electron micrographs of cultured PEG cells. A: infected cell 48 h post-infection (pi). The viral inclusions (arrow) were detected inside the cytoplasm. Nucleus (Nu). Bar = 440 nm; B: infected cell 48 h pi; viral inclusions (arrow) and strands forming (Sf) in cellular cytoplasm. Bar = 500 nm; C: infected cell 72 h pi; cytoplasmic vesicles and viral particles (arrows) near the plasma membrane. Bar = 250 nm. D: the viral particles near Negri body-like (NB) structures Bar = 440 nm.

3.5. Genetic identification

Firstly, to identify exactly the virus genotype the fragment of N gene was amplificated and sequenced. The bat virus primers including the primers for six genotypes of rabies and rabies-related viruses [Heaton, 1997] were synthesized to identify a virus genome. The amplicon of the expected length was obtained by PCR with the primers 5′-ATG-TAACACCCCTACAATGG-3′ and 5′-CAATTTGCACACATTTTGTG-3′, and then the nucleotide sequence of amplicon was determined by sequencing. The obtained nucleotide sequence was found to have 95% homology with Irkut strain of bat lyssavirus isolated before from a bat in Eastern Siberia. Eearlier Irkut virus strain had been isolated from a dead Greater Tubenosed Bat *(Murina leucogaster)* in Irkutsk [Botvinkin et al., 2003]. The homology level of this nucleotide sequence with European bat lyssavirus 1 (EBLV-1) is substantially less (from 77 to 76% of identity) and even less with EBLV-2, Duvenhage virus and Rabies virus. The complete sequence of N gene of Ozernoe strain determined in our study (GeneBank No FJ905105) has the 93% homology level with Irkut strain, 79% with EBLV-1 strain, 75% with Duvenhage virus, 77% with EBLV-2 and Khujand viruses, 76% with Rabies, Avaran and ABLV viruses, 75% with Lagos, 73% with West Caucasian and 72% with Mokola viruses (Tabl. 2). Since the Ozernoe strain is the first strain of the genotype 8 isolated from a dead human, we have identified its complete genome sequence. For this purpose, the primers for amplification of complete genome fragments were designed by comparison of complete genomes of the Irkut strain and strains of EBLV-1 of the lyssavirus subtype. Then the complete genome sequence of Ozernoe strain was obtained after sequencing and alignment of overlapping fragments (GenBank accession FJ905105). The lengths of each complete viral genome sequences were 11980 bases for Irkut and Ozernoe strains and corresponded to the standard rhabdovirus genome organization. Lyssavirus genome consists of negative-sense, single-stranded RNA that encodes five viral proteins: nucleoprotein N, phosphoprotein P, matrix protein M, glycoprotein G and polymerase L. Comparison with other lyssavirus sequences demonstrates variation in levels of homology: the nucleoprotein was the most conserved, and the phosphoprotein - the most variable genes (Table 2).

The comparison of complete genomes of Ozernoe and Irkut strains confirmed that they are closely related. The complete genome sequence of Ozernoe strain was 92% identical to the complete genome of Irkut strain, 77-78% to the EBLV-1 genome, and 75% to the EBLV-2 genome. Moreover, the virus proteins sequences are more homologous than the corresponding genes. For example, the N and L genes of Ozernoe strain are 92% identical to Irkut strain sequences, as well as 79% and 77%, respectively, to EBLV-1. At the same time, the corresponding nucleoprotein and polymerase sequences have 98% and 92% homology. Phosphoproteins were found to show the most striking difference with 95% and 70% homology, respectively. Phylogenetic analysis of complete-genome nucleotide sequences of all lyssavirus genotypes showed that Irkut and Ozernoe strains are located on the same branch of the phylogenetic tree, have a common ancestor and form one cluster.

Accession, bat lyssavirus	Maximum identity,%					
		Coding regions of genes				
	Complete genome	N gene	P gene	M gene	G gene	L gene
EF614260.1, Irkut	92%	93%	92%	92	91	92
EF157976.1, EBLV 1 isolate RV9	77%	79	73	80	74	78
EU293120.1, Duvenhage isolate 94286SA	75%	77	70	79	72	76
EF614259.1, Avaran	75%	76	69	78	72	75
EF157977.1, EBLV 2 isolate RV1333	75%	77	69	80	72	75
EF614261.1, Khujand	75%	76	69	78	72	75
AF418014.1, Australian bat lyssavirus	75%	76	68	76	71	74
JQ685919.1, Rabies isolate NJ2262	75%	75	68	74	71	75
EU293108.1, Lagos isolate 0406SEN	75	75	72	72	74	71
EU293117, Mokola isolate 86100CAM	73	74	74	73	69	71
GU170201, Shimoni	77	76	83	74	65	72
EF614258.1, West Caucasian bat virus	70	73	74	73	75	72

Table 2. Comparison of strain Ozernoe homology with other Lyssaviruses.

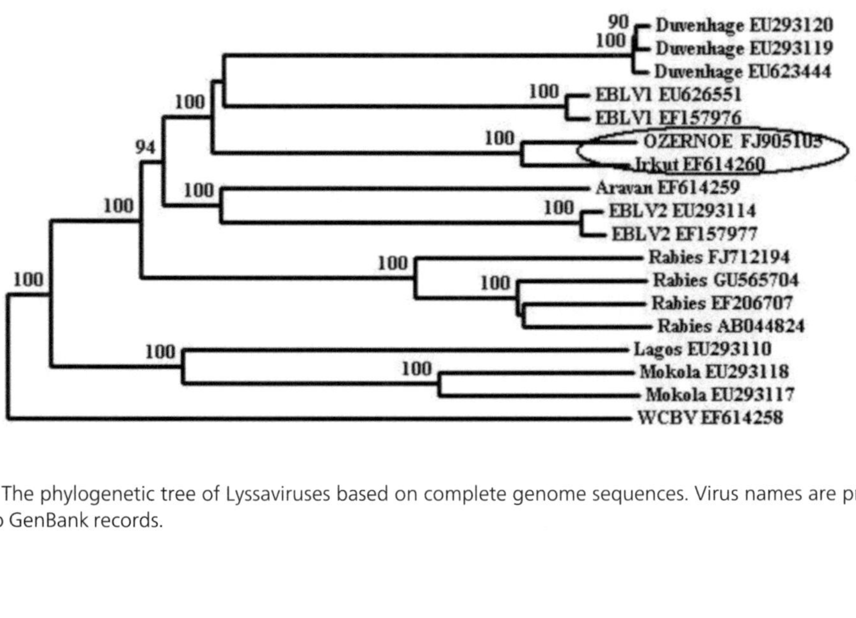

Figure 4. The phylogenetic tree of Lyssaviruses based on complete genome sequences. Virus names are provided according to GenBank records.

4. Discussion

Though human lyssavirus infection cases are rare at Eurasian continent, the minor cases have appeared again and again during the last decades. As a rule, such cases appear unexpectedly, diagnose with delay and end in fatal outcome. For example, the lyssavirus infection case with fatal outcome was described in Scotland in 2003 for the first time in 100 years [Nathwani et al., 2003]. Also, 2 cases of rabies have been confirmed in the United Kingdom in Daubenton's bats (*Myotis daubentonii*): the first in 1996 in Newhaven and the second in September, 2002 in Lancashire; both cases were caused by European bat Lyssavirus (EBLV) type 2a [Whitby et al., 2000; Johnson et al., 2002]. In Europe 3 human deaths from rabies caused by EBLV have been reported [Lumio et al., 1986; Roine et al., 1988; Rabies Bulletin Europe, 1987]. One can say that at present epizootic foci of Lyssaviruses are active and under certain conditions on epidemeological situations the lyssavirus infection cases could take place.

In our study we have shown the first fatal case of lyssavirus infection in Siberia and Russian Far East. The data of epidemiological anamnesis (the patient's underlip was wounded by bat), clinical picture of infection (hypersalivation, chocking, baryphonia, acute meningoencephalitis) as well as the virlogical, morphological and molecular genetic data have given the evidence that this case belonged to lyssavirus infection. The brief description of this case was presented earlier in the Journal "Rabies Bulletin Europe" [Leonova et al., 2009].

We have paid attention to the short incubation period (4 weeks), rapid infection development and fast (in 10 days) fatal outcome. First of all, such infection development could be assosiated with injury localization (head). Thus, the infection fatal case described in Scotland and caused by EBLV-2 was attributed with the bite of patient's finger. The incubation period lasted 19 weeks and fatal outcome came in 14 days after the beginning of disease [Nathwani et al., 2003]. Another fatal case of human rabies caused by Duvenhage bat lyssavirus in Kenya has also indicated about the significance of injury localization [van Thiel et al., 2009]. After the contact with bat the patient has pointed to the small double parallel bleeding wounds at right part of the nose. Though the wounds were disinfected (rinsed with water and soap and treated with alcohol), the patient has got ill in short incubation period (23 days) and died at 20th day of the disease in spite of intensive therapy.

The mother of patient Zh. said that the underlip of her daughter had two typical parallel scratches that were made by bat with the anterior teeth. It means that the saliva of infected animal was in the wound. It should be noted that the appearance of the drops of blood indicated blood vessel damage in dermal layer. But the patients could be mistaken during the contact with bat and told about scratching with leg claws which couldn't form double strip (the bat leg has only one claw) in contrast to skin damage by teeth. The character of skin damage by anterior teeth in a form of double strip should always be the fact of possible virus injection with bat saliva into human blood and requires the drastic measures for the rabies infection prevention.

Therefore, such head injury followed by the vessel damage is considered to have the third severity level which requires the introduction of antirabic immunoglobulin around the wound as well as a specific vaccination regardless the time of antirabic treatment seeking according to the recent criteria of World Health Organization (WHO) Expert Consulation on Rabies. Despite the wound on the underlip made by bat the patient was not vaccinated against rabies as a preventive measure. Representatives of the health care service in the Primorye Territory did not expect that an accidental contact of a human with bat would cause a typical rabies clinical picture.

The evidence of crossimmunity between classical rabies virus of genotype 1 and Lyssaviruses of genotypes 5 and 6 (EBLV types 1 and 2) was obtained; however, definitive proof of cross-protection is lacking [Badrane et al., 2001]. In spite of this fact, we are sure that in cases of possible infection the emergency vaccinal prevention against the rabies should be carried out. About this suggestion the IIFT results of blood sera of patient triply vaccinated against rabies could indicate because they demonstrated the high levels of sera specificity to Ozernoe strain antigen. Moreover, it is known that human diploid cells vaccine protects against classic rabies virus strains and Duvenhage virus, but not Mokola virus and Lagos bat virus; Duvenhage virus is neutralized by RIG, but Mokola and Lagos bat viruses are not [Fekadu et al., 1988; Hanlon et al., 2001]. So, based on the cases described above the vaccine against classic rabies could be used for disease prevention caused not only by rabies virus (genotype 1) but by EBLV (types 1 and 2) and Duvenhage virus. Apparently, it could be attributed to fact that Lyssavirus species segregate into two phylogroups. Phylogroup 1 includes Rabies virus (RABV), Duvenhage virus (DUVV), European bat lyssaviruses, type 1 and 2 (EBLV-1 and 2, respectively), and Australian bat lyssavirus (ABLV). Also, Aravan virus (ARAV), Khujand virus (KHUV) and Irkut virus (IRKV) cross-react serologically with the members of phylogroup 1. Phylogroup 2 includes Lagos bat virus (LBV), Mokola virus (MOKV) and Shimoni bat virus (SHIBV). West Caucasian bat virus (WCBV) does not cross-react serologically with any of the two phylogroups (http://www.who-rabies-bulletin.org/about_rabies/classification.aspx). Certainly, the exact experimental proofs of cross-reacting protection between different Lyssavirus genetic variants should be known to general practitioners to make rapid and correct decision about vaccinal prevention of rabies infection of different etiology. Especially, it is very important in cases with peripheral localization of injury place when a lot of time is available for virus elimination with specific antibodies after patient's vaccination.

Unfortunately, the bat species was not identified, because the killed bat was tortured by a dog. The residents of Ozernoe said that dog had died one month later. The dog, as the bat, was not examined. Other cases indicating a spread of the virus were not registered. However, the doctor working in the neighbouring village found a bat at the medical station. The cases when bats enter into houses are not rare and usually not hazardous for human health. At the same time, during the investigation of houses and nonresidential premises in Ozernoe we did not found any permanent inhabitations of bats. We have suggested that it is possible for bats from nearby forests to enter periodically into the houses.

There are 15 known species of chiropteran in the Far East. The most of them are referred to nonmigratory species; they do not fly far wintering in caves near summer habitats forming large assemblages. Some bat species from southern regions of Primorye Territory spend winters in the balks [Tiunov, 1997].

In Eastern Siberia lyssavirus isolated for the first time from a bat (*Murina leucogaster*) was reported in September, 2002. The bat, which looked healthy, entered into the house in Irkutsk. It was caught and observed. On the tenth day of its observation the symptoms of disease appeared which has resulted in fatal outcome. The virus called Irkut [Botvinkin et al., 2003] was isolated from the brain of the dead animal. During the strain isolation the infected suckling mice had 18 days of the incubation period, and among these mice only one fell ill. At the second passage the incubation period varied from 9 to 18 days. Moreover, it should be noted that the bat infected with Irkut strain wounded the girl, but the illness did not develop due to the timely vaccination against rabies.

Both cases in Irkutsk and Primorye Territory confirm that usually sick animals enter into human dwellings. First of all such animals are of a special danger and require to take measures which protect people from the possible accidental contacts with them. Other cases of lyssavirus infection in Europe reported by Botvinkin et al. (2003) look very similar to these ones.

Unfortunately, the final diagnosis in studied case of infection was stated postmortem. The isolation of Ozernoe strain revealed the following facts to pay attention to: a short incubation period up to 6-7 days; the examined suckling mice of a mouse family fell ill at the same time. If the suckling mice were challenged intracerebrally, the virus titre in the brain of the dead patient was evaluated as 3.7 lg LD_{50}. In the first passage the titre of Ozernoe strain in the mice challenged intracerebrally reached 6 lg LD_{50}. Haemagglutinins were found not only in brain of the infected mice, but also in the brain of the dead patient. These data indicate a high virus concentration which caused profound brain damages and the overall visceral injury followed by impairment of vital functions and resulted in the imminent fatal outcome. The postmortem analysis indicated the changes characteristic for rabies: extensive destructive changes of neurons, formation of many neuronophagic nodules like "rabies nodules", an evident spongy endema of the medullary substance. At the same time, a clearly defined inflammatory reaction around blood vessels was not found. This fact together with the found changes in lymphoid organs indicated the immunodeficiency state, which was undoubtedly associated with the virus infection.

The presence of extracellular viral particles with morphology similar to the structures of Rabies virus on cell surface membranes and spreads forming the electron-dense substance in cellular cytoplasm were revealed during the ultrastructural study. Extracellular viral particles in the environment were distinctly observed and had the morphological signs typical for the group of enveloped viruses with spikes on the surfaces [Iseni, 1998]. The oval and dense bodies (with diameter about 2550 nm) were determinated in cytoplasm and mainly in extracellular environment of PEG cells culture infected by strain Ozernoe. These structures were described earlier as Negri bodies in neurons infected by Rabies virus [Velandia et al., 2007].

To identify exactly the virus genotype the fragment of N gene was amplificated and sequenced. Moreover, the search for homologous sequences in GeneBank using BLAST program has given the absolute evidence that the closest relative of Ozernoe strain is Irkut strain isolated earlier from the bat in Eastern Siberia. Since the Ozernoe strain is the first strain of the genotype 8 isolated from a dead human, we have determined its complete genome sequence. The primers for amplification of genome fragments were designed by comparison of Irkut strain complete genome and EBLV-1 strains of the lyssavirus subtype. The comparison of complete genomes sequences of Ozernoe and Irkut strains confirmed that they are closely related. The virus proteins are more homologous than the corresponding genes. For example, N and L genes of Ozernoe strain are 92% identical to Irkut strains, as well as 79% and 77% to EBLV-1, respectively. At the same time, the corresponding nucleoprotein and polymerase have 98% and 92% homology, and the phosphoproteins show the most striking difference with 95% and 70% homology, respectively.

Irkut and Ozernoe strains are located on the same branch of the phylogenetic tree and form one cluster. The divergence time was estimated to be about 650 years that was calculated upon the rate of evolution within the range from 1.5×10^{-4} to 4.3×10^{-4} dS/site/year [Badrane, Tordo, 2001; Hughes, 2008]. It is interesting to note that Irkut and Ozernoe strains are so closely related despite of their divergence time and distance between their isolation places (about 3,000 km).

So we have demonstrated a real possibility of hazardous lyssavirus infection occurrence in cases when humans accidentally meet chiropteran. This is the first confirmed fatal case of lyssavirus infection on the territory of the Asian continent.

5. Conclusion

The clinical and epidemiological characteristics of fatal human case of lyssavirus infection identified fort he first time in the Asian part of Russia were provided. The evidence that this case belongs to Lyssavirus infection in the terms of etiology was obtained based on the data of epidemiological anamnesis, clinical picture of infection as well as the virological, morphological, and molecular genetic studies. The pathologic diagnosis was the acute stage of meningoencephalitis as underlying disease with complications of edema, swelling and dislocation of brain, the formation of neuronophagic nodules like "rabies nodules" mainly in the subcortical brain as well as bilateral hypostatic pneumonia and parenchymatous degeneration of myocardium, liver and kidney. The study by electron microscopy revealed that the viral particles of 100 nm in diameter could also be associated with the vesicles close to the endoplasmic reticulum or Golgi apparatus. The complete genome sequence of Ozernoe strain is 92% identical to the complete genome of Irkut strain and 77-78% to EBLV-1 genome. The phylogenetic analysis based on the complete genome sequences revealed that Ozernoe strain, isolated from the brain of the dead patient, and Irkut strain, isolated in Irkutsk from the brain of a bat, are located on the same branch of the phylogenetic tree and have the common ancestor. So the real possibility of serious Lyssavirus infection in cases when people have accidentally encountered with chiropteran was demonstrated.

This case has ended in fatal outcome because of the fact that doctors have never registered patients with a lyssavirus infection in the Far East before. Therefore, it was difficult to make the right decision for emergency vaccination against rabies after the accidence as it is usually done in the cases of classical rabies. The exact diagnosis was not get, the clinical course of infection was rapid and following remedial actions have been unsuccessful.

Acknowledgements

The authors thank the infectious disease specialists, neurologists from clinical hospitals of Primorsky Krai, actively involved in clinical and epidemiological description of the case.

This work was supported by Grant ISTC N° 4006.

Author details

Galina N. Leonova[1], Larisa M. Somova[1], Sergei I. Belikov[2], Il'ya G. Kondratov[2], Natalya G. Plekhova[1], Natalya V. Krylova[1], Elena V. Pavlenko[1], Mikhail P. Tiunov[3] and Sergey E. Tkachev[4]

1 Institute of Epidemiology and Microbiology, Siberian Branch of the Russian Academy of Medical Sciences, Vladivostok, Russia

2 Limnological Institute, Siberian Branch of the Russian Academy of Sciences, Irkutsk, Russia

3 Biology-soil Institute, Far Eastern Branch of Russian Academy of Sciences, Vladivostok, Russia

4 Institute of Chemical Biology and Fundamental Medicine, Siberian Branch of the Russian Academy of Sciences, Novosibirsk, Russia

References

[1] Badrane, H., & Tordo, N. (2001). Host switching in Lyssavirus history from the Chiroptera to the Carnivora orders. J. Virol. Sep., , 75(17), 8096-104.

[2] Badrane, H., Bahloul, C., Perrin, P., & Tordo, N. (2001). Evidence of two lyssavirus phylogroups with distinct pathogenicity and immunogenicity. J. Virol., , 75, 3268-76.

[3] Botvinkin, A. D., Kuzmin, I. V., & Rybin, S. N. (1996). The unusual bat lyssavirus Aravan from Central Asia. Myotis., , 34, 101-4.

[4] Botvinkin, A. D., Poleschuk, E. M., Kuzmin, I. V., Borisova, T. I., Gazaryan, S. V., Yager, P., & Rupprecht, C. E. (2003). Novel lyssavirus isolated from bats in Russia. Emerg. Inf. Dis.,, 9, 1623-1625.

[5] Botvinkin, A. D., Selnicova, O. P., Antonova, L. A., et al. (2005). Human Rabies case caused from a bat bite in Ukraine. Rab.Bull.Europe., p. 3.

[6] Boulger, L. R., & Porterfield, J. S. (1958). Isolation of a virus from Nigerian fruit bats. Trans. R. Soc. Trop. Med. Hyg., , 52, 421-4.

[7] Bourhy, H., Kissi, B., Lafon, M., Sacramento, D., & Tordo, N. (1992). Antigenic and molecular characterization of bat rabies virus in Europe. J Clin Microbiol., , 30, 2419-26.

[8] Rab, Bull., & Europe, . (2008). (1-4), 1-4.

[9] Familusi, J. B., Osunkoya, B. O., Moore, D. L., Kemp, G. E., & Fabiyi, A. (1972). A fatal human infection with Mokola virus. Am. J. Trop. Med. Hyg., , 21, 959-63.

[10] Fekadu, M., Shaddock, J. H., Sanderlin, D. W., & Smith, J. S. (1988). Efficacy of rabies vaccines against Duvenhage virus isolated from European house bats (Eptesicus serotinus), classic rabies and rabies-related viruses. Vaccine , 6, 533-539.

[11] Felsenstein, J. (1985). Phylogenies and the comparative method". American Naturalist , 125, 1-15.

[12] Fraser, G. C., Hooper, P. T., Lunt, R. A., Gould, A. R., Gleeson, L. J., Hyatt, A. D., Russell, G. M., & Kattenbelt, J. A. (1996). Encephalitis caused by a lyssavirus in fruit bats in Australia. Emerg. Infect. Dis., , 2, 327-31.

[13] Fooks, A. R., Mc Elhinney, L. M., Pounder, D. J., et al. (2003). Case report isolation of a European bad lyssavirus type-2a from a fatal Human case of Rabies Encephalitis. J. Med. Virol.;71, , 2(2), 281-289.

[14] Gribencha S.V.(2008). Rabies. In: Lvov D.K., editor. Meditsinskaya Virusologia (Medical Virology) [in Russian]. Moscow: "Med. Inform. Agenstvo":, 586-594.

[15] Hanlon, C. A., De Mattos, C. A., De Mattos, C. C., Niezgoda, M., Hooper, D. C., et al. (2001). Experimental utility of rabies virus-neutralizing human monoclonal antibodies in post-exposure prophylaxis. Vaccine , 19, 3834-3842.

[16] Heaton, P., Johnstone, P., Mc Elhinney, L., Cowley, R., O'Sullivan, E., & Whitby, J. (1997). Heminested PCR assay for detection of six genotypes of rabies and rabies related viruses. J. Clin. Microbiol., , 35, 2762-6.

[17] Hillis, D. M., & Bull, J. J. (1993). An empirical test of bootstrapping as a method for assessing confidence in phylogenetic analysis. Systematic Biology , 42, 182-192.

[18] Hughes, G. J. A., reassessment, of., the, emergence., time, of., European, bat., & lyssavirus, type.. (2008). Infect. Genet. Evol., , 8, 820-824.

[19] Iseni, F., Barge, A., Baudin, F., Blondel, D., & Ruigrok, R. W. H. (1998). Characterization of rabies virus nucleocapsids and recombinant nucleocapsid-like structures. J. Gen. Virol., , 79, 2909-2919.

[20] Ito, S., & Karnovsky, M. J. (1968). Formaldehyde-glutaraldehyde fixatives containing trinitrocompounds. J. Cell Biol., 39:168.

[21] Johnson, N., Selden, D., Parsons, G., & Fooks, A. R. (2002). European bat lyssavirus type 2 in a bat in Lancashire. Vet. Rec.; , 151, 455-6.

[22] Kemp, G. E., Causey, O. R., Moore, D. L., Odelola, A., & Fabiyi, A. (1972). Mokola virus. Further studies on IBAN 27377, a new rabies-related etiologic agent of zoonosis in Nigeria. Am. J. Trop. Med. Hyg., , 21, 356-9.

[23] Kimura, M. (1980). A simple method for estimating evolutionary rates of base substitutions through comparative studies of nucleotide sequences. Journal of Molecular Evolution , 16, 111-120.

[24] King, A. A., Meredith, C. D., & Thomson, G. R. (1994). The biology of Southern African Lyssavirus variants. In: Rupprecht C.E., Dietzschold B., Koprowski H., editors. Lyssaviruses. Berlin:Springer-Verlag; , 267-295.

[25] Kuzmin, I. V., Botvinkin, A. D., Rybin, S. N., & Bayaliev, A. B. (1992). Lyssavirus with usual antigenic structure isolated from bat in southern Kyrghyzstan. Vopr. Virusol., 5-6:256-259.

[26] Kuzmin, I. V., Botvinkin, A. D., & Khabilov, T. K. (2001). The lyssavirus was isolated from a whiskered bat in northern Tajikistan. Plecotus et al. , 4, 75-81.

[27] Kuzmin, I. V., Hughes, G. J., Botvinkin, A. D., et al. (2005). Phylogenetic relationships of Irkut and West Caucasian bat viruses within the Lyssavirus genus and suggested quantitative criteria based on the N gene sequence for lyssavirus genotype definition. Virus Res., 111, , 1(1), 28-43.

[28] Kuzmin I.V., Wu Xianfu, Tordo Noel, Rupprecht C.E.(2008). Complete genomes of Aravan, Khujand, Irkut and West Caucasian bat viruses, with special attention to the polymerase gene and non-coding region. Virus Res., , 136, 81-90.

[29] Leonova, G. N., Belikov, S. I., Kondratov, I. G., Krylova, N. V., Pavlenko, E. V., Romanova, E. V., Chentsova, I. V., & Petukhova, S. A. (2009). A fatal case of bat lyssavirus infection in Primorye Territory of the Russian Far East. J. "Rabies-Bulletin-Europe" Information Surveillance Report December 2009., 33(4-October)

[30] Lumio, J., Hillbom, M., Roine, R., Ketonen, L., Haltia, M., Valle, M., Neuvonen, E., & Lähdevirta, J. (1986). Human rabies of bat origin in Europe. Lancet., 1:378.

[31] Mc Call, J. M., Epstein, J. H., Neill, A. S., Heel, K., Field, H., Barret, J., Smith, G. A., Selvey, L. A., Rodwell, B., & Lunt, R. (2000). Potential exposure to Australian bat lyssavirus, Queensland, 1996-1999. Emerg. Infect. Dis., , 6, 259-264.

[32] Meredith, C. D., Rossouw, A. P., & Koch, H. V. P. (1971). An unusual case of human rabies thought to be chiropteran origin. S. Afr. Med. J., , 45, 767-769.

[33] Nathwani, D., Mc Intyre, P. G., White, K., Shearer, A. J., Reynolds, N., Walker, D., Orange, G. V., & Fooks, A. R. (2003). Fatal Human Rabies Caused by European Bat Lyssavirus Type 2a Infection in Scotland. Clin. Inf. Dis., , 37, 598-601.

[34] Pearse A.G.E.(1968). Histochemistry, theoretical and applied. 3rd edn., Churchill Livingstone, London, 660.

[35] Pieter-Paul, A. M., van Thiel, Rob. M. A., de Bie, Filip., Eftimov, Robert., Tepaske, Hans. L., Zaaijer, Gerard. J. J., van Doornum, Martin., Schutten, Albert. D. M. E., Osterhaus, Charles. B. L. M., Majoie, Eleonora., Aronica, Christine., Fehlner-Gardiner, Alex. I., Wandeler, Piet. A., & Kager, . (2009). Fatal Human Rabies due to Duvenhage Virus from a Bat in Kenya: Failure of Treatment with Coma-Induction, Ketamine, and Antiviral Drugs www.plosntds.orgJuly, e428., 3(7)

[36] Roine, R. O., Hillbom, M., Valle, M., et al. (1988). Fatal encephalitis caused by a bat-borne rabies related virus. Brain, , 111, 1505-16.

[37] Schneider, L. G., & Cox, J. H. (1994). Bat lyssaviruses in Europe. In: Rupprecht C.E., Dietzschold B., Koprowski H., editors. Lyssaviruses. Berlin: Springer-Verlag, , 207-218.

[38] Selimov, M. A., Tatarov, A. G., Botvinkin, A. D., Klueva, E. V., Kulikova, L. G., & Khismatullina, N. A. (1989). Rabies-related Yuli virus; identification with a panel of monoclonal antibodies. Acta Virol., , 33, 542-545.

[39] Selimov, M. A., Smekhov, A. M., Antonova, L. A., Shablovskaya, E. A., King, A. A., & Kulikova, L. G. (1991). New strains of rabies-related viruses isolated from bats in the Ukraine. Acta Virol., , 35, 226-231.

[40] Shaw, K. L., Lindemann, D., Mulligan, M. J., & Goepfert, P. A. (2003). Foamy virus envelope glycoprotein is sufficient for particle budding and release. J. Virol., 77, , 4(4), 2338-2348.

[41] Shope, R. E., Murphy, F. A., Harrison, A. K., Causey, O. R., Kemp, G. E., Simpson, D. I., & Moore, D. L. (1970). Two African viruses serologically and morphologically related to rabies virus. J. Virol., , 6, 690-692.

[42] Sureau, P., Tignor, G. H., & Smith, A. L. (1980). Antigenic characterization of the Bangui strain (ANCB 672d) of Lagos bat. Ann. Virol., , 131, 25-32.

[43] Swofford, D. L., Waddell, P. J., Huelsenbeck, J. P., Foster, P. G., Lewis, P. O., & Rogers, J. S. (2001). Bias in phylogenetic estimation and its relevance to the choice between parsimony and likelihood methods. Syst. Biol. , 50(4), 525-39.

[44] Tajima, E., & Nei, M. (1984). Estimation of evolutionary distances between nucleotide sequences. Mol. Biol. Evol. , 1, 269-285.

[45] Tiunov M.P.(1997). Rukokrylye Dalnego Vostoka (Chiropters of the Russian Far East) [in Russian]. Vladivostok: "Dalnauka", 126 p.

[46] Van der Merwe, M. (1982). Bats as vectors of rabies. S. Afr. J. Sci., , 78, 421-422.

[47] Velandia, M. L., Perez-Castro, R., Hurtado, H., & Castellanos, J. E. (2007). Ultrastructural description of rabies virus infection in cultured sensory neurons. Mem. Inst. Oswaldo Cruz., Rio de Janeiro, , 102(4), 441-447.

[48] Warrell, M. J., & Warrell, D. A. (2004). Rabies and other lyssavirus diseases. Lancet , 363, 959-969.

[49] Weekley, B. (1975). Electron Microscopy for Beginners [Russian translation], Moscow: "Mir", 320 p.

[50] WHO Expert Consulation on Rabies: first report.(2004). WHO technical report series, N 931: 18.

[51] Whitby, J. E., Heaton, P. R., Black, E. M., Wooldridge, M., Mc Elhinney, L. M., & Johnstone, P. (2000). First isolation of a rabies-related virus from a Daubenton's bat in the United Kingdom. Vet Rec., , 147, 385-8.

[52] World Health Organization.(1987). Bat rabies in the USSR. Rabies Bulletin Europe, , 4, 12-4.

Chapter 14

Pathogenesis of Encephalitis Caused by Persistent Measles Virus Infection

Tomoyuki Honda, Misako Yoneda, Hiroki Sato and Chieko Kai

Additional information is available at the end of the chapter

http://dx.doi.org/10.5772/54434

1. Introduction

Demyelinating encephalitis is a type of encephalitis in which the insulating myelin sheath surrounding nerve fibers is damaged. Most types of demyelinating encephalitis are known to be caused by viral infection, and therefore the nature of viral persistence in the central nervous system (CNS) has become crucial to understanding the pathogenesis of associated diseases. Subacute sclerosing panencephalitis (SSPE) is a progressive fatal demyelinating disease caused by infection with high levels of neuronal measles virus (MV) in the CNS. Thus, MV infection provides one of the main paradigms of persistent viral infection that causes encephalitis. Many reviews have been published explaining how MV establishes a persistent infection in the CNS [1, 2, 3]. A number of studies on SSPE using cDNA cloning and sequencing techniques have revealed that MV genomes are present in samples obtained from SSPE patients. This demonstrates the presence of mutations that may lead to MV persistence in the CNS. However, no study has been able to explain how persistent MV is reactivated and results in subsequent pathogenesis of the CNS. In this review, we describe a brief overview of MV and SSPE. We will attempt to focus on host cell modifications related to MV persistence, and on reactivation mechanisms of MV during persistent infections. We will then discuss the pathogenesis of persistent MV infections in patients to highlight molecular events that lead to the manifestation of SSPE symptoms. These key advances in the understanding of MV persistence will provide novel insights into the elucidation of SSPE pathogenesis.

2. Measles and the CNS sequelae

Measles. Measles is a highly contagious respiratory disease caused by MV. More than 10 million people worldwide are affected by MV each year, resulting in several hundred thousand deaths [4]. Clinical symptoms of infection are fever, cough, conjunctivitis, rash, and Koplik spots. Immunosuppression for many weeks after apparent recovery is also a characteristic of MV infection. CNS involvement in measles is a common feature, although most patients do not present with clinical evidence of encephalitis. However, transient electroencephalography abnormalities are observed in approximately 50% of patients [5]. Measles can induce encephalitis in at least four different paradigms: primary measles encephalitis (PME); acute post-infectious measles encephalomyelitis (APME); measles inclusion-body encephalitis (MIBE) and SSPE. PME and MIBE are caused by an active or ongoing MV infection, but SSPE and APME are not. APME, which occurs in approximately 0.1% of MV cases (with a lethality of approximately 20%), develops shortly after infection, but active virus is not observed in the CNS. In APME and SSPE, neuropathological demyelination has been observed to develop.

SSPE. SSPE is a progressive fatal neurological disease that causes widespread demyelination of the CNS and infection of neurons. This is followed by infection of oligodendrocytes, astrocytes and endothelial cells [6]. It takes approximately 6–8 years after an acute MV infection for the first symptoms of SSPE to appear [7, 8]. In the early stages, affected children present with poor school performance. Motor regression is eventually seen in 100% of affected individuals, and then the disease progresses to a vegetative state [9]. Serum and cerebrospinal fluid (CSF) contain high, or very high, titers of antibodies against MV [10, 11]. Intranuclear and/or intracytoplasmic inclusion bodies are often present [12, 13]. Infiltrating mononuclear cells are first apparent in the meninges, and perivascular cuffs and infiltrates can become extensive. Some infected neurons and oligodendrocytes contain fibrillary tangles similar to those seen in other neurodegenerative diseases [14, 15].

MV. MV is a negative-sense, single-stranded RNA virus that belongs to the genus *Morbillivirus*, family *Paramyxoviridae*. The virus is composed of six structural proteins: nucleoprotein (N), phosphoprotein (P), matrix protein (M), fusion protein (F), hemagglutinin (H), and large protein (L). Among these structural proteins, the N, P, and L proteins are essential for viral replication and transcription. MV genomic RNA is packaged into ribonucleoprotein (RNP) complexes, consisting of the N protein and a viral RNA-dependent RNA polymerase (RdRp). The RdRp is composed of the P and L proteins, both of which are responsible for replication and transcription of the MV genome. In addition to these structural proteins, the P gene of MV encodes accessory proteins, C and V.

MV persistence. MV produces not only an acute lytic infection, but also an occasional persistent infection. A growing body of evidence supports the persistence of MV in the infected host. As an example, a boy who had been treated for granulomatous disease using stem cell therapy died owing to MV complications [16]. Because neither the patient nor the stem cell donor had recently been exposed to MV or been vaccinated, it is most likely that MV persisted in either the donor or the patient and was reactivated. It is possible that a MV infection can persist throughout a patient's lifetime without triggering overt disease [17]. It is also possible that reactivation of a persistent MV infection can sometimes cause SSPE long after the acute infection [18].

http://dx.doi.org/10.5772/54434

SSPE virus strains. The sequences of viral genomes from SSPE cases are typically not related to current circulating wild-type viruses, but instead to those in circulation when patients developed an acute MV infection. This is confirmation that SSPE is caused by a persistent MV infection [19, 20]. Genetic analyses have also revealed that persistent MVs derived from SSPE cases (SSPE virus strains, SSPEVs) contain numerous mutations. The existence of characteristic mutations common to SSPEVs has been suggested [21, 22]. The M gene of SSPEVs appears to be particularly vulnerable to mutation, and its expression is restricted. In many SSPEVs, an A-to-G hypermutation occurs in the genome and destroys the M protein-coding frames. Although hypermutation of the M gene results in the defective expression of the M protein, replacement of the M gene did not confer a neurovirulent phenotype in hamsters [23]. Hypermutations in the M gene likely slow down the migration of the virus and thereby prolong infection. A mutated M protein interacts at low affinity, or not at all, with RNP complexes and is associated with the accumulation of nucleocapsids inside infected cells [24]. Other changes in SSPEV structural proteins have been found in the F and H proteins. The F proteins of some SSPEVs have been demonstrated to contribute to neurovirulence in animals by showing hyperfusion activity [23, 25]. The H protein also contributed to neurovirulence to some extent [23, 25], although it is not required for trans-synaptic transmission [26].

3. Host cell modifications in MV persistence

Modifications in MV-infected cells. The growth of RNA viruses depends on the mRNA translation machinery of the cells. Many viruses modify the host cell machinery to favor translation of their own mRNA. During the acute phase of MV infection, the virus induces suppression of protein synthesis (designated "shut-off") in host cells and viral mRNAs are preferentially translated [27]. The phosphorylation of eukaryotic initiation factor (eIF) 2α and the binding of the N protein to eIF3-p40, which are cellular initiation factors required for cap dependent tranlation, are involved in the induction of shut-off [27, 28]. The La protein is involved in the preferential translation of viral mRNAs [29]. All these modification are found in the acute MV infection (Figure 1A). A persistent MV infection becomes clinically apparent many years after the acute infection. There are no apparent symptoms in the time between acute infection, and the onset of SSPE clinical symptoms; this would indicate that replication of the persistently infecting MV is in equilibrium with replication of the host cells. Some as yet unidentified modifications might be involved in disease progression during MV persistence (Figure 1B). These need to be investigated to understand the mechanisms of persistence and pathogenicity.

Modulation of gene expression patterns in MV-infected cells. Several studies examining gene expression in MV-infected cells have been reported [30-32]. MV infection of dendritic cells up-regulates a broad array of interferon (IFN)-αs, but fails to up-regulate double-stranded RNA-dependent protein kinases [31]. MV infection of human peripheral blood mononuclear cells (PBMCs) modulates the activity of NF-κB transcription factors [30]. MV infection also induces expression of molecules involved in defense against endoplasmic reticulum (ER) stress and apoptosis in PBMCs and human lung epithelial cells [30, 32]. All these molecules affected in MV-infected cells might be involved in SSPE pathogenesis. As an example, long-term administration of IFNs is one type of SSPE therapy [33]. NF-κB may be a determinant of multiple sclerosis (MS) susceptibility, a chronic demyelinating disease of the CNS in humans [34]. As glial cells appear to be vulnerable to ER stress, altered expression of the molecules involved in ER stress can perturb myelination by oligodendrocytes [35]. Apoptotic processes have also been suggested to contribute to MS, where local tissue damage involves apoptosis of oligodendrocytes and neurons [36].

Lipid metabolism in cells persistently infected with MV. Most studies examining gene expression in MV-infected cells have been performed in non-neuronal cells. Because modulation in gene expression is cell-type dependent [37], studies using neuronal cells are more informative. The molecules affected during persistent infection might be different from those in the acute infection. Two studies using neuronal cells persistently infected with MV revealed alterations in lipid metabolism, such as decreased cholesterol synthesis and impaired β-oxidation, that were associated with MV persistence [38, 39]. Myelination is a complex process that requires a precise stoichiometry for gene dosage, along with protein and lipid synthesis. An alteration in lipid metabolism during persistent MV infection would affect the maintenance of myelin in the CNS.

4. Reactivation mechanisms of persistent MV

It is known that persistent MV infection is asymptomatic but can eventually result in SSPE [2]. The latent MV should be reactivated at the onset of disease, resulting in clinical signs of SSPE (Figure 1C). However, the molecular mechanisms of MV persistence and reactivation are yet to be elucidated.

Heat shock protein 72 (hsp72). One potential molecule involved in MV reactivation is hsp72. Hsp72 binds to two conserved motifs in the variable tail of the N protein, known as box 2 (amino acids 489–506) and box 3 (amino acids 517–525) [40]. The tail of the N protein is within the same area where the XD domain of the P protein (amino acids 459–507) binds to the N protein [41]. *In vivo* models using mice expressing hsp72, or hyperthermal preconditioned mice, have revealed that hsp72 levels can serve as a host determinant of viral neurovirulence in mice. This indicates the direct influence of hsp72 on viral gene expression [42, 43]. Hsp72 induction by some type of reactivation event might enhance the replication of persistent MV in the CNS, resulting in the onset of clinical symptoms. Accumulation of the H protein inside the cell during persistent MV infection might be such a reactivation event, as antibodies against the MV can decrease cell surface expression of viral glycoproteins, which has been suggested to contribute to the establishment of MV persistence [44, 45]. Indeed, overexpression of the H protein leads to induction of hsp72 (Figure 2).

http://dx.doi.org/10.5772/54434

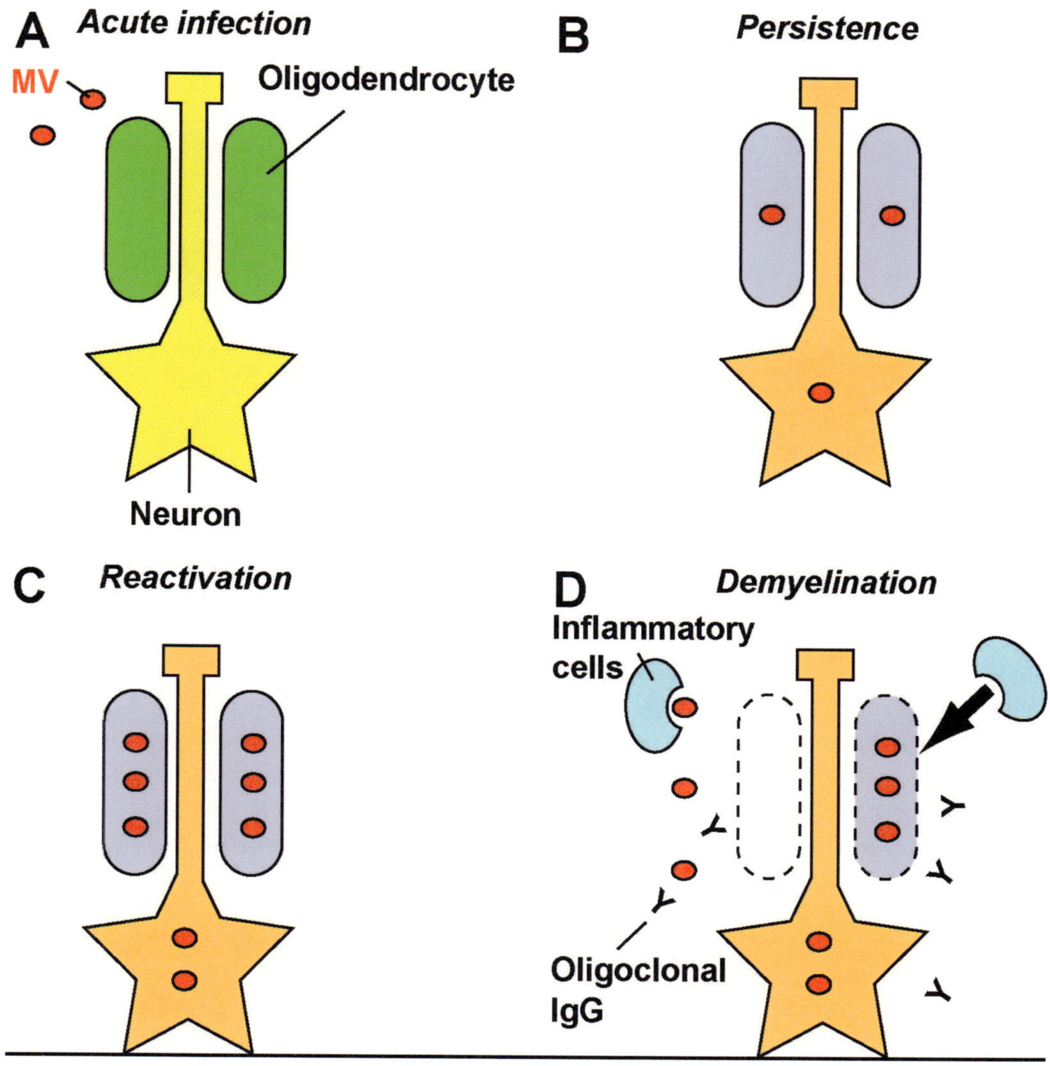

Figure 1. A model for the pathogenesis of persistent MV infection. (A) Acute infection. MV enters the CNS and infects neurons and oligodendrocytes. (B) Persistent infection. MV establishes a persistent infection in the CNS. MV replication is attuned to the host cells, with minor or reversible modifications of the cells. Minor or reversible modifications, such as alterations in lipid metabolism, in MV-infected cells might be involved in a progressive infection. (C) Reactivation. Some reactivation events stimulate the latent MV, leading to rapid replication in the CNS. (D) Demyelination. Reactivated MV destroys host cells, including oligodendrocytes, and drives damaging inflammatory responses, resulting in demyelination. Damaging resulting from MV infection can lead to a spreading of epitopes that generate autoimmune responses. The oligoclonal IgG found in the SSPE brain and the CSF, which is directed against MV, possibly cross-reacts with myelin proteins. Activated autoreactive T cells, or T cells activated by viral antigens can cross the blood-brain barrier and enter the brain parenchyma. These infiltrating inflammatory cells induce extensive lesions in the CNS.

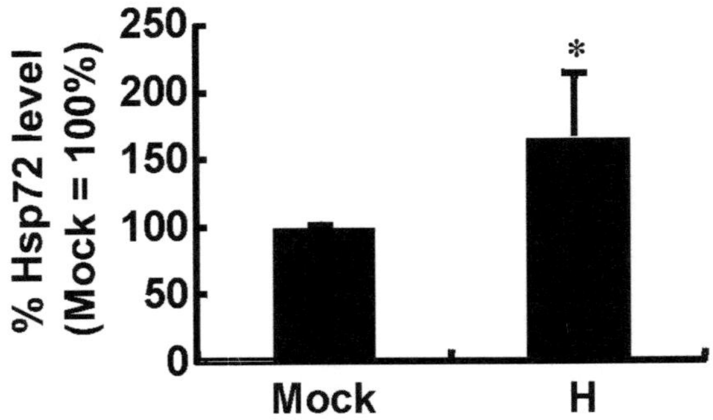

Figure 2. Hsp72 induction by the H protein. 293T cells were mock-transfected, or transfected with the H protein. At 24 h post-transfection, cells were harvested, and quantitative analysis of hsp72 was performed using quantitative real-time RT-PCR. Values are expressed as mean plus S.E. and compared with those from mock-transfected cells. * $p < 0.05$.

Peroxiredoxin 1 (Prdx1). Prdx1, another potential molecule involved in SSPE, has recently been identified as a critical component during MV replication and transcription [46]. It was shown to bind to the same area of the N protein as the P protein (box 2), and competes with binding of the P protein. A reduction in Prdx1 expression appears to result in a steeper MV transcription gradient, as it has less of an effect on the N protein expression compared with the L protein expression. The binding affinity of Prdx1 to the N protein is approximately 40-fold lower than that for the P protein. This would suggest that Prdx1 may only play a role in MV RNA synthesis during the early stages of infection, when the amount of cellular Prdx1 is much greater than that of the viral P protein [46]. Likewise, Prdx1 might play a role in the reactivation of latent MVs that are attuned to host cells. Recent studies have implicated Prdx as a target of age-related modifications [47]. Age-related modifications, such as hyperoxidization, likely affect Prdx1 thereby influencing MV transcription, and may explain why it takes several years after an acute MV infection for the first symptoms of SSPE to appear.

Post-translational modifications. Generally, infectious virus cannot be recovered from the CNS at autopsy, or from a biopsy of SSPE cases. In SSPE, MV-specific inclusions are present in the cytoplasm and nuclei of infected cells, and the incidence of certain types of inclusion bodies decline with prolonged duration of the disease [12, 13]. The N protein is most abundantly expressed in infected cells, and a major component of MV-specific inclusions. The N protein has been shown to be modified post-translationally by phosphorylation [48, 49]. The phosphorylation at serine residues 479 and 510 in the tail of the N protein has been shown to play an important role in viral replication and transcription [48]. Some reactivation events might stimulate host cell kinases responsible for these phosphorylations. Other post-translational modifications could possibly be involved in the reactivation of latent MV.

5. Pathogenesis of persistent MV infection

MV infection induces clinically significant immunosuppression, which can continue for many weeks after an apparent recovery from measles [50, 51]. Long-lived cytokine imbalances and direct effects on the proliferation of lymphocytes are reportedly implicated with the immunosuppression. In contrast, a persistent brain infection leads to a hyperimmune antibody response, a pathogenic feature of SSPE [10, 11]. For example, there are extremely high titers of neutralizing antibodies in the serum and CSF against viral structural proteins. The immune system would appear to be involved in SSPE pathogenesis (Figure 1D).

Direct cytopathic effects. Persistent MV infection might destroy infected cells, including oligodendrocytes, and damage inflammatory responses, thereby resulting in demyelination. Consistent with this idea, there is a strong correlation among the extent of viral fusion activity, cytopathic effects of MV, and severity of neurovirulence in a hamster model [23]. More commonly, T and B cells may directly attack viral antigens expressed on persistently infected glial cells and destroy these cells. Damage resulting from MV infection can lead to a spreading of epitopes that may result in the generation of autoimmune responses [52]. In SSPE patients, brain-antigen-reactive T cells are found in the periphery [53].

Autoantigen. Autoimmune responses to myelin proteins are considered to be possible causes of some demyelinating diseases including SSPE. The level of antibodies against CD9, a glycoprotein that is abundant at the surface of myelin, is elevated and reaches a peak that coincides with the appearance of brain atrophy in SSPE patients [54]. It has also been suggested that autoimmunity could arise as a result of cross-reactivity between viral and myelin antigens [55, 56]. Myelin basic protein (MBP)-homologous sequences in the N and C proteins may account not only for encephalomyelitis in humans, but also for cross-reactions as detected by delayed skin tests with MBP in measles-sensitized guinea pigs [57].

Superantigen. Another mechanism has been proposed that implicates superantigens in the etiology of autoimmune demyelinating diseases [58]. Superantigens activate T cells through the variable domain of the T cell receptor β chain. This distinctive mode of T cell activation, together with the ability of superantigens to bind to a wide variety of major histocompatibility complex molecules outside the antigen groove, leads to one superantigen activating a whole class of T cells irrespective of antigen specificity. Activated T cells can cross the blood-brain barrier and enter the brain parenchyma. A few cells homing to the brain have been shown to be enough to induce extensive lesions in the CNS [58]. Once activated, autoreactive T cells enter the brain and initiate inflammatory lesions. The permeability of the blood-brain barrier increases, leading to an influx of soluble factors, such as tumor necrosis factor, into the CNS. All these events will result in extensive CNS lesions. Exogenous superantigens can be produced by bacteria, mycoplasma or viruses [59], and therefore the existence of superantigens during persistent MV infection should be investigated in future studies.

6. Conclusion

Many previous studies have demonstrated that changes in host cell homeostasis contribute to the pathogenesis of persistent MV infections. Rapid replication of MV that has been quiescent for years is triggered by some reactivation event(s) and results in hyper-reactive immune responses. Demyelination in persistent MV infections is due to a complex combination of viral cytopathic effects on neuronal cells and immune-mediated mechanisms. Although the pathogenesis of persistent MV infection remains to be fully elucidated, some of the key advances outlined in this review will provide novel insights into the understanding of human demyelinating encephalitis, and other encephalitis types induced by viruses.

Acknowledgements

This work was supported by Grants-in-Aid for Scientific Research (KAKENHI) from the Japan Society for the Promotion of Science (JSPS), and in part by Global COE Program "Center of Education and Research for the Advanced Genome-Based Medicine: For personalized medicine and the control of worldwide infectious diseases", Ministry of Education, Culture, Sports, Science and Technology, Japan.

Author details

Tomoyuki Honda[1,2], Misako Yoneda[1], Hiroki Sato[1] and Chieko Kai[1*]

*Address all correspondence to: ckai@ims.u-tokyo.ac.jp

1 Laboratory Animal Research Center, Institute of Medical Science, The University of Tokyo, Minato-ku, Tokyo, Japan

2 Department of Viral Oncology, Institute for Virus Research, Kyoto University, Sakyo-ku, Kyoto, Japan

References

[1] Rima BK & Duprex WP. Molecular mechanisms of measles virus persistence. Virus Res 2005;111(2):132-147.

[2] Reuter D & Schneider-Schaulies J. Measles virus infection of the CNS: human disease, animal models, and approaches to therapy. Med Microbiol Immunol 2010;199(3):261-271.

[3] Schneider-Schaulies J, et al. Measles infection of the central nervous system. J NeuroVirol 2003;9:247-252.

[4] Moss WJ & Griffin DE. Global measles elimination. Nat Rev Microbiol 2006;4(12): 900-908.

[5] Gibbs FA., et al. Electroencephalographic abnormality in "uncomplicated" childhood diseases. JAMA 1959;171(8):1050-1055.

[6] Kirk J, Zhou AL, McQuaid S, Cosby SL, & Allen IV. Cerebral endothelial cell infection by measles virus in subacute sclerosing panencephalitis: ultrastructural and in situ hybridization evidence. Neuropathol Appl Neurobiol 1991;17(4):289-297.

[7] Modlin JF, Jabbour JT, Witte JJ, & Halsey NA. Epidemiologic studies of measles, measles vaccine, and subacute sclerosing panencephalitis. Pediatrics 1977;59(4): 505-512.

[8] Tuncay R, et al. MRI in subacute sclerosing panencephalitis. Neuroradiology 1996;38(7):636-640.

[9] Akram M, Naz F, Malik A, & Hamid H. Clinical profile of subacute sclerosing panencephalitis. J Coll Physicians Surg Pak 2008;18(8):485-488.

[10] Connolly JH, Allen IV, Hurwitz LJ, & Millar JH. Measles-virus antibody and antigen in subacute sclerosing panencephalitis. Lancet 1967;1(7489):542-544.

[11] Tourtellotte WW, Parker JA, Herndon RM, & Cuadros CV. Subacute sclerosing panencephalitis: brain immunoglobulin-G, measles antibody and albumin. Neurology 1968;18(1 Pt 2):117-121.

[12] Tomoda A, Miike T, Miyagawa S, Negi A, & Takeshima H. Subacute sclerosing panencephalitis and chorioretinitis. Brain Dev 1997;19(1):55-57.

[13] Lewandowska E, Lechowicz W, Szpak GM, & Sobczyk W. Quantitative evaluation of intranuclear inclusions in SSPE: correlation with disease duration. Folia Neuropathol 2001;39(4):237-241.

[14] McQuaid S, Allen IV, McMahon J, & Kirk J. Association of measles virus with neurofibrillary tangles in subacute sclerosing panencephalitis: a combined in situ hybridization and immunocytochemical investigation. Neuropathol Appl Neurobiol 1994;20(2):103-110.

[15] Ikeda K, et al. Numerous glial fibrillary tangles in oligodendroglia in cases of subacute sclerosing panencephalitis with neurofibrillary tangles. Neurosci Lett 1995; 194(1-2):133-135.

[16] Freeman AF, et al. A new complication of stem cell transplantation: measles inclusion body encephalitis. Pediatrics 2004;114(5):e657-660.

[17] Katayama Y, Hotta H, Nishimura A, Tatsuno Y, & Homma M. Detection of measles virus nucleoprotein mRNA in autopsied brain tissues. J Gen Virol 1995;76 (Pt 12): 3201-3204.

[18] Haase AT, Ventura P, Gibbs CJ, & Tourtellotte WW. Measles virus nucleotide sequences: detection by hybridization in situ. Science 1981;212(4495):672-675.

[19] Jin L, Beard S, Hunjan R, Brown DW, & Miller E. Characterization of measles virus strains causing SSPE: a study of 11 cases. J Neurovirol 2002;8(4):335-344.

[20] Rima BK, et al. Temporal and geographical distribution of measles virus genotypes. J Gen Virol 1995;76 (Pt 5):1173-1180.

[21] Ayata M, Hirano A, & Wong TC. Structural defect linked to nonrandom mutations in the matrix gene of biken strain subacute sclerosing panencephalitis virus defined by cDNA cloning and expression of chimeric genes. J Virol 1989;63(3):1162-1173.

[22] Cattaneo R, Schmid A, Billeter MA, Sheppard RD, & Udem SA. Multiple viral mutations rather than host factors cause defective measles virus gene expression in a subacute sclerosing panencephalitis cell line. J Virol 1988;62(4):1388-1397.

[23] Ayata M, et al. The F gene of the Osaka-2 strain of measles virus derived from a case of subacute sclerosing panencephalitis is a major determinant of neurovirulence. J Virol 2010;84(21):11189-11199.

[24] Patterson JB, et al. Evidence that the hypermutated M protein of a subacute sclerosing panencephalitis measles virus actively contributes to the chronic progressive CNS disease. Virology 2001;291(2):215-225.

[25] Cattaneo R & Rose JK. Cell fusion by the envelope glycoproteins of persistent measles viruses which caused lethal human brain disease. J Virol 1993;67(3):1493-1502.

[26] Young VA & Rall GF. Making it to the synapse: measles virus spread in and among neurons. Curr Top Microbiol Immunol 2009;330:3-30.

[27] Inoue Y, Tsukiyama-Kohara K, Yoneda M, Sato H, & Kai C. Inhibition of host protein synthesis in B95a cells infected with the HL strain of measles virus. Comp Immunol Microbiol Infect Dis 2009;32(1):29-41.

[28] Sato H, et al. Measles virus N protein inhibits host translation by binding to eIF3-p40. J Virol 2007;81(21):11569-11576.

[29] Inoue Y, et al. Selective translation of the measles virus nucleocapsid mRNA by la protein. Front Microbiol 2011;2:173.

[30] Bolt G, Berg K, & Blixenkrone-Møller M. Measles virus-induced modulation of host-cell gene expression. J Gen Virol 2002;83(Pt 5):1157-1165.

[31] Zilliox MJ, Parmigiani G, & Griffin DE. Gene expression patterns in dendritic cells infected with measles virus compared with other pathogens. Proc Natl Acad Sci U S A 2006;103(9):3363-3368.

[32] van Diepen A, et al. Quantitative proteome profiling of respiratory virus-infected lung epithelial cells. J Proteomics 2010;73(9):1680-1693.

[33] Gutierrez J, Issacson RS, & Koppel BS. Subacute sclerosing panencephalitis: an update. Dev Med Child Neurol 2010;52(10):901-907.

[34] Yan J & Greer JM. NF-kappa B, a potential therapeutic target for the treatment of multiple sclerosis. CNS Neurol Disord Drug Targets 2008;7(6):536-557.

[35] D'Antonio M, Feltri ML, & Wrabetz L. Myelin under stress. J Neurosci Res 2009;87(15):3241-3249.

[36] Mc Guire C, Beyaert R, & van Loo G. Death receptor signalling in central nervous system inflammation and demyelination. Trends Neurosci. 2011;34(12):619-628

[37] Sato H, et al. Measles virus induces cell-type specific changes in gene expression. Virology 2008;375(2):321-330.

[38] Takahashi M, Watari E, Shinya E, Shimizu T, & Takahashi H. Suppression of virus replication via down-modulation of mitochondrial short chain enoyl-CoA hydratase in human glioblastoma cells. Antiviral Res 2007;75(2):152-158.

[39] Robinzon S, et al. Impaired cholesterol biosynthesis in a neuronal cell line persistently infected with measles virus. J Virol 2009;83(11):5495-5504.

[40] Taylor MJ, et al. Identification of several different lineages of measles virus. J Gen Virol 1991;72 (Pt 1):83-88.

[41] Bourhis JM, et al. The intrinsically disordered C-terminal domain of the measles virus nucleoprotein interacts with the C-terminal domain of the phosphoprotein via two distinct sites and remains predominantly unfolded. Protein Sci 2005;14(8): 1975-1992.

[42] Carsillo T, Carsillo M, Niewiesk S, Vasconcelos D, & Oglesbee M. Hyperthermic preconditioning promotes measles virus clearance from brain in a mouse model of persistent infection. Brain Res 2004;1004(1-2):73-82.

[43] Carsillo T, Traylor Z, Choi C, Niewiesk S, & Oglesbee M. hsp72, a host determinant of measles virus neurovirulence. J Virol 2006,80(22):11031-11039.

[44] Joseph BS & Oldstone MB. Immunologic injury in measles virus infection. II. Suppression of immune injury through antigenic modulation. J Exp Med 1975;142(4): 864-876.

[45] Fujinami RS & Oldstone MB. Alterations in expression of measles virus polypeptides by antibody: molecular events in antibody-induced antigenic modulation. J Immunol 1980;125(1):78-85.

[46] Watanabe A, et al. Peroxiredoxin 1 is required for efficient transcription and replication of measles virus. J Virol 2011;85(5):2247-2253.

[47] Wang Q, et al. Differential proteomics analysis of specific carbonylated proteins in the temporal cortex of aged rats: the deterioration of antioxidant system. Neurochem Res 2010;35(1):13-21.

[48] Hagiwara K, et al. Phosphorylation of measles virus nucleoprotein upregulates the transcriptional activity of minigenomic RNA. Proteomics 2008;8(9):1871-1879.

[49] Prodhomme EJ, et al. Extensive phosphorylation flanking the C-terminal functional domains of the measles virus nucleoprotein. J Proteome Res 2010;9(11):5598-5609.

[50] Moss WJ, Ota MO, & Griffin DE. Measles: immune suppression and immune responses. Int J Biochem Cell Biol 2004;36(8):1380-1385.

[51] Schneider-Schaulies S & ter Meulen V. Measles virus and immunomodulation: molecular bases and perspectives. Expert Rev Mol Med 2002;4(13):1-18.

[52] Miller SD, et al. Persistent infection with Theiler's virus leads to CNS autoimmunity via epitope spreading. Nat Med 1997;3(10):1133-1136.

[53] Johnson RT, et al. Measles encephalomyelitis--clinical and immunologic studies. N Engl J Med 1984;310(3):137-141.

[54] Shimizu T, et al. Elevated levels of anti-CD9 antibodies in the cerebrospinal fluid of patients with subacute sclerosing panencephalitis. J Infect Dis 2002;185(9):1346-1350.

[55] Oldstone MB. Molecular mimicry and autoimmune disease. Cell 1987;50(6):819-820.

[56] Wucherpfennig KW & Strominger JL. Molecular mimicry in T cell-mediated autoimmunity: viral peptides activate human T cell clones specific for myelin basic protein. Cell 1995;80(5):695-705.

[57] Jahnke U, Fischer EH, & Alvord EC. Sequence homology between certain viral proteins and proteins related to encephalomyelitis and neuritis. Science 1985;229(4710): 282-284.

[58] Brocke S, Veromaa T, Weissman IL, Gijbels K, & Steinman L. Infection and multiple sclerosis: a possible role for superantigens? Trends Microbiol 1994;2(7):250-254.

[59] Kotzin BL, Leung DY, Kappler J, & Marrack P. Superantigens and their potential role in human disease. Adv Immunol 1993;54:99-166.

Chapter 15

Viral Encephalitis with Focus on Human Enteroviruses

Po-Ying Chia and Justin Jang Hann Chu

Additional information is available at the end of the chapter

http://dx.doi.org/10.5772/52574

1. Introduction

The field of infectious diseases is an exciting field with new agents emerging continuously. The emergence of new diseases is partly contributed by our growing population, expansion of residential areas into previously uninhabited areas and increase in global travel. Most of the emerging new infections are due to RNA viruses and nearly half have been described to cause encephalitis or significant neurological symptoms [1].

This review will focus on encephalitis caused by enteroviruses. Encephalitis is basically inflammation of the brain. Several viruses can result in encephalitis and some viruses, such as Enterovirus 71 (EV71), have been documented to cause epidemics.

2. Virology of enterovirus

Enteroviruses are single-stranded, positive-sense RNA viruses belonging to the *Picornaviridae* family. They are associated with various human and animal diseases, and are traditionally classified into 4 groups, namely, Coxsackie A viruses, Coxsackie B viruses, echoviruses and polioviruses, depending on the clinical presentation. Recently, however, enteroviruses have been named numerically e.g. EV70 and EV71 in recognition of the similarities among the 4 groups noted on genomic studies [2].

RNA viruses are known for their high spontaneous mutation rate, which is attributed to the absence of proof reading in viral RNA polymerases. This invariably leads to the emergence of new enteroviruses and consequently, new clinical presentations. Enterovirus 71 was first described in California USA in 1969 [3] and will arguably be the next most important enterovirus after the eradication of poliovirus.

The enterovirus is a small, non-enveloped spherical particle around 30nm in diameter. The viral genomic RNA is encapsidated within the capsid shell comprising the VP1-4 capsid proteins. The capsid proteins are arranged into a symmetrical icosahedral lattice. These capsid proteins recognize receptors on host cells and demonstrate antigenicity. The viral genome is translated into a polyprotein around 250kDa which then undergoes cleavage via the viral proteases. The viral non-structural proteins 2A-C and 3A-D are essential for the replication of the virus within infected cells [4].

Phylogenetic studies of enterovirus 71 have identified 3 genotypes and numerous subtypes. The 3 genotypes are A, B and C, whereas the subtypes are classified numerically. Increased neurovirulence have been attributed to certain subtypes, such as genotype C1 [5]. Still, the exact pathogenesis for the variation in disease presentation is unknown.

3. Epidemiology

Herpes simplex virus holds the dubious honor of being the commonest cause of acute focal encephalitis, and is thus the presumptive diagnosis in patients with viral encephalitis. However, prospective studies have shown that about 9% have a different etiology and may be due to enteroviruses [6, 7]. Enteroviruses have a worldwide distribution, but recent outbreaks of EV71 have been centered in Asia, particularly East and Southeast Asia [8-16]. Enterovirus 71 is not the only enterovirus that involves the central nervous system (CNS). In a Canadian survey of enteroviral infections of the CNS from 1973 to 1981, coxsackie-virus A9, B1, B2, B3 and B5, echoviruses type 6, 7, 9, 11, 30, poliovirus type 2 were isolated as well [17]. The incidence of encephalitis specifically in enterovirus infections is reported to be at 3% [18], with the majority presenting meningitis.

Clinically evident infection occurs mainly in children with few cases reported in adults [19]. There is a male preponderance [19]. In children, the infection usually presents as hand, foot and mouth disease (HFMD). Yet from the late 1990s onwards, increasingly severe cases caused by enterovirus have been documented, particularly involving EV71. In adults, there have been a few case reports occurring after immunosuppressive therapy such as rituximab [20]. Rituximab is a chimeric anti-CD20 monoclonal antibody that can cause profound B-cell lymphopenia and antibody deficiency. There are 3 main different clinical neurological complications of EV71 infection; 1.flaccid paralysis and encephalitis [3, 21], 2.HFMD and meningoencephalitis [22-24] and 3.HFMD or herpangina and rhombencephalitis with neurogenic pulmonary edema [16, 25-27].

The incidence of CNS complications in enterovirus infection has been reported to range from 2-10% [28]. Even so, according to a prospective study of 773 children [5] and retrospective study of 423 patients [19], it can go as high as to 19-42%, respectively. Of the 773 children, EV71 was isolated in 277 (41%) and out of the 277 children, a further 28 had coinfections with a second virus (other enteroviruses, adenovirus and unidentified virus) [5]. Coxsackie A virus was isolated in 85 patients and out of these, 4 had coinfections as well. Other enteroviruses, adenoviruses or unidentified viruses were isolated in 58 [5].

http://dx.doi.org/10.5772/52574

While coinfections with other enteroviruses did not appear to increase the risk of neurological complications, an association was found between patients who were coinfected with dengue viruses and neurological symptoms [5]. Similarly, in the retrospective study of 423 patients, those with CNS involvement were more likely to have EV71 (21%) instead of coxsackie A virus infection (16%). In addition, rate of disease progression and severity was reported to be greater in EV71 infection [19].

4. Pathogenesis

The reservoir of human pathogenic enterovirus is humans and transmission of enteroviruses occurs through the fecal-oral route via droplets or in utero [28]. Infection starts in the gastrointestinal system with proliferation in the pharynx or intestinal lymph nodes before disseminating to the rest of the body.

In vitro studies of EV71 show that the virus binds to DLD-1 intestinal cells which express sialic acid (SA) linked glycan on the cell surface [29]. Decreasing O-linked glycans or glycolipids on the cell surface decreased EV71 infection of DLD-1 intestinal cells but this was not reproducible on decreasing N-linked glycans. SA linked glycans isolated from human milk also inhibited EV71 infection of DLD-1 intestinal cells [29], suggesting potential therapeutic use.

The first step for a virus to infect the CNS is to cross the blood brain barrier (BBB). The BBB serves as a physical barrier, consisting of endothelial cells joined to each other by tight junctions and surrounded by foot processes of astrocytes, preventing access to the CNS. The meninges, choroid plexus and ependymal cells lining the ventricles also prevent access. Within the CNS are also dendritic cells and macrophages that detect pathogens and contribute to the host defense response. In utero, the BBB has not fully matured and viruses crossing into the placental circulation can also result in CNS infection.

Several RNA viruses causing neurological symptoms e.g. poliovirus, enter the CNS through axonal transport from the peripheral nervous system (PNS), circumventing the blood brain barrier. Coxsackie-virus B3 on the other hand targets nestin^{+} myeloid cells which subsequently migrate through ependymal cell layer of the BBB into the CNS [30]. Other enteroviruses such as EV71 cross the BBB by binding to receptors e.g. P-selectin glycoprotein ligand-1, infecting cells (leucocytes and lymphocytes) that normally cross the BBB [31], hitchhiking their way into the CNS. Enterovirus 71 and coxsackie-viruses have also been shown to bind to scavenger receptor class B member 2 (SCARB2) found on fibroblasts and GPI-anchored protein decay-accelerating factor found on epithelial cells in the CNS, gaining entry into the CNS [28, 32]. SCARB2 participates in membrane transportation and the re-organization of endosomal and lysosomal compartments [33]. The coxsackievirus and adenovirus receptor (CAR) also facilitates viral entry in a caveolin-dependent or independent manner [32, 34] while human poliovirus receptor, an adhesion molecule, is used by human poliovirus in a caveolin independent manner but dynamin-dependent manner to gain entry [32, 35]. The receptors and varying method of entry in different cell types may explain for the tropism to a certain degree. Human poliovirus receptors are found in high levels in the anterior horn cells of the spinal cord, accounting for the predilection of poliovirus for infection anterior horn cells [36]. However, there are other factors that contribute to the tropism of the viruses such as cell proliferation. It has been reported that coxsackievirus 3B targets neural progenitor and stem cells and viral replication increases markedly during cell division and when the cells are arrested at the G_1 or G_1/S phase while viral replication is reduced in quiescent cells in the $G_0/G_2/M$ phase [37].

The human immune system consists of adaptive and innate immunity, both of which utilizes pattern recognition receptors (PRR) e.g. Toll-like receptor and RIG-I-like receptors that detect viral nucleic acids and initiate host defence [38], including modulating the release of chemokines, cytokines and interferons [39]. An appropriate host response to viral infection requires a complex interplay between the innate and adaptive immune system.

After entry into the CNS, glial cells which constitute part of the CNS innate immune system, detect the intracellular viral nucleic acid, and stimulate the release of IFN-1, causing apoptosis and inhibit viral replication. It is, however, important to note that collateral damage incurred upon activation of cytolytic T cells during an adaptive immune response within the CNS may be more damaging to neurons than the infection. Furthermore, both greater cytokine induced tissue destruction due to higher systemic levels of proinflammatory cytokines like IL-6, IL-1β, and TNF [40] and the pervasive infiltration of leukocytes into the CNS exacerbate the neuropathology linked to enteroviruses [41]. Due to this, the host may contain immune response towards viral infection within the CNS.

Even so, viruses have also evolved to escape host defence by producing viral proteins that inhibit host anti-viral response. For example, EV71 produces protein 3C which inhibits RIG-I like receptors and thus blocks host IFN-1, and protein 2C which inhibits IkB kinase beta phosphorylation, consequently blocking the TNF alpha activated NκB signaling pathway [42, 43]. *In vitro* studies also showed that protein 2C stimulates neuronal apoptosis via activation of the Abl-Cdk5 pathway [44]. Interestingly, *in vitro* studies of coxsackievirus A16 which is less neurovirulent than EV71 [45] may suggest that coxsackievirus A16 stimulates Abl to a smaller degree and does not stimulate Cdk5 [44]. Viruses can also dodge the adaptive immune system by binding to dendritic cell specific intercellular adhesion molecule-3-grabbing non-integrin (DC-SIGN). The DC-SIGN is a receptor present on macrophages and dendritic cells which recognizes and binds to pathogen associated molecular patterns (PAMPs) on viruses, bacteria and fungi. The binding itself stimulates phagocytosis and results in pathogen entry into dendritic cells and T-cells. Intracellular entry is not only mediated via DC-SIGN but also by other receptors such as CD36 and CD163. This results in suboptimal T and NK cell response as viral proteins inhibit IFN-1 synthesis and escape immune surveillance.

Neurological complications are reported at higher frequencies in younger children. The exact pathogenesis remains unknown, but research has elucidated a number of differences between patients who developed such complications and those who do not.

In a case-control study of 78 children who had EV71 infection, of which 31 children developed meningoencephalitis, expression of CD40-ligand on T cells was significantly lower in cases than in controls in the acute phase, but not in the convalescent phase of the disease [46]. CD40 ligand expression on T cells is recognized as a marker of T and B cell interaction [47]. Thus, a decrease in expression may suggest a decrease in stimulation of B cells, antibody class switching and antibody production. Yet, there was no significant difference in lymphocyte proliferation between cases and controls. In cases with meningoencephalitis, it was also noted that interleukin 4 production was significantly lower in cases than in controls during the acute phase, suggesting a decrease response from Th2 cells which stimulate the humoral immune system [46]. This suggests that a compromised immune status precipitates the fulminant progression of EV infections.

In the same study, significant polymorphism of the cytotoxic T lymphocyte antigen-4 (CTLA-4) was noted, with cases having more G/G genotype at position 49 of exon 1 than in controls. CTLA-4 is involved in T cell anergy and apoptosis, and different polymorphisms has been linked to infectious and autoimmune conditions [46].

In enterovirus infection, autophagocytosis is subverted and induced in infected neurons, allowing for intracellular replication of viral particles before host cell death occurs. Autophagy is usually a protective process that occurs in cells to sequester and breakdown unwanted organelles or protein aggregates. In poliovirus [48] and coxsackievirus B4 [49] infections, however, it has been induced to assist in virus replication instead. It is postulated that enterovirus utilizes the autophagosome membrane for viral replication and increase in viral replication is associated with autophagy induction [49]. The exact mechanism by which autophagocytosis increases viral replication is currently unclear.

Non-structural 3C protein of EV71 has been reported to block polyadenylation of host messenger RNA while non-structural 2A protein impedes the host cap-dependent translation and simultaneously stabilizes polysomes enhancing translation of viral messenger RNA [50]. Non-structural 2A protein thus boosts viral protein synthesis, and it has been shown to be necessary for host cell apoptosis as well [51]. Accordingly, it is assumed that by deactivating the host cell translation, enteroviruses may directly cause apoptotic cell death in neurons. Enteroviruses bring about both anti-apoptotic (non-structural 3A and 2B proteins) and pro-apoptotic effects (VP2, non-structural 2A and 3C proteins) on the host cell [52]. Viral non-structural protein 2B is also known to be a viroporin that increases permeability of host cell resulting in eventual cell death.

The highest rates of infections occur in young children below 4 years of age, with fatal infections most commonly occurring at the ages of 6-11 months [13, 16, 53]. This age period is also associated with a decline in maternal antibodies within the child. Enterovirus 71 infects human peripheral blood monocytes, and it is postulated that in the presence of sub-neutralizing amounts of anti-EV71 antibodies, infectivity is enhanced [54]. This is also known as antibody-dependent enhancement (ADE), widely described in dengue infection as well as other viral infections such as human immunodeficiency virus infection [55]. Heterotypic non-neutralizing antibodies bind to the virions, forming EV71-antiEV71 antibody complexes, which subsequently bind to Fc-R on human monocytes and therefore, enhancing infectivity. *In vitro* experiments have shown that the addition of immune sera from patients increased EV71 infection of THP-1 cells, a leukemia cell line of macrophage lineage with monocytic markers, whereas addition of Fc-RI (CD64) significantly inhibited the infection [54].

Furthermore, patients who suffer from neurogenic pulmonary edema have been reported to have lower absolute monocyte counts, CD4, CD8 and NK cells counts as compared to patients who had autonomic nerve system abnormalities and uncomplicated brainstem encephalitis [56].

5. Pathogenesis of neurogenic pulmonary edema

Patients with enterovirus encephalitis who suffer from pulmonary edema, pulmonary hemorrhage and cardiopulmonary collapse usually have fairly normal premorbid cardiac function with normal pulmonary artery pressures and vascular resistance [56]. Myocarditis is also not evident on autopsy reports [57].

Involvement of the medulla and hence, the vagal nucleus and medial reticular nuclei is postulated to cause pulmonary edema [58, 59]. Neurogenic pulmonary edema occurs when there is pulmonary edema and CNS disease in the absence of underlying cardiopulmonary disease [58]. While the pathogenesis is not clear, it is believed that an insult to the medulla results in torrential release of catecholamine. This in turn, causes a rapid increase in total peripheral vasoconstriction and systemic hypertension, shifting blood from the systemic circulation to the pulmonary circulation. Since the pulmonary circulation is usually a low resistance system, it is unable to adapt to the sudden increase in hydrostatic pressure. The results are protein rich pulmonary edema and pulmonary hemorrhages. The resulting "catecholamine storm" induces catecholamine cardiotoxicity as well including coagulative myocytolysis, myofibrillar degeneration, and cardiomyocytes apoptosis [60]. This neurogenic nature is validated by MRI findings of brainstem involvement [61] and postmortem examinations of mortality cases of enterovirus encephalitis in which pathological lesions were predominantly located in the brainstem and the spinal cord, rather than in the lung or heart [21, 27, 62].

6. Pathogenesis in chronic infection

Chronic infection by enterovirus has been reported [63] and it is postulated that the persistence of infection alters normal neural stem cell migration and or differentiation. Although viral latency has yet to be established, there is evidence for their persistence in infected cells for years [64-66]. Therefore, enteroviral RNA may be reactivated upon stimulation. In the case of hypogammaglobulinaemia, reactivated enterovirus is not inactivated and can spread freely. In the same degree, persistent meningoencephalitis has been reported in patients with agammaglobulinemia [67, 68]. In fact, the first case of enteroviral meningoencephalitis was reported in a patient with agammaglobulinemia [69].

7. Clinical signs and symptoms

Enteroviruses can cause a wide spectrum of clinical diseases, including but not limited to the common cold, gastroenteritis, hand, foot and mouth disease (HFMD), herpangina, myocarditis, severe neonatal sepsis-like disease, hepatoadrenal failure, aseptic meningitis, acute flaccid paralysis, meningoencephalitis, encephalitis, neurogenic pulmonary edema, pulmonary hemorrhage and shock induced sudden death especially in the young age group [13, 62, 70]. The neurological presentations include aseptic meningitis, benign intracranial hypertension, acute flaccid paralysis, opsoclonus-myoclonus syndrome, Guillain-Barre syndrome, transverse myelitis, encephalitis, cerebellitis, brainstem encephalitis, rhombencephalitis and encephalomyelitis [13, 25, 26, 71-76].

Clinical manifestations can be classified according to 5 grades. In grade I, patients demonstrate clinical signs of HFMD and/or herpangina with erythematous vesicles on palms, soles, elbows and trunk and oral ulcers on mucosa of lips as well as palate. The majority of patients will display grade I symptoms as seen in the 1998 Taiwan epidemic where 5506 out of 5632 patients were classified to have grade I symptoms [61]. In grade II, patients suffer from fever, photophobia, vomiting, headache, and abdominal pain. Patients who initially exhibit grade II symptoms may subsequently progress onto grade III. The disease may take a fulminant course in patients younger than 2 years of age, deteriorating directly to grade IV in a short period of time. In grade III, patients may demonstrate lethargy, apathy, drowsiness, tachycardia, cranial nerve involvement (VI-XII), myoclonic jerks, monoparesis or hemiparesis, conjugate gaze disturbances, dyspnea and ataxia. Patients with grade III symptoms that are younger than 2 years of age usually progress to grade IV while older patients tend to recover completely after 1-2 weeks. In grade IV, patients experience hypothermia, pulmonary edema, respiratory failure, neurogenic shock and semicoma. In the last stage, grade V, there is pulmonary hemorrhage, respiratory distress syndrome, cardiorespiratory failure, coma and death. According to symptomatology, encephalitis is suspected in grade III-IV.

HFMD and herpangina are generally mild, self-limiting illnesses that occur in infants and young children. The culprit virus for HFMD and herpangina is usually coxsackie-virus A16 or EV71 [8, 14, 19]. Despite this, a small percentage of patients can rapidly decompensate and die within days. In cases where neurological complications occur, the culprit viruses isolated are usually EV71 and coxsackie-virus A16 [19] in some instances other echovirus 7 [77, 78].

Patients who had CNS complications were usually younger and more likely to have symptoms of fever, vomiting, breathlessness and signs of shock that includes cold peripheries and poor urinary output [5]. The exact symptoms and signs depend on the extent of CNS involvement. For example, in EV71 encephalitis, clinical signs of lethargy and cranial nerve palsies such as conjugate gaze disturbance, dyspnea and tachycardia suggest involvement of the brain stem, [61] and this is further substantiated by the magnetic resonance imaging.

8. Investigations and diagnosis

In general, profound leucopenia is usually noted in patients with severe EV71 infections [56]. This is attributed to T-cell apoptosis as EV71 infection may increase FasL expression.

- Investigations: Lumbar puncture

A common investigation in the presence of neurological symptoms would be a lumbar puncture. In aseptic meningitis, there is usually lymphocytic cerebrospinal fluid (CSF) pleocytosis [20] and normal glucose levels [79]. Yet in some of the patients, neutrophilia was observed with low glucose levels less than half of that of plasma glucose instead [5].

- Investigations: Magnetic resonance imaging

Magnetic resonance imaging of the brain is also a useful investigation. Reports of magnetic resonance imaging of polioencephalitis are rare as poliovirus is currently rarely seen in developed countries. The few imaging reports of polioencephalitis reveal involvement of the midbrain and posterior medulla and pons [61].

During the 1998 Taiwan EV71 epidemic, magnetic resonance features were described by Shen et al [61]. Out of 15 patients classified in grade III with clinical encephalitis, 10 had abnormal magnetic resonance imaging scans. Of the patients with abnormal scans, all 10 demonstrated hyperintense lesions of the posterior medulla and pons on T2 weighted images but not on T1 weighted images, which implies acute inflammation. The majority showed involvement of the mesencephalon and dentate nuclei of cerebellum, and in severe cases, the ventral horns of the spinal cord and deep supratentorial nuclei as well [61]. The inclusion of the brainstem is supported by pathological findings on autopsy [26, 80], with inflammation limited to the gray matter of the spinal cord and medulla as well as the tegmentum of the midbrain and pons [80]. It is of note that EV71 and poliovirus affect the same areas of the brain and the areas of involvement demonstrated on the nuclei correlated with the clinical symptoms and signs. A marked difference would be that although the inflammation of inferior olives is reported in EV71 infection, it is absent in bulbar poliomyelitis [80].

Newer techniques in magnetic resonance imaging such as fluid attenuated inversion recovery and diffusion weighted imaging allow detection of subtle meningeal and cortical abnormalities that can occur in meningoencephalitis [81]. Consequently, in patients stable enough to undergo scans, magnetic resonance imaging can reveal areas of CNS involvement. This allows greater diagnostic accuracy and perhaps predicts the need for cardiothoracic support before patients deteriorate too rapidly.

9. Diagnostic methods

Diagnosis normally depends on (a) rise in virus specific acute and convalescent antibody titers, (b) isolation of the virus via viral cultures from throat swabs, stool specimens and CSF samples (c) visual identification of virus via (i) electron microscopy (ii) unique histological

http://dx.doi.org/10.5772/52574

features and/or (iii) histochemical staining, (d) in situ hybridization assays or (e) polymerase chain reaction (PCR) to amplify viral nucleic acids [82, 83]. Since some enteroviruses such as coxsackievirus A [84] do not grow in standard cell cultures [85], the extensive use of PCR with its generally high specificity and sensitivity has greatly improved diagnosis for numerous pathogens. The overall sensitivity, specificity, positive and negative predictive values have been reported to be 85.7%, 93.9%, 61.7% and 98.3%,respectively, using viral culture as the gold standard [86]. However, the majority of clinically suspected viral encephalitis are still of unknown etiology. It is presumed as well that enterovirus will be detectable in the gastrointestinal (GI) tract, but in the case of chronic encephalitis, by the time the disease surfaces, the virus may have cleared from the GI tract and be undetectable in the stool. Additionally, due to low viral concentration, detection of viral RNA in the CSF early after manifestation may be challenging as well.

In EV71 encephalomyelitis, inflammation is stereotypical. Common areas of involvement are the spinal cord, brainstem, hypothalamus, cerebellar dentate nucleus, cerebral cortex and meninges. The anterior pons, corpus striatum, temporal lobe, hippocampus and cerebellar cortex are spared. These areas of involvement facilitate the differentiation of encephalitis due to EV71 from Japanese encephalitis virus [87]. The nature of the lesions, however, is non-specific, with inflammatory infiltration of perivascular and parenchymal tissue, edema, necrosis, stimulation of microglial cells and phagocytic destruction of neurons[83].

The tests currently available have a low diagnostic yield, even in the case of PCR which has high specificity and high sensitivity. This is shown in a meta-analysis conducted in 2010 which reviewed 41 studies on the etiology of encephalitis [88]. In 26 of the studies, more than 50% of the cases were of unknown etiology [88]. Identifying the viral etiological agent enables effective preventive measures and treatments to be implemented.

The European Union Concerted Action on Virus Meningitis and Encephalitis conducted a multicenter retrospective study to evaluate the Amplicor Enterovirus PCR test [86]. 476 CSF samples were collected from 9 laboratories in 5 European countries and analysed via cultures and PCR [86]. Out of 476 samples, 50 were positive via cultures and 66 via PCR. Relative increase in rate of positivity via PCR in relation to culture is thus 32%. Among the 50 samples positive by cultures, 38 were positive while 12 were negative by PCR. On repeat testing of the 12 samples that were culture positive but PCR negative with a different set of primers and probes, 4 of the samples became PCR positive [86]. On the other hand, in the 66 samples positive via PCR, 28 were negative via cultures [86]. Interestingly, in samples from patients with meningitis following the case definition of CSF pleocytosis (more than 10 leukocytes/mm3), 25 were positive via cultures and 45 via PCR, thus there were samples from patients who did not satisfy the criteria for pleocytosis and yet had enterovirus infection.

The California Encephalitis Project (CEP) conducted from 1998-2000 evaluated samples from 334 patients with case definition of encephalitis, which is encephalopathy requiring hospitalization plus one of the following: fever, seizure, focal neurologic findings, cerebrospinal fluid pleocytosis and electroencephalographic or neuroimaging findings consistent with encephalitis [89]. Encephalopathy is defined as depressed or altered level of consciousness lasting 24 hours, lethargy and/or change in personality [89]. 9% of the cases had a confirmed viral agent, 3% a confirmed bacterial agent, 1% a confirmed parasitic agent, 10% a non-infectious etiology and 12% a possible etiology identified. 3% had a non-encephalitis infection identified. Nevertheless, CEP is not population based and the study group consisted of diagnostically challenging cases. Therefore, the rate of unknown etiology cases may be an overestimate when extrapolated to the general population.

Diagnostic strategies that have emerged recently include MassTagPCR, panmicrobial DNA microarrays and high-throughput DNA pyrosequencing [82]. MassTag PCR is a multiplex PCR assay utilizing primer pairs targeting highly conserved gene sequences that represent a wide variety of potential pathogens. The primer pairs have been tagged with MassCodes that are used to identify the etiological agent. There are different MassTag PCR systems with different primers for different clinical specimens and presentations. Clinical use of this method has demonstrated effectiveness in identification of pathogens [90-93]. Panmicrobial DNA microarrays utilize a single chip with numerous highly conserved gene sequences, permitting the swift identification of pathogens similar to that of MassTag PCR [94, 95]. Clinical use of this diagnostic method has also demonstrated efficacy in pathogen identification [96-98].

High-throughput DNA pyrosequencing on the other hand, does not make use of highly conserved gene sequences. Instead, it uses random primers to amplify all RNA after removing human chromosomal DNA from the sample [99]. Amplification products are then sequenced via pyrosequencing wherein DNA polymerases synthesize complementary strands to the amplified products and each enzymatic attachment of a complementary nucleotide results in an emission of a light signal. The light signal is recorded and the sequences are identified and subsequently analyzed to look for pathogens. This technique allows for identification of novel pathogens [100].

10. Treatment

At present, only herpes simplex encephalitis, one of the more prevalent infective encephalitis, has a specific treatment validated by scientific research. It is treated with aciclovir [101]. Effective treatment is lacking for other viruses and mainly symptomatic in nature.

Currently, intravenous immunoglobulin (IVIG) is administered to patients with severe HFMD [5]. Enteroviruses are cleared from the host by antibody-mediated mechanisms (22), and IVIG is an effective treatment option. Various routes of administration have been documented including intravenous, intrathecal and intraventricular with different degrees of success [102-104].

11. Potential treatments in the future – vaccines

However, the best defence would be prevention through vaccination, especially in the case of rabies, polio, mumps and measles. Vaccination may be an option to prevent infection by enteroviruses as well, but the potential ADE phenomenon is an important consideration in the development of a safe and effective vaccine. The genetic diversity of enterovirus strains therefore complicates the development of vaccines [105].

12. Potential treatments in the future – anti-virals

Ribavirin, a broad-spectrum antiviral synthesized by ICN pharmaceuticals, Inc., USA inhibits the replication of a variety of enteroviruses. Studies on EV71-infected mice has shown that ribavirin can reduce mortality by reducing the viral loads in tissues. The required dosage of ribavirin is close to the initial dose of the drug administered intravenously to treat patients with encephalitis caused by Nipah virus [106]. Given these results, ribavirin may be, in combination with interferon, deployed to combat potentially fatal EV71 infection. Interferon has a synergist effect and this combination is already adopted as a standard therapy for HCV-infected patients [107].

Pyridyl imidazolidinone is a novel class of EV71 inhibitor [108]. It was first identified using computer-assisted drug design. It targets EV71 capsid protein VP1 and time course experiments on one of the pyridyl imidazolidinones, BPR0Z-194, have shown that viral replication is effectively inhibited in early stages, suggesting that the compound inhibits adsorption of virions and/or viral RNA uncoating [108]. Resistant strains do exist, and sequence analysis has demonstrated that a single amino acid alteration at position 192 of VP1 confers resistance to BPR0Z-194 [108].

Pleconaril, an anti-viral produced by Sterling-Winthrop, Inc., USA incorporates itself into the capsid of enteroviruses and blocks the virus from docking to cellular receptors and uncoating to release RNA into the cell. It targets VP1 and has already passed the last stage of clinical trials [109]. Results are promising with pleconaril showing antiviral effects for most enteroviruses [109, 110]. Presently, there is an ongoing study on the efficacy of pleconaril in enteroviral sepsis syndrome in neonates [111]. The National Health Research Institutes (NHRI) in Taiwan has reported a number of virtual compounds with similar stable conformations and preliminary studies have identified a few promising imidazolidinone derivatives.

13. Potential treatments in the future – RNA interference

Another promising therapy is the use of RNA interference (RNA-i) in silencing viral gene expression [28, 112]. As aforementioned, viruses penetrate the BBB and the very nature of the BBB makes it difficult for large and charged molecules to cross it. RNA-i on the other hand, are small and have the potential to cross the BBB and exert a therapeutic effect. RNA-i can bind to specific viral mRNA, causing degradation and preventing the translation and synthesis of viral proteins that enable the virus to inhibit the host IFN-1 response [112]. To synthesize RNA-i for therapeutic use, the viral proteins and subsequent viral mRNA have to be identified in advance. *In vitro* experiments performed have shown effective inhibition of EV71 infection [113] however *in vivo* experiments utilizing murine models have yet to replicate similar results [114].

14. Prognosis

There are cases where spontaneous recoveries do not occur and neurological symptoms persist. A retrospective study of 105 patients from 1966 to 1972, with documented enterovirus infection and CNS complications, revealed that half, 9 out of 18, of the children not lost to follow up still displayed signs after 1-5 years [78]. Magnetic resonance imaging of two cases with neurological sequelae demonstrated hypointense lesions on T1-weighted images and hyperintense lesions on T2-weighted images, implying tissue destruction [61]. In a more recent retrospective study of 177 cases with enterovirus isolated via throat swab or stool specimen, 92 patients (52%) had nervous system involvement, out of which 13 patients (7%) had persistent neurological deficits at discharge [19]. Out of the 92 patients with neurological involvement, 67 (73%) had EV71 isolated and of the 13 patients with deficits at discharge, 11 (85%) had EV71 isolated. The persistent neurological deficits ranged from dysphagia and weakness to lack of regular, spontaneous respiration despite presence of brain function [19]. Studies have also linked EV71 CNS infections to increased symptoms of inattention, hyperactivity, oppositional defiance, internalizing problems, and greater likelihood of the diagnosis of attention deficit hyperactivity disorder [115].

Overall, mortality rates for HFMD is reported to be at 0.05% in China [19]. In the aforementioned retrospective study of 177 cases, 5 mortalities were reported and in all these 5 cases, EV71 was isolated [19]. Of the 5 mortalities, 2 were attributed to neurogenic pulmonary edema, 2 to shock and 1 to brain-death. Mortalities in EV71 infection is generally due to neurogenic pulmonary edema secondary to medulla destruction [13, 80, 116, 117]. In Taiwan, the Department of Health has recorded a decrease of incidence in recent years, however the mortality rate is still high (9 deaths in 1999, 41 deaths in 2000, 58 deaths in 2001) [60].

15. Conclusion

The reemergence and emergence of viral infections with involvement of the neurological system is a challenge to public health officers, clinicians and researchers. Enterovirus infection is a major concern with changing circulating genotypes in Asia. While CNS complications of encephalitis are being increasingly reported in enterovirus infections, further research is needed to understand whether this is due to increased virulence or due to undetected immune system defects. The epidemiology continuously evolves with shifting population and hence, there is also a need to have better diagnostic methods and treatment options.

http://dx.doi.org/10.5772/52574

16. Acknowledgements

This study is supported by the Singapore Ministry of Health's National Medical Research Council under its Individual Research Grant (IRG11may096).

Author details

Po-Ying Chia[1] and Justin Jang Hann Chu[2*]

*Address all correspondence to: miccjh@nus.edu.sg; poying.chia@mohh.com.sg

1 Tan Tock Seng Hospital, Singapore

2 Laboratory of Molecular RNA Virology and Antiviral Strategies, Yong Loo Lin School of Medicine, Department of Microbiology, National University of Singapore, Singapore

References

[1] Olival, K.J. and P. Daszak, The ecology of emerging neurotropic viruses. J Neurovirol, 2005. 11(5): p. 441-6.

[2] Oberste, M.S., et al., Molecular evolution of the human enteroviruses: correlation of serotype with VP1 sequence and application to picornavirus classification. J Virol, 1999. 73(3): p. 1941-8.

[3] Schmidt, N.J., E.H. Lennette, and H.H. Ho, An apparently new enterovirus isolated from patients with disease of the central nervous system. J Infect Dis, 1974. 129(3): p. 304-9.

[4] Kitamura, N., et al., Primary structure, gene organization and polypeptide expression of poliovirus RNA. Nature, 1981. 291(5816): p. 547-53.

[5] Ooi, M.H., et al., Human enterovirus 71 disease in Sarawak, Malaysia: a prospective clinical, virological, and molecular epidemiological study. Clin Infect Dis, 2007. 44(5): p. 646-56.

[6] Whitley, R.J., et al., Diseases that mimic herpes simplex encephalitis. Diagnosis, presentation, and outcome. NIAD Collaborative Antiviral Study Group. JAMA, 1989. 262(2): p. 234-9.

[7] Whitley, R.J., et al., Herpes simplex encephalitis: vidarabine therapy and diagnostic problems. N Engl J Med, 1981. 304(6): p. 313-8.

[8] Chan, K.P., et al., Epidemic hand, foot and mouth disease caused by human enterovirus 71, Singapore. Emerg Infect Dis, 2003. 9(1): p. 78-85.

[9] Kim, K.H., Enterovirus 71 infection: An experience in Korea, 2009. Korean J Pediatr, 2010. 53(5): p. 616-22.

[10] McMinn, P., et al., Phylogenetic analysis of enterovirus 71 strains isolated during linked epidemics in Malaysia, Singapore, and Western Australia. J Virol, 2001. 75(16): p. 7732-8.

[11] Fujimoto, T., et al., Outbreak of central nervous system disease associated with hand, foot, and mouth disease in Japan during the summer of 2000: detection and molecular epidemiology of enterovirus 71. Microbiol Immunol, 2002. 46(9): p. 621-7.

[12] Tu, P.V., et al., Epidemiologic and virologic investigation of hand, foot, and mouth disease, southern Vietnam, 2005. Emerg Infect Dis, 2007. 13(11): p. 1733-41.

[13] Chen, S.C., et al., An eight-year study of epidemiologic features of enterovirus 71 infection in Taiwan. Am J Trop Med Hyg, 2007. 77(1): p. 188-91.

[14] Yang, F., et al., Survey of enterovirus infections from hand, foot and mouth disease outbreak in China, 2009. Virol J, 2011. 8: p. 508.

[15] Podin, Y., et al., Sentinel surveillance for human enterovirus 71 in Sarawak, Malaysia: lessons from the first 7 years. BMC Public Health, 2006. 6: p. 180.

[16] Ho, M., et al., An epidemic of enterovirus 71 infection in Taiwan. Taiwan Enterovirus Epidemic Working Group. N Engl J Med, 1999. 341(13): p. 929-35.

[17] Thivierge, B. and G. Delage, [Infections of the central nervous system caused by enterovirus: 223 cases seen at a pediatric hospital between 1973 and 1981]. Can Med Assoc J, 1982. 127(11): p. 1097-102.

[18] Koskiniemi, M., et al., Epidemiology of encephalitis in children: a 20-year survey. Ann Neurol, 1991. 29(5): p. 492-7.

[19] Xu, W., et al., Distribution of enteroviruses in hospitalized children with hand, foot and mouth disease and relationship between pathogens and nervous system complications. Virol J, 2012. 9(1): p. 8.

[20] Servais, S., et al., Enteroviral meningoencephalitis as complication of Rituximab therapy in a patient treated for diffuse large B-cell lymphoma. Br J Haematol, 2010. 150(3): p. 379-81.

[21] Nagy, G., et al., Virological diagnosis of enterovirus type 71 infections: experiences gained during an epidemic of acute CNS diseases in Hungary in 1978. Arch Virol, 1982. 71(3): p. 217-27.

[22] Zheng, Z.M., et al., Enterovirus 71 isolated from China is serologically similar to the prototype E71 BrCr strain but differs in the 5'-noncoding region. J Med Virol, 1995. 47(2): p. 161-7.

[23] Samuda, G.M., et al., Monoplegia caused by Enterovirus 71: an outbreak in Hong Kong. Pediatr Infect Dis J, 1987. 6(2): p. 206-8.

[24] Hagiwara, A., et al., Genetic and phenotypic characteristics of enterovirus 71 isolates from patients with encephalitis and with hand, foot and mouth disease. Arch Virol, 1984. 79(3-4): p. 273-83.

[25] Chang, L.Y., et al., Clinical features and risk factors of pulmonary oedema after enterovirus-71-related hand, foot, and mouth disease. Lancet, 1999. 354(9191): p. 1682-6.

[26] Huang, C.C., et al., Neurologic complications in children with enterovirus 71 infection. N Engl J Med, 1999. 341(13): p. 936-42.

[27] Lum, L.C., et al., Neurogenic pulmonary oedema and enterovirus 71 encephalomyelitis. Lancet, 1998. 352(9137): p. 1391.

[28] Denizot, M., J.W. Neal, and P. Gasque, Encephalitis due to emerging viruses: CNS innate immunity and potential therapeutic targets. J Infect, 2012.

[29] Yang, B., H. Chuang, and K.D. Yang, Sialylated glycans as receptor and inhibitor of enterovirus 71 infection to DLD-1 intestinal cells. Virol J, 2009. 6: p. 141.

[30] Tabor-Godwin, J.M., et al., A novel population of myeloid cells responding to coxsackievirus infection assists in the dissemination of virus within the neonatal CNS. J Neurosci, 2010. 30(25): p. 8676-91.

[31] Yamayoshi, S., et al., Scavenger receptor B2 is a cellular receptor for enterovirus 71. Nat Med, 2009. 15(7): p. 798-801.

[32] Coyne, C.B. and J.M. Bergelson, Virus-induced Abl and Fyn kinase signals permit coxsackievirus entry through epithelial tight junctions. Cell, 2006. 124(1): p. 119-31.

[33] Yamayoshi, S., K. Fujii, and S. Koike, Scavenger receptor b2 as a receptor for hand, foot, and mouth disease and severe neurological diseases. Front Microbiol, 2012. 3: p. 32.

[34] Patel, K.P., C.B. Coyne, and J.M. Bergelson, Dynamin- and lipid raft-dependent entry of decay-accelerating factor (DAF)-binding and non-DAF-binding coxsackieviruses into nonpolarized cells. J Virol, 2009. 83(21): p. 11064-77.

[35] Brandenburg, B., et al., Imaging poliovirus entry in live cells. PLoS Biol, 2007. 5(7): p. e183.

[36] Gromeier, M., et al., Expression of the human poliovirus receptor/CD155 gene during development of the central nervous system: implications for the pathogenesis of poliomyelitis. Virology, 2000. 273(2): p. 248-57.

[37] Feuer, R., et al., Cell cycle status affects coxsackievirus replication, persistence, and reactivation in vitro. J Virol, 2002. 76(9): p. 4430-40.

[38] Kawai, T. and S. Akira, Toll-like receptor and RIG-I-like receptor signaling. Ann N Y Acad Sci, 2008. 1143: p. 1-20.

[39] Hosking, M.P. and T.E. Lane, The role of chemokines during viral infection of the CNS. PLoS Pathog, 2010. 6(7): p. e1000937.

[40] Lin, T.Y., et al., Proinflammatory cytokine reactions in enterovirus 71 infections of the central nervous system. Clin Infect Dis, 2003. 36(3): p. 269-74.

[41] Feuer, R., et al., Viral persistence and chronic immunopathology in the adult central nervous system following Coxsackievirus infection during the neonatal period. J Virol, 2009. 83(18): p. 9356-69.

[42] Zheng, Z., et al., Enterovirus 71 2C protein inhibits TNF-alpha-mediated activation of NF-kappaB by suppressing IkappaB kinase beta phosphorylation. J Immunol, 2011. 187(5): p. 2202-12.

[43] Lei, X., et al., The 3C protein of enterovirus 71 inhibits retinoid acid-inducible gene I-mediated interferon regulatory factor 3 activation and type I interferon responses. J Virol, 2010. 84(16): p. 8051-61.

[44] Chen, T.-C., et al., Enterovirus 71 triggering of neuronal apoptosis through activation of Abl-Cdk5 signalling. Cellular Microbiology, 2007. 9(11): p. 2676-2688.

[45] Chang, L.Y., et al., Comparison of enterovirus 71 and coxsackie-virus A16 clinical illnesses during the Taiwan enterovirus epidemic, 1998. Pediatr Infect Dis J, 1999. 18(12): p. 1092-6.

[46] Yang, K.D., et al., Altered cellular but not humoral reactions in children with complicated enterovirus 71 infections in Taiwan. J Infect Dis, 2001. 183(6): p. 850-6.

[47] Grewal, I.S. and R.A. Flavell, The role of CD40 ligand in costimulation and T-cell activation. Immunol Rev, 1996. 153: p. 85-106.

[48] Jackson, W.T., et al., Subversion of Cellular Autophagosomal Machinery by RNA Viruses. PLoS Biol, 2005. 3(5): p. e156.

[49] Yoon, S.Y., et al., Coxsackievirus B4 uses autophagy for replication after calpain activation in rat primary neurons. J Virol, 2008. 82(23): p. 11976-8.

[50] Rhoades, R.E., et al., Enterovirus infections of the central nervous system. Virology, 2011. 411(2): p. 288-305.

[51] Shih, S.R., et al., Viral protein synthesis is required for Enterovirus 71 to induce apoptosis in human glioblastoma cells. J Neurovirol, 2008. 14(1): p. 53-61.

[52] Whitton, J.L., C.T. Cornell, and R. Feuer, Host and virus determinants of picornavirus pathogenesis and tropism. Nat Rev Microbiol, 2005. 3(10): p. 765-76.

[53] Chang, L.Y., et al., Risk factors of enterovirus 71 infection and associated hand, foot, and mouth disease/herpangina in children during an epidemic in Taiwan. Pediatrics, 2002. 109(6): p. e88.

[54] Wang, S.M., et al., Enterovirus 71 infection of monocytes with antibody-dependent enhancement. Clin Vaccine Immunol, 2010. 17(10): p. 1517-23.

[55] Takada, A. and Y. Kawaoka, Antibody-dependent enhancement of viral infection: molecular mechanisms and in vivo implications. Rev Med Virol, 2003. 13(6): p. 387-98.

[56] Wang, S.M., et al., Pathogenesis of enterovirus 71 brainstem encephalitis in pediatric patients: roles of cytokines and cellular immune activation in patients with pulmonary edema. J Infect Dis, 2003. 188(4): p. 564-70.

[57] Wu, J.M., et al., Cardiopulmonary manifestations of fulminant enterovirus 71 infection. Pediatrics, 2002. 109(2): p. E26-.

[58] Brown, R.H., Jr., et al., Medulla oblongata edema associated with neurogenic pulmonary edema. Case report. J Neurosurg, 1986. 64(3): p. 494-500.

[59] Baker, A.B., Poliomyelitis. 16. A study of pulmonary edema. Neurology, 1957. 7(11): p. 743-51.

[60] Fu, Y.C., et al., Cardiac complications of enterovirus rhombencephalitis. Arch Dis Child, 2004. 89(4): p. 368-73.

[61] Shen, W.C., et al., MR imaging findings of enteroviral encephaloymelitis: an outbreak in Taiwan. AJNR Am J Neuroradiol, 1999. 20(10): p. 1889-95.

[62] Wang, S.M., et al., Clinical spectrum of enterovirus 71 infection in children in southern Taiwan, with an emphasis on neurological complications. Clin Infect Dis, 1999. 29(1): p. 184-90.

[63] Valcour, V., et al., A case of enteroviral meningoencephalitis presenting as rapidly progressive dementia. Nat Clin Pract Neurol, 2008. 4(7): p. 399-403.

[64] Dunn, J.J., et al., Stable enterovirus 5' nontranslated region over a 7-year period in a patient with agammaglobulinemia and chronic infection. J Infect Dis, 2000. 182(1): p. 298-301.

[65] Feuer, R., et al., Coxsackievirus replication and the cell cycle: a potential regulatory mechanism for viral persistence/latency. Med Microbiol Immunol, 2004. 193(2-3): p. 83-90.

[66] Galbraith, D.N., C. Nairn, and G.B. Clements, Evidence for enteroviral persistence in humans. J Gen Virol, 1997. 78 (Pt 2): p. 307-12.

[67] Rudge, P., et al., Encephalomyelitis in primary hypogammaglobulinaemia. Brain, 1996. 119 (Pt 1): p. 1-15.

[68] McKinney, R.E., Jr., S.L. Katz, and C.M. Wilfert, Chronic enteroviral meningoencephalitis in agammaglobulinemic patients. Rev Infect Dis, 1987. 9(2): p. 334-56.

[69] Quartier, P., et al., Enteroviral meningoencephalitis in X-linked agammaglobulinemia: intensive immunoglobulin therapy and sequential viral detection in cerebrospinal fluid by polymerase chain reaction. Pediatr Infect Dis J, 2000. 19(11): p. 1106-8.

[70] Choi, C.S., et al., Clinical manifestations of CNS infections caused by enterovirus type 71. Korean J Pediatr, 2011. 54(1): p. 11-6.

[71] McMinn, P., et al., Neurological manifestations of enterovirus 71 infection in children during an outbreak of hand, foot, and mouth disease in Western Australia. Clin Infect Dis, 2001. 32(2): p. 236-42.

[72] Chang, L.Y., et al., Transmission and clinical features of enterovirus 71 infections in household contacts in Taiwan. JAMA, 2004. 291(2): p. 222-7.

[73] Melnick, J.L., Enterovirus type 71 infections: a varied clinical pattern sometimes mimicking paralytic poliomyelitis. Rev Infect Dis, 1984. 6 Suppl 2: p. S387-90.

[74] Chumakov, M., et al., Enterovirus 71 isolated from cases of epidemic poliomyelitis-like disease in Bulgaria. Arch Virol, 1979. 60(3-4): p. 329-40.

[75] Ishimaru, Y., et al., Outbreaks of hand, foot, and mouth disease by enterovirus 71. High incidence of complication disorders of central nervous system. Arch Dis Child, 1980. 55(8): p. 583-8.

[76] Alexander, J.P., Jr., et al., Enterovirus 71 infections and neurologic disease--United States, 1977-1991. J Infect Dis, 1994. 169(4): p. 905-8.

[77] Lum, L.C., et al., Echovirus 7 associated encephalomyelitis. J Clin Virol, 2002. 23(3): p. 153-60.

[78] Zuckerman, M.A., et al., Fatal case of echovirus type 9 encephalitis. J Clin Pathol, 1993. 46(9): p. 865-6.

[79] Tyler, K.L., Emerging viral infections of the central nervous system: part 1. Arch Neurol, 2009. 66(8): p. 939-48.

[80] Wong, K.T., L.C. Lum, and S.K. Lam, Enterovirus 71 infection and neurologic complications. N Engl J Med, 2000. 342(5): p. 356-8.

[81] Zimmerman, R.D., MR imaging findings of enteroviral encephalomyelitis: an outbreak in Taiwan. AJNR Am J Neuroradiol, 1999. 20(10): p. 1775-6.

[82] Wilson, M.R. and K.L. Tyler, Issues and updates in emerging neurologic viral infections. Semin Neurol, 2011. 31(3): p. 245-53.

[83] Wong, K.T., Emerging and re-emerging epidemic encephalitis: a tale of two viruses. Neuropathol Appl Neurobiol, 2000. 26(4): p. 313-8.

[84] Rotbart, H.A., et al., Factors affecting the detection of enteroviruses in cerebrospinal fluid with coxsackievirus B3 and poliovirus 1 cDNA probes. J Clin Microbiol, 1985. 22(2): p. 220-4.

[85] Chonmaitree, T., et al., Comparison of cell cultures for rapid isolation of enteroviruses. J Clin Microbiol, 1988. 26(12): p. 2576-80.

[86] van Vliet, K.E., et al., Multicenter evaluation of the Amplicor Enterovirus PCR test with cerebrospinal fluid from patients with aseptic meningitis. The European Union

Concerted Action on Viral Meningitis and Encephalitis. J Clin Microbiol, 1998. 36(9): p. 2652-7.

[87] Wong, K.T., et al., Enterovirus 71 encephalomyelitis and Japanese encephalitis can be distinguished by topographic distribution of inflammation and specific intraneuronal detection of viral antigen and RNA. Neuropathol Appl Neurobiol, 2012.

[88] Granerod, J., et al., Challenge of the unknown. A systematic review of acute encephalitis in non-outbreak situations. Neurology, 2010. 75(10): p. 924-32.

[89] Fowlkes, A.L., et al., Enterovirus-associated encephalitis in the California encephalitis project, 1998-2005. J Infect Dis, 2008. 198(11): p. 1685-91.

[90] Lamson, D., et al., MassTag polymerase-chain-reaction detection of respiratory pathogens, including a new rhinovirus genotype, that caused influenza-like illness in New York State during 2004-2005. J Infect Dis, 2006. 194(10): p. 1398-402.

[91] Briese, T., et al., Diagnostic system for rapid and sensitive differential detection of pathogens. Emerg Infect Dis, 2005. 11(2): p. 310-3.

[92] Palacios, G., et al., MassTag polymerase chain reaction for differential diagnosis of viral hemorrhagic fever. Emerg Infect Dis, 2006. 12(4): p. 692-5.

[93] Dominguez, S.R., et al., Multiplex MassTag-PCR for respiratory pathogens in pediatric nasopharyngeal washes negative by conventional diagnostic testing shows a high prevalence of viruses belonging to a newly recognized rhinovirus clade. J Clin Virol, 2008. 43(2): p. 219-22.

[94] Wang, D., et al., Microarray-based detection and genotyping of viral pathogens. Proc Natl Acad Sci U S A, 2002. 99(24): p. 15687-92.

[95] Wang, D., et al., Viral discovery and sequence recovery using DNA microarrays. PLoS Biol, 2003. 1(2): p. E2.

[96] Chiu, C.Y., et al., Utility of DNA microarrays for detection of viruses in acute respiratory tract infections in children. J Pediatr, 2008. 153(1): p. 76-83.

[97] Ksiazek, T.G., et al., A novel coronavirus associated with severe acute respiratory syndrome. N Engl J Med, 2003. 348(20): p. 1953-66.

[98] Urisman, A., et al., Identification of a novel Gammaretrovirus in prostate tumors of patients homozygous for R462Q RNASEL variant. PLoS Pathog, 2006. 2(3): p. e25.

[99] Gunson, R.N., T.C. Collins, and W.F. Carman, Practical experience of high throughput real time PCR in the routine diagnostic virology setting. J Clin Virol, 2006. 35(4): p. 355-67.

[100] Quan, P.L., et al., Astrovirus encephalitis in boy with X-linked agammaglobulinemia. Emerg Infect Dis, 2010. 16(6): p. 918-25.

[101] Pouplin, T., et al., Valacyclovir for herpes simplex encephalitis. Antimicrob Agents Chemother, 2011. 55(7): p. 3624-6.

[102] Erlendsson, K., T. Swartz, and J.M. Dwyer, Successful reversal of echovirus encephalitis in X-linked hypogammaglobulinemia by intraventricular administration of immunoglobulin. N Engl J Med, 1985. 312(6): p. 351-3.

[103] Johnson, P.R., Jr., K.M. Edwards, and P.F. Wright, Failure of intraventricular gamma globulin to eradicate echovirus encephalitis in a patient with X-linked agammaglobulinemia. N Engl J Med, 1985. 313(24): p. 1546-7.

[104] Dwyer, J.M. and K. Erlendsson, Intraventricular gamma-globulin for the management of enterovirus encephalitis. Pediatr Infect Dis J, 1988. 7(5 Suppl): p. S30-3.

[105] Hsu, B.M., C.H. Chen, and M.T. Wan, Genetic diversity of epidemic enterovirus 71 strains recovered from clinical and environmental samples in Taiwan. Virus Res, 2007. 126(1-2): p. 69-75.

[106] Li, Z.H., et al., Ribavirin reduces mortality in enterovirus 71-infected mice by decreasing viral replication. J Infect Dis, 2008. 197(6): p. 854-7.

[107] Poordad, F. and D. Dieterich, Treating hepatitis C: current standard of care and emerging direct-acting antiviral agents. J Viral Hepat, 2012. 19(7): p. 449-64.

[108] Shih, S.R., et al., Mutation in enterovirus 71 capsid protein VP1 confers resistance to the inhibitory effects of pyridyl imidazolidinone. Antimicrob Agents Chemother, 2004. 48(9): p. 3523-9.

[109] Pevear, D.C., et al., Activity of pleconaril against enteroviruses. Antimicrob Agents Chemother, 1999. 43(9): p. 2109-15.

[110] Romero, J.R., Pleconaril: a novel antipicornaviral drug. Expert Opin Investig Drugs, 2001. 10(2): p. 369-79.

[111] National Institute of Allergy and Infectious Diseases (NIAID). A Double-Blind, Placebo-Controlled, Virologic Efficacy Trial of Pleconaril in the Treatment of Neonates With Enteroviral Sepsis Syndrome, in ClinicalTrials.gov.

[112] Tan, E.L. and Chu, J.J., RNA interference (RNAi) - An antiviral Strategy for Enteroviruses. . J Antivir Antiretrovir S2. doi:10.4172/jaa.S2-001, 2011.

[113] Tan, E.L., et al., Enhanced potency and efficacy of 29-mer shRNAs in inhibition of Enterovirus 71. Antiviral Res, 2007. 74(1): p. 9-15.

[114] Tan, E.L., et al., Inhibition of enterovirus 71 in virus-infected mice by RNA interference. Mol Ther, 2007. 15(11): p. 1931-8.

[115] Gau, S.S., et al., Attention-deficit/hyperactivity-related symptoms among children with enterovirus 71 infection of the central nervous system. Pediatrics, 2008. 122(2): p. e452-8.

[116] Wang, S.M. and C.C. Liu, Enterovirus 71: epidemiology, pathogenesis and management. Expert Rev Anti Infect Ther, 2009. 7(6): p. 735-42.

http://dx.doi.org/10.5772/52574

[117] Chan, L.G., et al., Deaths of children during an outbreak of hand, foot, and mouth disease in sarawak, malaysia: clinical and pathological characteristics of the disease. For the Outbreak Study Group. Clin Infect Dis, 2000. 31(3): p. 678-83.